儿科与新生儿学聚焦

Paediatrics and Neonatology

IN*focus*

Paediatrics and Neonatology in Focus,1st edition
Ros Thomas, David Harvey
ISBN: 0-443-07436-4

Authorized translation from English Language edition published by the Proprietor.
ISBN: 981-259-559-7

Elsevier (Singapore) Pte Ltd.
3 Killiney Road, #08-01 Winsland House I, Singapore 239519
Tel: (65)6349-0200, Fax: (65)6733-1817

First Published 2006
2006 年初版

北京市版权局著作权合同登记号：01-2006-1179

儿科与新生儿学聚焦

Paediatrics and Neonatology

IN *focus*

原著 Roslyn Thomas
David Harvey

主译 刘锦纷

译者 刘锦纷 蔡小满 孙彦隽

北京大学医学出版社
Peking University Medical Press

ERKE YU XINSHENGERXUE JUJIAO

图书在版编目（CIP）数据

儿科与新生儿学聚焦 /（英）托马斯（Thomas, R.），（英）哈维（Harvey, D.）著；刘锦纷，蔡小满，孙彦隽译.
北京：北京大学医学出版社，2006.6
书名原文：Paediatrics and Neonatology in Focus
ISBN 7-81071-988-2

I.儿… II.①托… ②哈… ③刘… ④蔡… ⑤孙…
III.①小儿疾病－基本知识②新生儿疾病－基本知识
IV. R72

中国版本图书馆 CIP 数据核字（2006）第 015834 号

儿科与新生儿学聚焦

译　　者：刘锦纷　蔡小满　孙彦隽
出版发行：北京大学医学出版社 (电话：010-82802230)
地　　址：(100083) 北京市海淀区学院路 38 号　北京大学医学部院内
网　　址：http://www.pumpress.com.cn
E-mail：booksale@bjmu.edu.cn
印　　刷：莱芜市圣龙印务有限责任公司
经　　销：新华书店
责任编辑：畅晓燕　　责任校对：杜悦　　责任印制：郭桂兰
开　　本：889mm × 1194mm　1/32　印张：13　字数：419 千字
版　　次：2006 年 6 月第 1 版　2006 年 6 月第 1 次印刷
书　　号：ISBN 7-81071-988-2 /R・988
定　　价：95.00 元

注意

医学是一个不断进步的领域。由于新的研究与临床经验不断扩展着我们的知识，我们在遵守标准的安全预防措施的同时，也有必要在治疗和用药方面做出适当的变动。建议读者对每一用药都要检查其生产厂家所提供的最新产品信息，以确定药物的推荐剂量、服用方法、持续时间及相关禁忌证。根据自己的经验和患者的病情，决定每一位病人的服药剂量和最佳治疗方法，是经治医师的责任。不论是出版商还是著者，对于由于本出版物引起的任何个人或财产的损伤或损失，均不承担任何责任。

出版者

译者前言

《儿科与新生儿学聚焦》这本书包含了大量的临床照片，行文言简意赅，通过各个独立章节图文并茂地描述了一些临床常见和罕见的疾病。这使读者对知识的理解更为直接，有助于医学生及相关医学人员凭借此书来识别和诊断疾病。

这种图片和文字说明相结合的图集，对医学生、儿科医生或者非儿科专业的医生来说，具有较大的积极意义。大量的图片使本书的可读性和趣味性更强，避免了大篇幅文字对读者形成的阅读压力，使人有兴趣继续阅读或者时常加以翻阅。由于本书以精练的语言文字配合图片进行概要性的阐述，相信这有利于我们的儿科同仁们在门诊、手术或者午休等间隙时间，见缝插针地进行阅读，不断地加深印象。

刘锦纷

上海交通大学医学院附属上海儿童医学中心

著者前言

我们希望这本有关儿科和新生儿学的图集可以激励医学生、护士、助产士进一步钻研这个令人激动的专业。对于那些已经接受过儿科学和儿童健康方面职业培训的人员而言，书中列举的问题可以作为对自身知识掌握程度的测试，并对下一个检查难点进行准备。

为了能够让读者在等待下一个演讲、辅导课、门诊病人以及院内呼机传呼或病人按铃召唤期间可对该书进行浏览，书中每页的主题都彼此独立，内容布局简洁明了。我们无意让该书成为一本包罗万象的教科书，而是集中于可以用临床照片和X线片演示的疾病，因此我们相信它可以成为激起你求知欲的一个有用的辅助工具。

Roslyn Thomas
David Harvey

目录

Contents

胎斑

发病率	几乎普遍存在于非高加索人群的新生儿中。尤其在亚洲婴儿中多见，但也偶见于黑发的高加索婴儿中。
临床特征	局部青灰色或蓝色色素沉着，多见于腰骶部（图1），但也可出现于躯干和肢体的任何部位（图 2）。可能被误认为是瘀伤。
预后	随着婴儿的长大，胎斑会变得越来越不明显。

中毒性红斑（新生儿荨麻疹，嗜酸性皮疹）

发病率	除了早产儿外，极其常见。多数足月儿在生后1周也会出现。
病理学	充满嗜酸性细胞的小囊泡。
临床特征	分布广泛的、高于皮面的红斑样皮疹（图 3），通常于生后1周内出现。是一种中央为白色丘疹，周围有一红晕的独立的皮肤损伤。
意义	除了可能会被误认为脓斑外，没有什么重要意义。病因尚不明。
治疗	不需要处理，皮疹会自行消退。

粟粒疹（乳白斑）

发病率	很常见，约 40% ~ 50% 的新生儿会出现。
病理学	是一种肥大的皮脂腺。
临床特征	粟粒疹是良性的白色丘疹，可见于鼻部和脸颊部（图 4）。
治疗	不需要特殊处理，会自行消退。有时会被误诊为感染。

Mongolian blue spot

Incidence — Almost universal in non-Caucasian neonates. Particularly obvious in Asian infants and occasionally also occurs in Caucasian infants with dark hair.

Clinical features — Slate grey or bluish pigmentation, usually in the lumbosacral region (Fig. 1), but may occur anywhere on the trunk or limbs (Fig. 2). May be mistaken for bruising by the inexperienced.

Prognosis — Becomes less obvious as the infant grows older.

Erythema toxicum (urticaria of newborn, eosinophil rash)

Incidence — Extremely common, except in preterm infants. Majority of term infants are affected in the first week of life.

Aetiology — Vesicles are full of eosinophils.

Clinical features — Widespread, fluctuating erythematous maculopapular rash (Fig. 3), usually beginning after birth at any time in the first week. Individual lesions consist of a white central papule surrounded by an erythematous flare.

Significance — None, except may occasionally be mistaken for septic spots. Aetiology unknown.

Management — None required, as rash disappears spontaneously.

Milia (milk spots)

Incidence — Very common, seen in 40-50% newborn infants.

Pathology — Milia are hypertrophic sebaceous glands.

Clinical features — Milia are fine white spots seen on the nose and cheeks (Fig. 4).

Management — Disappear spontaneously, but occasionally mistaken for infection. No treatment required.

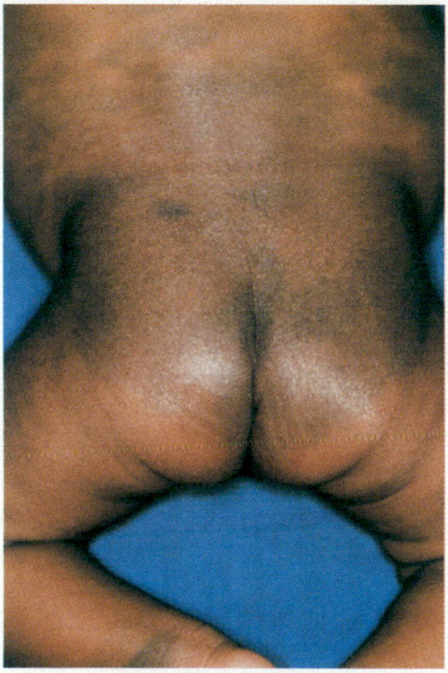

图 1 典型的位于腰骶部的胎斑
Typical Mongolian blue spot in lumbosacral region

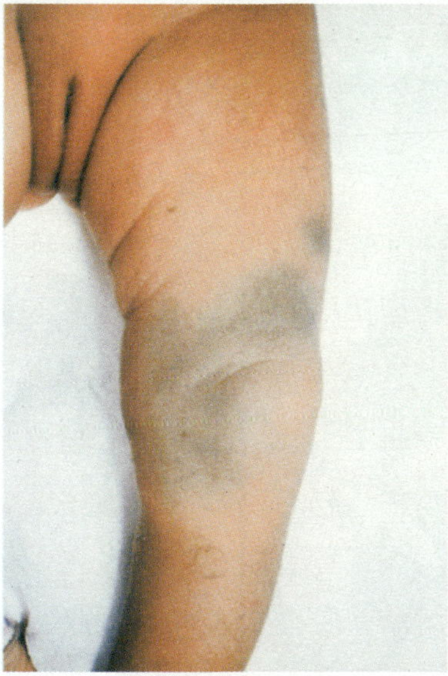

图 2 位于膝部周围的胎斑
Mongolian blue spot around the knee

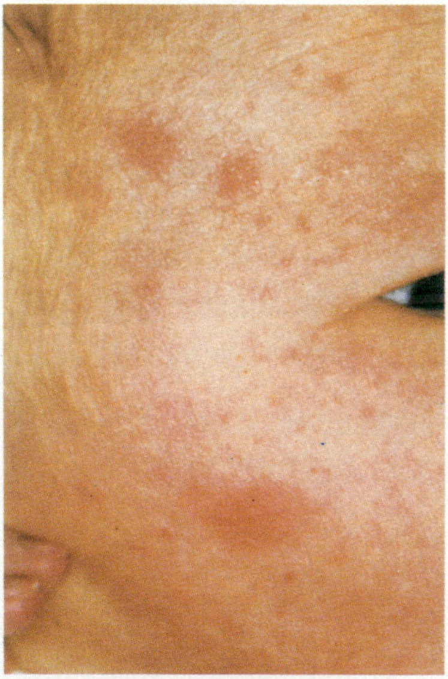

图 3 脸部的中毒性红斑
Erythema toxicum on the face

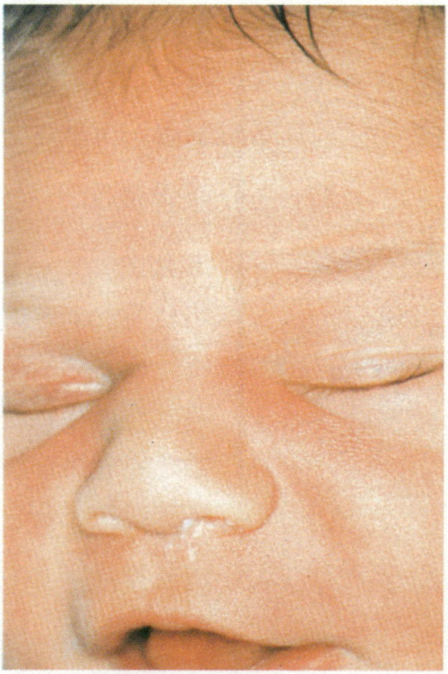

图 4 鼻部的粟粒疹
Milia on nose

上皮珠

临床特征 经常以成串的白色小斑块出现在口腔硬腭和软腭交汇处的中线部位（图 5），又称作爱泼斯坦小结 (Epstein's pearls)。也可见于牙龈和阴茎包皮处。

病理学 上皮珠是一种表皮囊肿。

病程和预后 不需要特殊处理，会自行消退。

早生乳牙

发病率 很罕见，但常出现于有早生乳牙家族史的人群中。

临床特征 一般出现于下中切牙的部位（图 6）。通常是松动的附着在牙龈上。

治疗 应早期拔除，以免牙齿误吸入食管和气道，或引起舌部溃疡。拔除早生乳牙不会影响今后的出牙。

舌下囊肿

临床特征 是位于舌下的黏液潴留性囊肿（图 7）。与下颌下腺和舌下腺导管相比，还有可能会发生更深部位的囊肿。

治疗 通常会自行消失。但较大的囊肿可能会对喂养带来困难，所以这时就需要外科手术治疗（袋形缝术）。

骶骨浅凹

临床特征 常见于骶骨部位（图 8），通常末端封闭。一般通过视诊可以排除有无瘘管，此时运用超声检查可能有所帮助。触诊时可在基底部摸到凸起的尾骨。

合并症 通常会合并有其他中线部位的异常（如：脂肪瘤、多毛痣或者血管瘤）出现在背部较高位置，并可伴有马尾神经丛的异常。

治疗 倘若排除了瘘管，那么无需处理。

Epithelial pearls

Clinical features Often occur in clusters as white spots in the mouth (Fig. 5) in midline at junction of hard and soft palate (Epstein's pearls). May also occur on alveolar margin or prepuce.

Pathology Epithelial pearls are epidermal cysts.

Course and prognosis They disappear spontaneously. No treatment is required.

Natal teeth

Incidence Uncommon, but there is often a family history of natal teeth.

Clinical features Commonly occur in the central lower incisor region (Fig. 6). Usually only loosely attached.

Management Best removed early in order to prevent aspiration, or ulceration of the tongue. Extraction will not deplete permanent dentition.

Ranula

Clinical features Mucous retention cyst under the tongue (Fig. 7). Deeper cysts may occur in relation to submandibular or sublingual ducts.

Management Often disappear spontaneously. Large cysts may occasionally interfere with feeding, and surgery may then be indicated (marsupialization).

Sacral pits and dimples

Clinical features Common over the sacrum (Fig. 8). Usually blind-ending. Fistulae can usually be excluded by inspection, ultrasound may be helpful. A prominent coccyx can often be palpated in the base.

Associations Other midline abnormalities (e.g. lipomas, hairy naevi or haemangiomata) may occur higher on the back and may be associated with tethering of cauda equina (diastatomyelia).

Management None required, providing a fistula has been excluded.

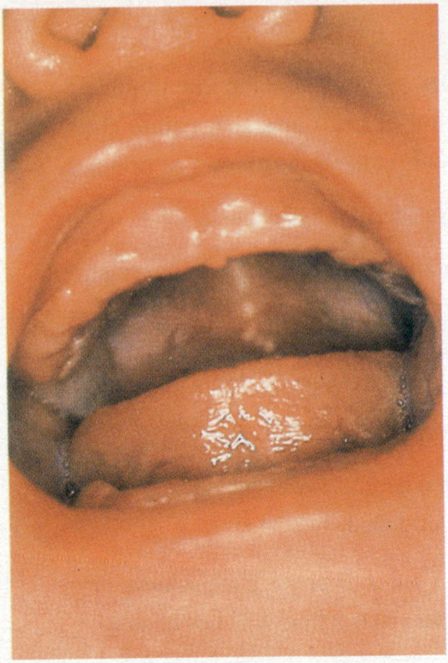

图5　位于腭中线的上皮珠
Epithelial pearls in the midline of the palate

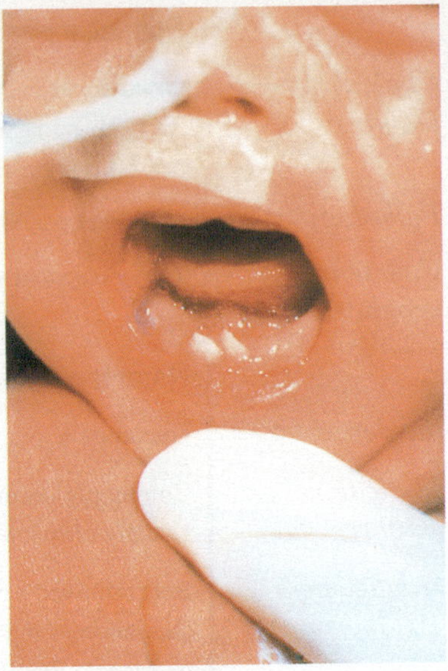

图6　早生乳牙
Natal teeth

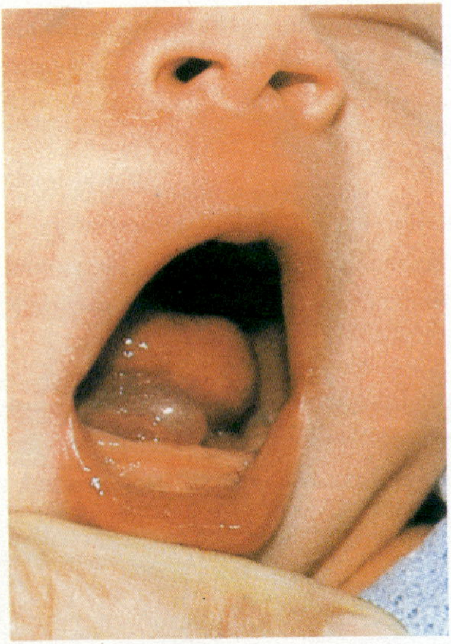

图7　舌下囊肿
Ranula

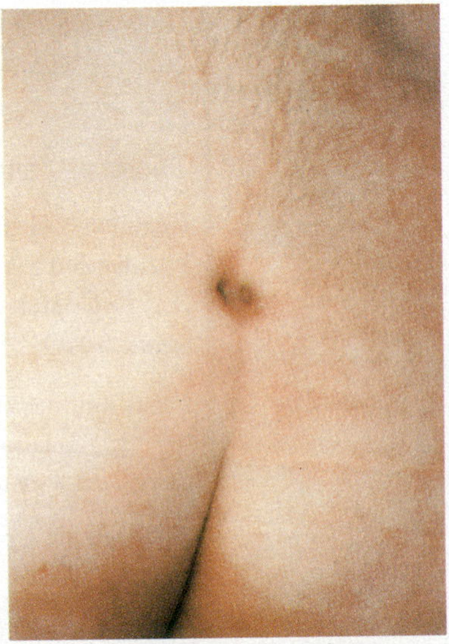

图8　位于骶骨上方的浅凹
A dimple over the sacrum

激素表现

临床特征 大约30% ~ 40%的新生儿（包括男婴）都会有可触及的乳腺结节（男性乳房发育），这是由于母亲妊娠后期分泌的雌激素、孕酮、催乳素通过胎盘对胎儿的影响。通常在出生后最初几周可存在乳腺增大，并伴有泌乳现象（witch乳）。在新生女婴的外阴后部通常会有黏膜息肉。一些女婴在出生后几天内会出现阴道分泌黏液和阴道流血的现象（图9）。

治疗 不需要处理。外阴息肉会在几周内自行萎缩。乳房组织会在几个月内逐步复原。父母大可不必因为这些而为孩子的生理性征有所顾虑，并且还应该被告知不要去挤压孩子的乳房。仅在发生乳腺炎时才需应用抗生素，但该情况较为罕见。

胎脂

临床特征 足月新生儿皮肤上黏稠的像油膏样的白色物质。常出现在面部、耳部、颈部和腹股沟皮肤皱褶处（图10），但偶尔也会在全身大量结块。如果在分娩过程中出现胎儿窘迫，胎脂会被胎粪沾污。

血管现象

发病率 很常见。

病因学 是血管舒缩不稳定的一种良性表现。

临床特征 在出生后数天内出现外周性发绀很常见，发生在肢体末端和口周。但是不会有中央性发绀。该处皮肤极少会出现“五颜六色”的变化。如果有，其肤色变化的分界线会很明显（图11）。

治疗 无需处理。

Hormonal manifestations

Clinical features

Some 30-40% of newborn infants, including male infants, have palpable breast nodules (gynaecomastia) due to placental transfer of maternal oestrogen, progesterone and prolactin. Breast enlargement, often with lactation (witch's milk) is present during the first weeks of life. A tag of mucous membrane is often present in the posterior vulval region of newborn female infants. Discharge of mucus or vaginal bleeding (Fig. 9), occurs in some infants a few days after birth.

Management

No treatment is required. Vulval tags shrivel up within a few weeks. Gradual involution of breast tissue occurs over a few months. Parents can be reassured about the physiological nature of these events and advised not to squeeze the breasts. Antibiotics are only necessary if the breast becomes infected (mastitis), which is rare.

Vernix caseosum

Clinical features

Slimy, ointment-like white substance on skin of some term infants at birth. It is usually found on the face, ears and in folds of neck or groin (Fig. 10), but is occasionally liberally caked all over the body. Vernix is sometimes stained by meconium if there was fetal distress before birth.

Vascular phenomena

Incidence

Very common.

Aetiology

Innocent manifestation of vasomotor instability.

Clinical features

Peripheral cyanosis is very common in the first few days after birth. It occurs in the extremities and around the mouth. There is no central cyanosis. Harlequin colour change is a very rare, but dramatic colour change with vivid midline demarcation of colour (Fig. 11).

Management

None required.

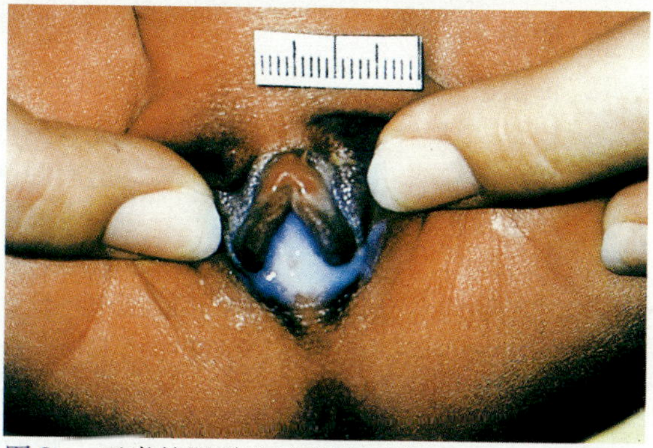

图 9　正常的阴道分泌黏液现象
Normal mucoid vaginal discharge

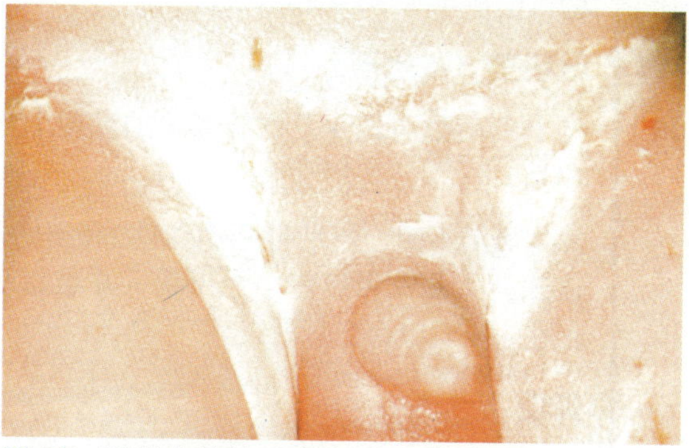

图 10　腹股沟处的胎脂
Vernix caseosum in the groin

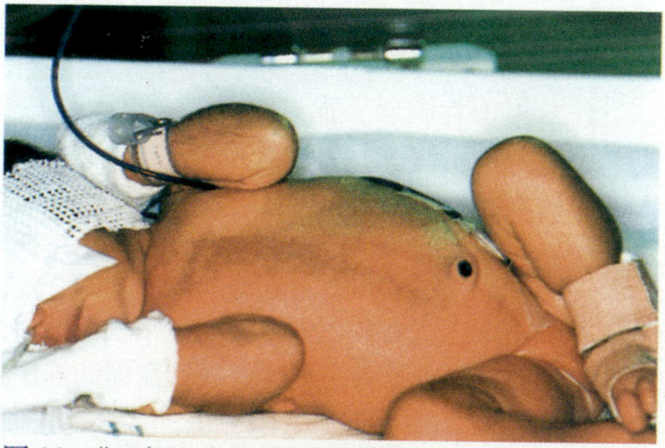

图 11　“五颜六色”的血管现象
Harlequin vascular phenomenon

脐带

临床特征

饱满而半透明的脐带包含两根动脉和一根静脉（图12）。单根脐动脉可能会合并其他先天畸形。脐带会在出生后7～10天内通过干性坏疽而脱落，有时会残留潮湿的基底部。脐部有分泌物或蜂窝织炎伴脐部周围红肿，则提示有感染，需要全身应用抗生素。血清血液性分泌物或脐带基底部出现肉质隆起则提示可能有脐部肉芽肿，或很少情况下是卵黄管残留物或永久性脐尿管。

治疗

肉芽肿通常会自行脱落，或局部应用硝酸银。局部应用抗生素可能会导致脐带脱落延迟。脐带附着超过3周可能会合并慢性肉芽肿病。

吸吮垫（吸吮茧）

临床特征

是出生后数周新生儿唇缘较厚的黏膜上皮细胞（图13）。

治疗

发生原因不明，但是与吮吸的压力和损伤无关，因为这在新生儿吮吸前就已经出现，并且常在出生时便存在。吸吮垫会自行消失。

粪便

临床特征

胎粪是新生儿排出的一种较黏稠、油腻的墨绿色粪便（图14）。胎粪是无嗅的，含有黏液、上皮碎片以及由胃肠道分泌的胆汁。如果在分娩过程中发生胎儿窘迫，那么胎儿在宫内就会排出胎粪。胎粪吸入会导致肺炎，引起严重的呼吸困难。如果在出生时发现羊水中有胎粪，那么在第一次自主呼吸前用力的吸引并进行复苏是有必要的。生后48小时内如果没有胎粪排出则提示可能存在肠道梗阻。随着喂养的开始，粪便的颜色、硬度也会随之改变，在出生后数天会变成绿色的、含有黏液的、更软的粪便。母乳喂养的孩子，其粪便通常是软的或半成形的，但有时会是液体状、芥末黄色并带有淡淡甜味的粪便。排便的次数不定，但一般在每餐喂食中或喂食后会有一次排便。人工喂养的孩子通常会排出较硬的、深褐色粪便，并且次数会少于母乳喂养的孩子。

Umbilical cord

Clinical features

Fleshy translucent cord containing two arteries and one vein (Fig. 12). A single umbilical artery may be associated with other congenital abnormalities. The cord separates within 7-10 days by dry gangrene or with a residual moist base. Frank discharge or cellulitis with a red flare around the umbilicus indicates infection and requires systemic antibiotics. Serosanguineous discharge or a fleshy protuberance from the base may be an umbilical granuloma or rarely a vitello-intestinal remnant or persistent urachus.

Management

Granulomas usually resolve spontaneously or with local application of silver nitrate. Topical antibiotics may actually delay separation. Adherence of umbilical cord beyond 3 weeks may be associated with chronic granulomatous disease.

Sucking pad (sucking callous)

Clinical features

Thickened epithelium of mucous membranes of lips (Fig. 13) in first few weeks of life.

Management

The cause is unknown, but they are not related to pressure or trauma as they occur before suckling and are often present at birth. Sucking pads disappear spontaneously.

Stools

Clinical features

Meconium is sticky, tarry, greenish-black stool (Fig. 14) passed by newborn infants. It is odourless, and contains mucus, epithelial debris and bile from the gastrointestinal tract. Meconium may be passed by the fetus before birth if there is fetal distress. Inhalation of meconium causes pneumonitis with severe respiratory distress. If meconium is present at birth, vigorous suction and resuscitation are indicated before the first spontaneous breath. Failure to pass meconium within 48 h of birth may indicate intestinal obstruction. After feeding, stools gradually change in colour and consistency, becoming softer, greenish in colour and mixed with mucus for a few days. Breast-fed stools are usually soft or semi-formed, but are sometimes liquid and mustard yellow in colour with a faint sweet odour.
Frequency varies, but often passed after or during each feed. Formula fed babies usually pass firmer, browner and less frequent stools than breast-fed infants.

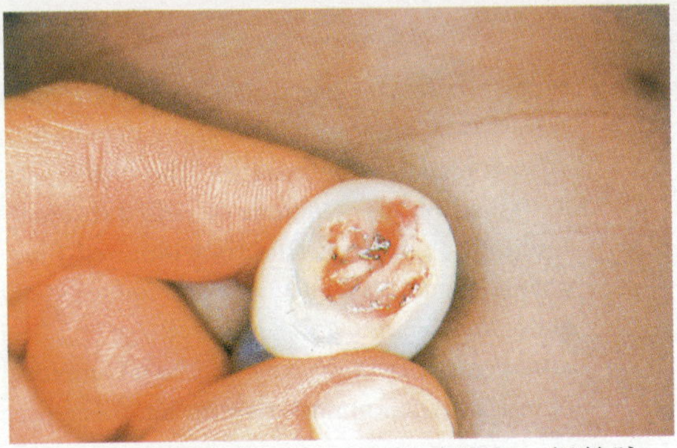

图 12　脐带的横断面显示两根动脉和一根静脉
Cut surface of umbilical cord showing two arteries and one vein

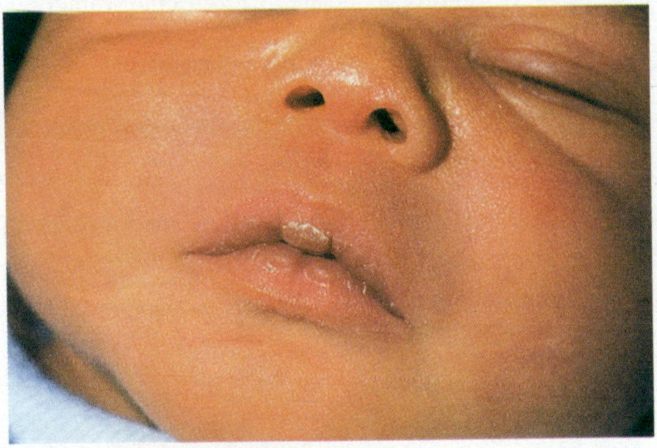

图 13　唇缘的吸吮垫
Sucking pad on lip

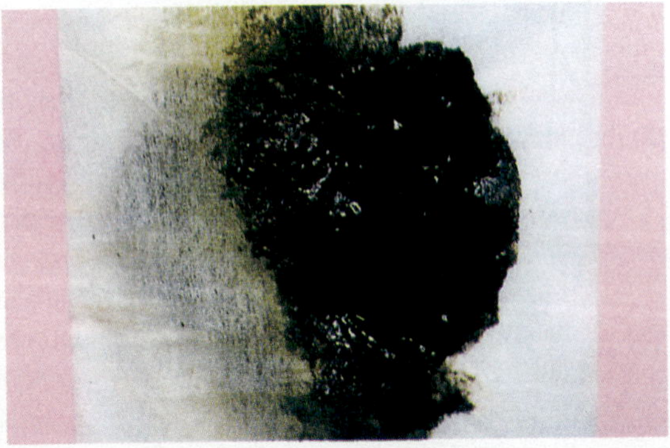

图 14　胎粪
Meconium

黄疸

发病率

非常普遍，约50%的足月儿以及80%的早产儿会在生后3～5天出现肉眼可见的黄疸。

病理学

- 出生后24～48小时出现的早期黄疸通常是由异常的溶血、感染或瘀伤而造成。
- 生理性黄疸是在出生48小时后出现，通常会在7～10天内减退。其主要成分是非结合胆红素，是由于红细胞破坏数量增加以及肝脏内葡萄糖醛酸酶不成熟所造成。
- 延迟性黄疸持续超过14天有时可见于正常足月儿或母乳喂养的婴儿，但是应该排除其他情况，尤其是甲状腺功能减退、半乳糖血症、肝病、红细胞酶缺乏和胆道闭锁。

临床特征

皮肤和结膜黄染（图15）。肝、脾大提示存在异常溶血、感染或代谢障碍，而在生理性黄疸中不存在肝脾大。

意义

非常严重的非结合血胆红素增多症可能会引起永久性的脑损伤（核黄疸），伴有手足徐动症样脑瘫和感觉神经性耳聋。

治疗

观察黄疸的临床变化和监测血清胆红素水平。如果在出生48小时内即出现黄疸，黄疸延续超过14天，或在任何一个阶段黄疸水平显著升高，则需要进一步调查原因。应避免脱水和应用硫胺类药物，它们会与胆红素竞争结合白蛋白。没有证据表明额外补液有利于或加速正常新生儿黄疸消退。某些婴儿如果血清胆红素水平较高可以应用光照疗法（图16）或采取换血措施。一些黄疸婴儿，尤其是那些患有严重猕猴溶血病（rhesus haemolytic disease）的婴儿在光照疗法的过程中会出现青铜综合征（图17）。

Jaundice

Incidence

Very common. About 50% of full-term infants and 80% of preterm infants are visibly jaundiced by 3-5 days of age.

Pathology

- Early jaundice occurring within 24-48 h of birth is usually due to abnormal haemolysis, infection, or bruising.
- Physiological jaundice appears after 48 h of age and usually subsides within 7-10 days. It is mainly unconjugated bilirubin due to increased red cell destruction and immaturity of hepatic enzymes.
- Prolonged jaundice lasting beyond 14 days is sometimes seen in normal preterm or breast-fed infants, but other conditions should be excluded, especially hypothyroidism, galactosaemia, liver disease, red cell enzyme defects and biliary atresia.

Clinical features

Yellow staining of the skin (Fig. 15) and conjunctivae. Hepatosplenomegaly indicates the presence of abnormal haemolysis, infection or a metabolic disorder, and is not found in physiological jaundice.

Significance

Very severe unconjugated hyperbilirubinaemia may cause permanent brain damage (kernicterus) with athetoid cerebral palsy and sensorineural deafness.

Management

Observe jaundice clinically and monitor plasma bilirubin level. Investigation may be required if jaundice appears earlier than 48 h, is prolonged beyond 14 days or is unusually high at any stage. Dehydration and drugs such as sulphonamides, which compete with bilirubin for albumin-binding, should be avoided. There is no evidence that extra fluids are needed or hasten the resolution of jaundice in normal infants. Phototherapy (Fig. 16) or exchange transfusion may be required in some infants with high levels of plasma bilirubin. Some jaundiced babies, particularly those with severe rhesus haemolytic disease develop a curious bronze colour under phototherapy (Fig. 17).

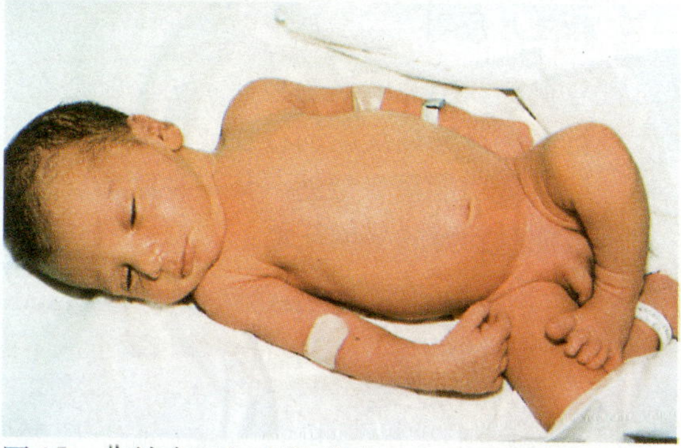

图 15　非结合胆红素性黄疸
Jaundice due to unconjugated bilirubinaemia

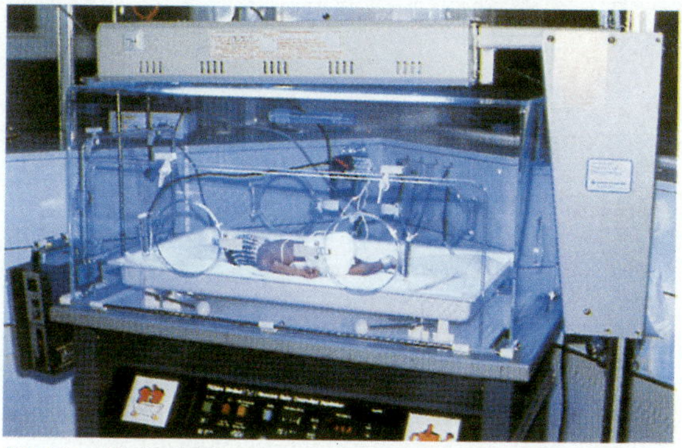

图 16　光照疗法
Phototherapy

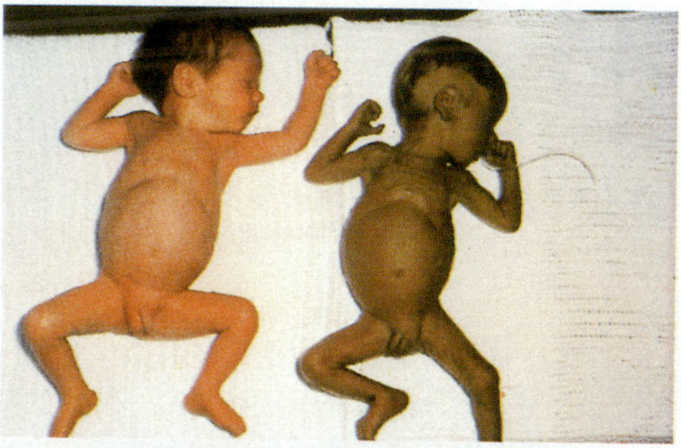

图 17　青铜综合征婴儿和正常婴儿
Bronze baby syndrome with a normal baby

新生儿反射

有很多新生儿的原始神经系统反射会在婴儿早期自行消失。原始反射的存在或缺失对于评估胎龄和神经系统功能很有帮助。某一种原始反射的延迟消失可能是脑瘫的早期征象。

临床特征

- 拥抱反射（moro reflex）或惊吓反射（startle reflex）：将婴儿置于仰卧位，将头部和躯干从下面托起。当头部和肩部突然回落到原水平时，婴儿会被诱发出一种上肢先迅速外展、伸直，随后缓慢外展、屈曲的惊吓反应（图18）。当快速地将婴儿放置于仰卧位时常常伴有哭闹。不对称拥抱反射的最常见原因是肱骨或锁骨骨折，或是臂丛神经麻痹（Erb 麻痹）。
- 抓握反射：当将手指放于新生儿指（趾）根部的掌面时，他的指（趾）会屈曲，是一种阳性反应（图19）。
- 吸吮反射（sucking reflex）和觅食反射（rooting reflex）：轻轻敲击口唇周围的面部或脸颊可以引出吸吮反射和觅食反射。
- 眉间轻叩：轻敲鼻根部可以引出瞬目反射。
- 牵引反射：握着新生儿的手腕，把他从仰卧位拉起，他的颈部和手臂会呈屈曲位。
- 放置反射：如果使新生儿的足背触及某平面的下缘，那么他的腿会屈曲，并自行将脚放于平面上。
- 踏步反射：如果使新生儿的一个足底触及平面，那么他会自动做出踏步走的动作（图20）。
- 侧弯反射：如果在新生儿后腰部的一侧轻划一下，那么他的臀部会自行弯向受刺激一侧。
- 不对称颈强直反射：如果新生儿的头部转向一侧，那么同侧的上下肢会伸直，而对侧的上下肢会屈曲。

意义

通过对原始反射的检查只能对新生儿的一般情况作一下了解。没有一个反射与某一特定的解剖异常或病理损伤有关。原始反射的存在或缺失必须结合病史、胎龄和其他神经学检查来综合考虑。

Neonatal reflexes

There is a large number of primitive neonatal neurological reflexes which disappear spontaneously during early infancy. Presence or absence may be useful in assessment of gestational age and neurological function. Delayed disappearance of certain primitive reflexes may be an early sign of cerebral palsy.

Clinical features

- Moro or startle reflex: the infant is held supine, with trunk and head being supported from below. When the head and shoulders are suddenly allowed to fall back, a startle response with rapid abduction and extension of the upper limbs followed by slower abduction and flexion is elicited. Often accompanied by a cry and may be demonstrated unintentionally when briskly placing an infant in the supine position (Fig. 18). The most common cause of an asymmetric Moro response is a fracture of the humerus or clavicle, or a brachial plexus palsy (Erb's palsy).
- Grasp reflexes: flexion of the digits is a positive response to a finger being placed on the palmar surface of the base of the fingers (Fig. 19) or the plantar surface of the toes.
- Sucking and rooting reflexes: stroking the face near the mouth or cheek causes a sucking and searching response.
- Glabellar tap: a blink of the eyelids is produced in response to tapping the base of the nose.
- Traction reflex: pulling the infant up from the supine position by the wrists results in flexion of the arms and neck.
- Placing reflex: if a foot is brought up under the edge of a surface, the leg is flexed and the baby places the foot on the surface.
- Walking reflex: when the sole of the foot is brought into contact with a surface, there is automatic walking (Fig. 20).
- Galant reflex: if the posterior loin is stroked, the baby swings the buttock towards that side.
- Asymmetric tonic neck reflex: if the head is turned laterally, there is extension of the arm and leg on the same side and flexion of the opposite arm and leg.

Significance

Only very general conclusions can be drawn from examination for primitive reflexes. None of the reflexes is associated with a particular anatomical or pathological lesion. Presence or absence must be considered in association with history, gestational age and other aspects of the neurological examination.

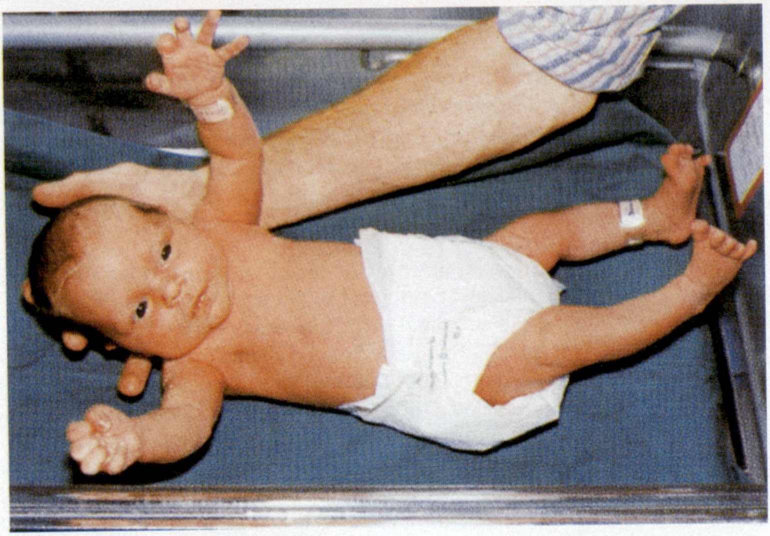

图 18　拥抱反射或惊吓反射
Moro or startle reflex

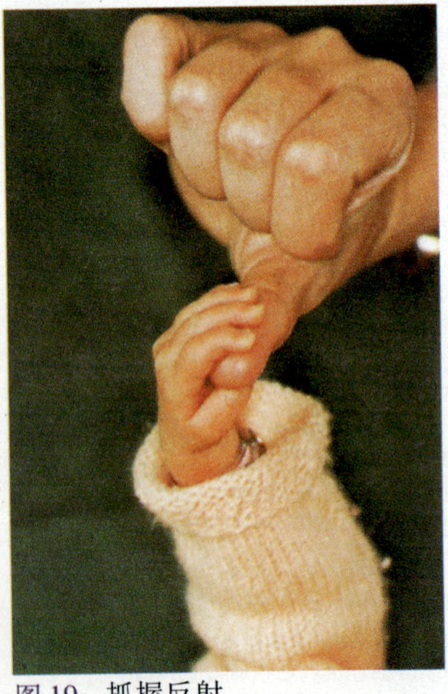

图 19　抓握反射
Grasp reflex

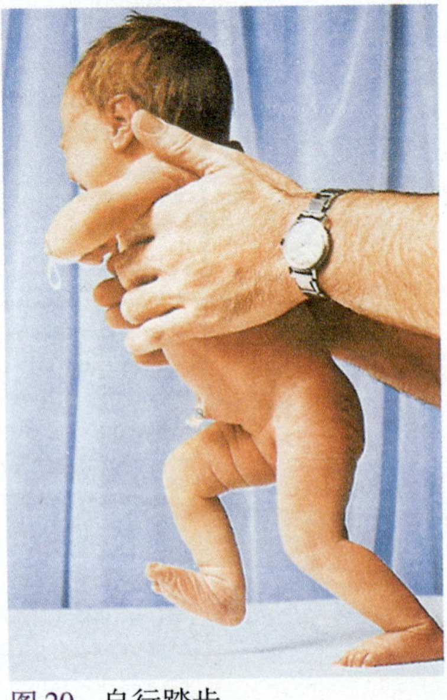

图 20　自行踏步
Automatic walking

先锋头

临床特征

发生于胎先露部位的头皮下水肿或瘀伤（图21），通常位于头部顶骨或枕骨处。出生后即刻肿胀最明显，但在数天内自行消退。

头颅血肿

临床特征

是在分娩过程中出现的柔软的肿胀或肿块，其形状和大小如同乒乓球，边界不清，但不会超越颅缝（图22）。它是由颅骨骨膜小血管破裂所造成。出现于胎先露的部位，多见于顶骨处，有时为双侧。头颅血肿在出生时并无显现，但由于进行性出血，在出生后数天表现最为明显。

病程和预后

头颅血肿会自行消退，有时会有血肿机化，但可能持续数周或数月才能完全消退。黄疸是常见的并发症。

产科操作

临床特征

产钳通常会在钳拉部位产生压迹和微小的瘀伤（图23），并且有可能造成面瘫或皮下脂肪坏死。这些并发症也可出现于顺产的新生儿，尤其是由于胎下降较慢引起产程较长的分娩过程中。皮下脂肪坏死可以发生在任何骨突出的部位，但多见于脸颊部。它通常表现为较硬的、表面发红的一块区域，有时会发生机化。人工破膜、胎儿头皮血采样和头皮电极都可能引起切割伤。当除去头皮夹的时候应特别小心，错误的拆离方法会导致头皮撕脱。当第二产程延长时，采取吸引术帮助分娩，即利用负压对头皮的吸引常常会引起瘀伤和头部髻样突出。有时还会引起先露部位更为严重的水疱、擦伤或撕裂伤（图24），偶尔还会引起严重的帽状腱膜下出血。

预后

一般情况下这些损伤是很轻微的，但可能会引起感染。大多数都能自行消退，而无明显的瘢痕和后遗症。

Caput succedaneum

Clinical features

Subcutaneous oedema and bruising of the presenting part (Fig. 21), usually the parietal or occipital region of the head. Swelling is maximal soon after birth, and disappears spontaneously within a few days.

Cephalhaematoma

Clinical features

Soft swelling or lump, often the size and shape of a table tennis ball, with a very discrete edge which never crosses suture lines (Fig. 22) which results from rupture of small vessels in the periosteum. Occurs over the presenting part, usually the parietal bone, is sometimes bilateral and associated with caput. Not apparent at birth, but with ongoing bleeding the maximal size occurs within a few days of birth.

Course and prognosis

Cephalhaematomas disappear spontaneously, sometimes accompanied by calcification, but may take several weeks or months to completely resolve. Jaundice is a common complication.

Obstetric manipulations

Clinical features

Forceps often result in pressure indentation or minor bruising (Fig. 23) and may cause facial palsy or subcutaneous fat necrosis. Both of these complications can also occur after a spontaneous vaginal delivery, particularly after a long labour with slow descent of the presenting part. Subcutaneous fat necrosis can occur over any bony prominence, but is most common on the cheek. It usually appears as an indurated, red area, sometimes followed by calcification. Artificial rupture of membranes, fetal scalp sampling and scalp electrodes may all cause incised wounds. Particular care should be taken when removing scalp clips, as incorrect detachment may result in a core of scalp being removed. Ventouse extraction, by applying suction to the scalp to assist delivery when there is delay in the second stage of labour, frequently causes bruising and a chignon-shaped caput. Sometimes it causes more serious blistering, abrasions or laceration of the presenting part (Fig. 24), and occasionally more serious subaponeurotic haemorrhage.

Prognosis

The lesions are usually trivial, but may become the site of infection. Most resolve spontaneously without significant scarring or more permanent sequelae.

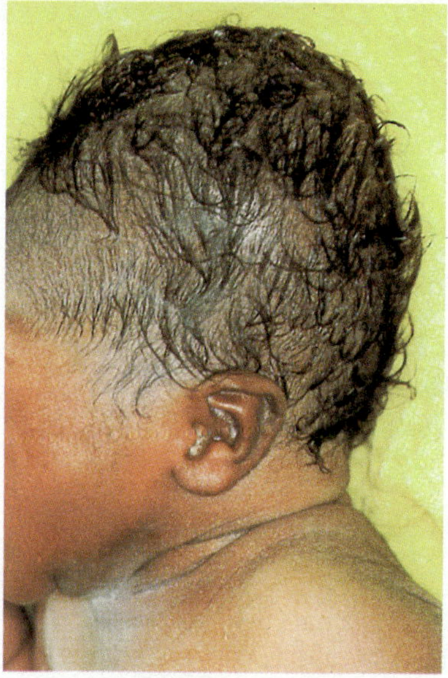

图 21　先露部位的头颅变形
Moulding and caput in vertex presentation

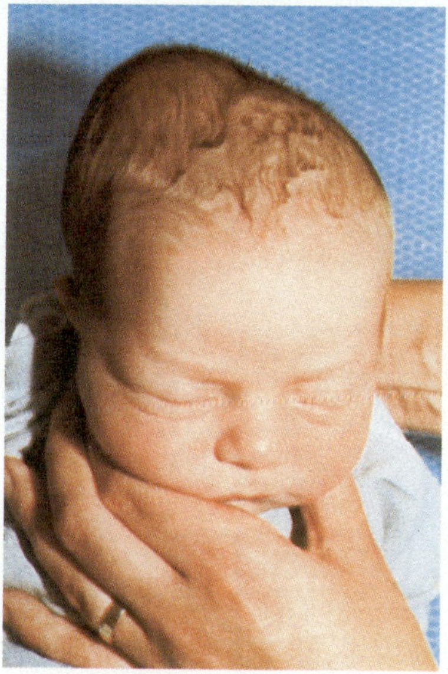

图 22　顶骨部位的头颅血肿
Parietal cephalhaematoma

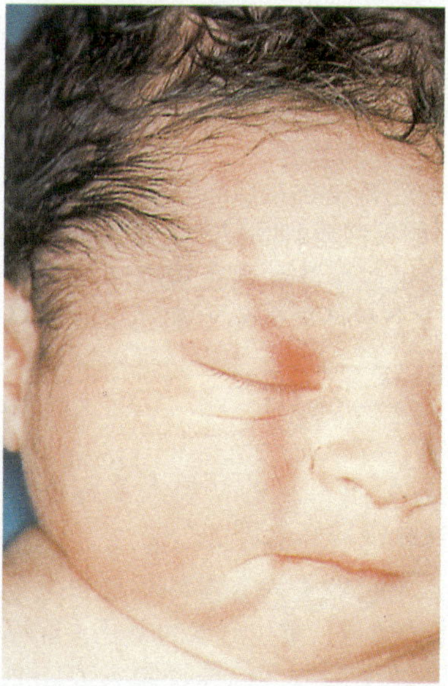

图 23　产钳压迹
Forceps mark

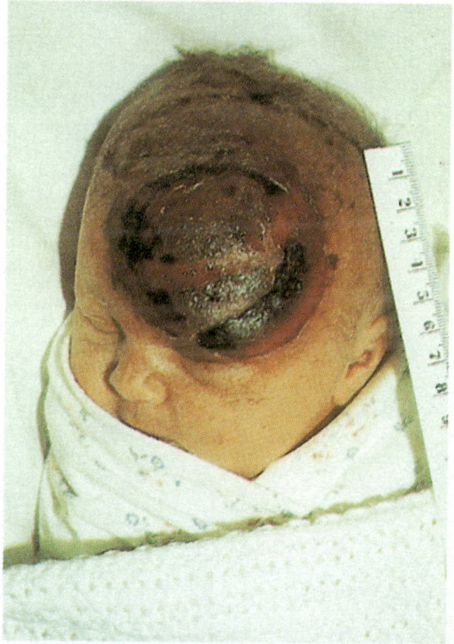

图 24　由于产程延长而用吸引术导致非常严重的擦伤
Very severe abrasion from a prolonged application of ventouse

面瘫

病因学　面瘫是由于面神经从腮腺穿出时受到压迫所造成。常发生于正常阴道分娩的新生儿，但有时产钳压迫也会造成面瘫。

临床特征　通常是单侧面部肌肉无力，导致嘴角向下歪斜（图25），并且有时会有流涎。会引起喂食困难和患侧眼睑不能闭合。

预后　大多都能在出生后数天至数周内自行恢复。

Erb 麻痹

病因学　通常是在臀位产或伴有肩先露的难产过程中由于对颈部的牵引而造成的臂丛上部神经受牵拉或撕裂。少数也可能是臂丛神经发育不全所造成，但这很难在新生儿期加以区别。

临床特征　受损侧的上臂和手部就好像“侍者讨小费姿势”（图26），表现为肩部外展无力或麻痹，肘部屈曲，腕关节伸展和后旋。

预后　麻痹或无力通常会在数周或数月后自行恢复，但偶尔会有持续性麻痹。如果恢复时间较长，那么被动的物理治疗和夜间夹板可以预防和阻止肌肉挛缩。少数情况下如果到6～9个月还未恢复，那么采取外科手术治疗会有所帮助。

体位畸形

发病率　体位畸形和压迫效应是很常见的，但大多程度较轻、病程短暂，并且无须特殊处理。

临床特征　面先露的新生儿，在生后数天内会保持头部和颈部伸展，呈现角弓反张的体位。臀位分娩的婴儿头部不会变形，但其腿部会在生后数天内保持髋关节屈曲位（图27）。许多正常婴儿都会有“畸形足”的表现（图 28），这完全可以通过被动运动来加以矫正，以达到足和踝部的充分活动。

Facial palsy

Aetiology

Facial palsy is due to compression of the facial nerve as it exits from the parotid gland. Often occurs after normal vaginal delivery, but is sometimes caused by pressure from forceps blades.

Clinical features

Weakness, usually unilateral, of facial muscles which may cause drooping of the mouth (Fig. 25) and sometimes dribbling. There is often feeding difficulty and inability to close the eye on the affected side.

Prognosis

Most resolve spontaneously within a few days or weeks after birth.

Erb's palsy

Aetiology

Stretching or tearing of the upper part of the brachial plexus, usually caused by neck traction during breech delivery or with shoulder dystocia. Occasionally may be due to hypoplasia of the brachial plexus, but this is difficult to distinguish in the neonatal period.

Clinical features

The affected arm and hand assume the waiter's tip position (Fig. 26), weakness or paralysis of abduction of shoulder, with flexion at elbow and extension and supination of wrist.

Prognosis

Weakness or paralysis usually responds spontaneously over a period of weeks or months, but paralysis is occasionally permanent. If resolution takes a long time, passive physiotherapy and night splints will prevent contractures. Occasionally surgery may be helpful if paralysis has not resolved by 6-9 months of age.

Postural deformities

Incidence

Postural and compressional effects are common but the majority are mild, transient and do not require treatment.

Clinical features

After a face or brow presentation, the infant may lie with head and neck extended in an opisthotonic posture for several days. After breech delivery, the head is not moulded and legs are often maintained in hip flexion for days (Fig. 27). In many normal infants, feet are often moulded into postural talipes (Fig.28) which can be fully reduced by passive manipulation, and there is a full range of foot and ankle movement.

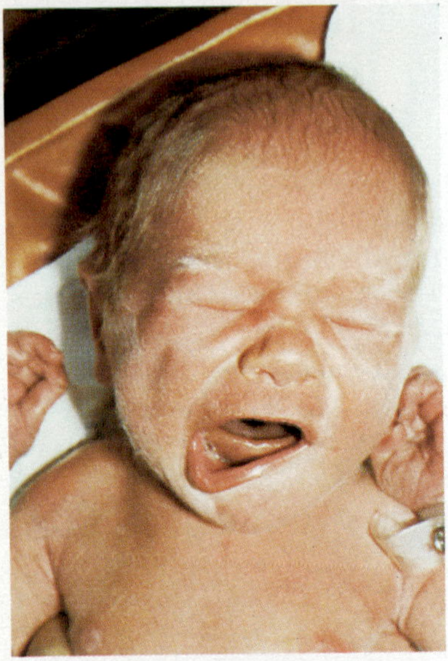

图 25 面瘫导致的嘴角下斜
Facial palsy affecting the lower lip

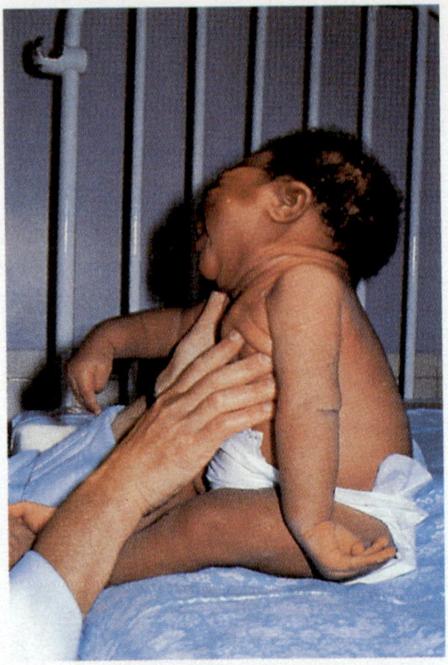

图 26 Erb 麻痹的“侍者讨小费姿势”
Erb's palsy with arm in waiter's tip position

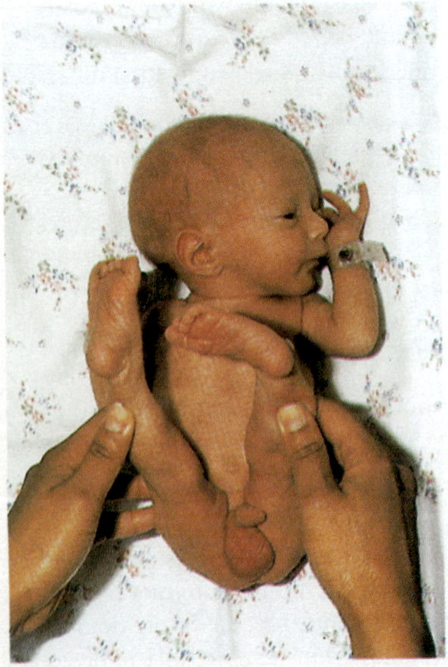

图 27 伸展的臀位
Extended breech position

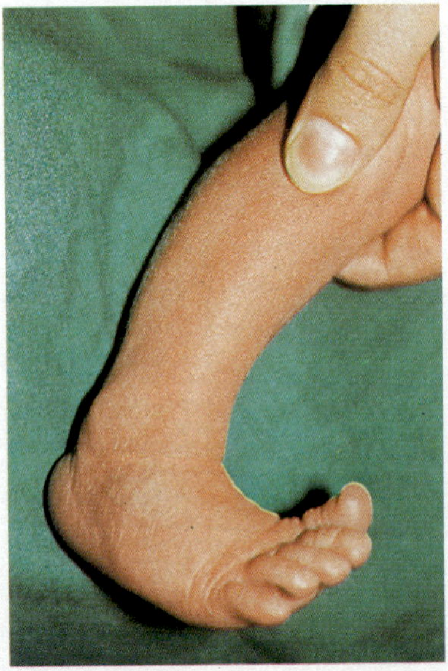

图 28 畸形足
Postural talipes

生后到 6 周

大运动

出生时，当把婴儿从仰卧位拉起时，有一个明显的头部运动迟滞。检查者的手放于婴儿的胸部，并将其托起，让其位于一个腹部向下的悬空位时（图29），他的背部拱起，臀部和膝部稍屈曲。到6周时，当婴儿在俯卧位时，他的头部可自行抬起，并且当将其从仰卧位拉起到坐位时，他对自己的头部运动有一定的控制能力。

精细运动和视觉

婴儿自出生时就有视觉，到 6 周时能够将视线集中到某一个物体上，并且可以在90度的范围内跟随物体水平移动。

听觉和说话

能对周围的噪音表示出惊吓的反应，并能被平和的声音所安抚。

社交行为

婴儿当被抱起哺乳时会停止哭闹。到5周时，婴儿也会对熟悉的声音和面孔做出微笑的反应。

3 ~ 6 个月

大运动

到6个月时，婴儿在俯卧位时，下肢能很好的踢动，前臂能撑起上身，抬起头部和胸部（图30），并开始侧着身打滚。他们还能够扶坐或靠坐。到4 ~ 8个月时，开始能够独坐。他们开始可以负重，并且如果有人扶着他们的手臂和胸部，他们就能够站立起来。

精细运动和视觉

婴儿会笨拙地用其手掌伸向、抓住物体，并最终握住小件物体。他们会将手中的物体放进嘴里，并且也开始会放开手中的物体。

听觉和说话

婴儿可以大笑，可以发出“咯咯”的欢乐声和一些没有含义的乱语。大约在 6 个月左右他们开始呀呀学语。还会对叫喊他们的名字做出反应。

社交行为

当给婴儿喂食时，他们会自己握着奶瓶。当你逗他们玩耍时，会与你一起嬉戏。他们会观察和玩弄自己的手和脚，并会将脚放入自己的嘴里（图 31）。

Birth to 6 weeks

Gross motor

At birth, there is marked head lag when the infant is pulled from the supine position. In ventral suspension with the examiner's hand supporting the chest (Fig. 29), the back is rounded and there is some flexion of the hips and knees. By 6 weeks of age, the infant can lift the head when placed in the prone position and there is some head control when pulled from supine to sitting.

Fine motor and vision

A baby can see at birth, but by 6 weeks can fix his vision on objects and will follow horizontally across to 90 degrees.

Hearing and speech

Response to noise will be indicated by startle or quietening to a soothing voice.

Social behaviour

The infant will stop crying when picked up to be nursed. Infants also begin to smile in response to familiar noises and faces by 5 weeks.

3-6 months

Gross motor

By 6 months, the infant in the prone position kicks well, pushes up from the forearms, lifting the head and chest (Fig. 30), and begins to roll from front to back. They can sit with support or leaning forward into the tripod position. The age of first sitting unsupported ranges from 4-8 months. They begin to weight-bear and to rise to the standing position when supported by the arms or chest.

Fine motor and vision

The infant will reach out for objects with a coarse palmar approach and will clasp and retain small objects placed in the hand. They place objects into the mouth and also begin to release objects.

Hearing and speech

The infant can laugh, gurgle and coo. Around 6 months, they usually begin to babble. They will turn when their name is called.

Social behaviour

The infant holds on to a bottle or feeding cup when fed and frolics when played with. They examine and play with their own hands and feet and place their feet into their mouths (Fig. 31).

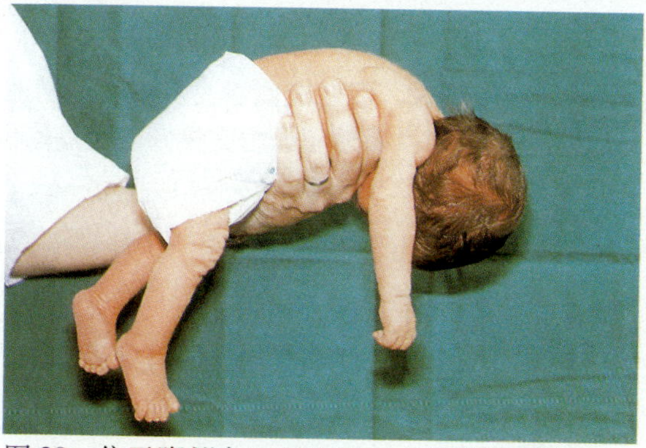

图 29　位于腹部向下悬空位时，其背部拱起
Ventral suspension showing rounded back

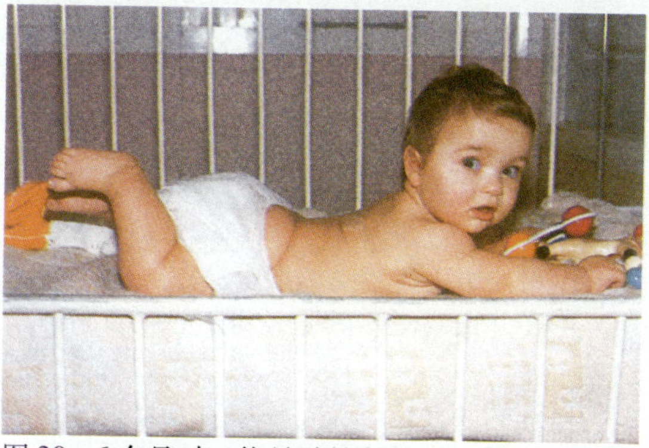

图 30　6 个月时，能前臂撑起上身
A press-up at 6 months

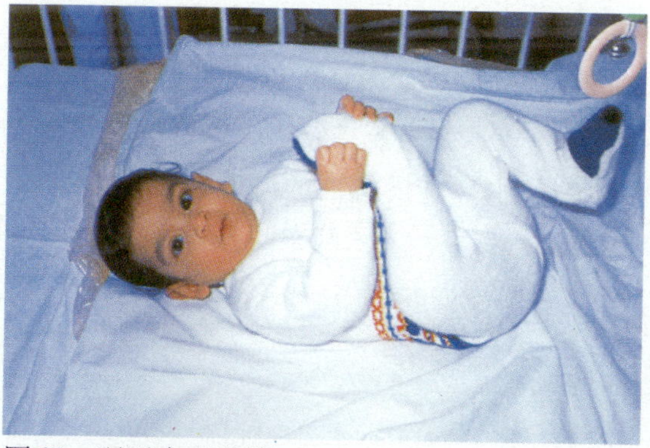

图 31　玩弄自己的脚
Playing with feet

6 ~ 9个月

大运动	到6个月时，婴儿能侧着身打滚。他们能挺直背部独坐。开始以手臂和腿为支撑做出爬行体位（图 32）。他们也开始用手和膝部爬行。
精细运动和视觉	他们可以用食指和拇指钳抓小件物体。并可将物体从一只手转移到另一只手（图 33）。
听觉和说话	到9个月时，他们开始用叫喊来吸引他人的注意力，并且开始发出没有意义的音节，像说“哒哒”和“吗吗”。
社交行为	孩子会转向说话的方向。当你将物体从他们的手中拿走时，他们会做出抵抗的反应。他们会努力伸手去拿他们够不到的东西。他们喜欢吃自己的手指。

9 ~ 12个月

大运动	大多数婴儿在9 ~ 10个月时都会爬行前进，但也有约10%的正常婴儿从未爬行前进过，而是滚动着向前或用手作为支撑推着身体前进（图34）。像这样的婴儿通常学步较晚，可能直到2岁才能学会独自走路。而其家族中的成员可能也有类似的正常运动发育的变异情况。9 ~ 12个月的孩子开始可以将自己拉起处于站立位，并可以扶着家具在房间里巡走。
精细运动和视觉	婴儿会用两块积木相互撞击出声。他们也能寻找掉落于地上的东西。
听觉和说话	到9 ~ 12个月，除了“哒哒”和“吗吗”以外，他们通常可发出1 ~ 2个可辨识的简单单词。
社交行为	他们喜欢模仿性的游戏，如拍手和挥手表示“再见”。但在1岁前当面对陌生人时，他们会害羞。

6-9 months

Gross motor

By 6 months, the infant can roll from front to back. They sit unsupported with a straight back. They begin to pivot around on their arms and legs into the crawling position (Fig. 32). They may also begin to crawl on hands and knees.

Fine motor and vision

Small objects are picked up between index finger and thumb in a pincer grasp. Objects are transferred from one hand to the other (Fig. 33).

Hearing and speech

By 9 months they shout to gain attention and vocalize non-specific syllables such as 'dada' and 'mama'.

Social behaviour

The baby turns when being talked to and resists when objects are taken from them. They try to reach objects out of their reach. They like to feed themselves with their fingers.

9-12 months

Gross motor

Most infants are crawling by 9-10 months of age. About 10% of normal infants never crawl, but move around by rolling, paddling or bottom shuffling (Fig. 34). Such children are often late walkers, and other family members may have also exhibited this normal variant of motor development. These children may not walk alone until 2 years of age. Children of 9-12 months begin to pull themselves to standing and to cruise around the room holding on to furniture.

Fine motor and vision

The infant will bang two cubes together. They also look for fallen objects.

Hearing and speech

By 9-12 months, they usually have one or two recognizable single words in addition to 'dada' and 'mama'.

Social behaviour

They enjoy imitative games such as clapping hands and waving goodbye, but are shy with strangers until the end of the first year.

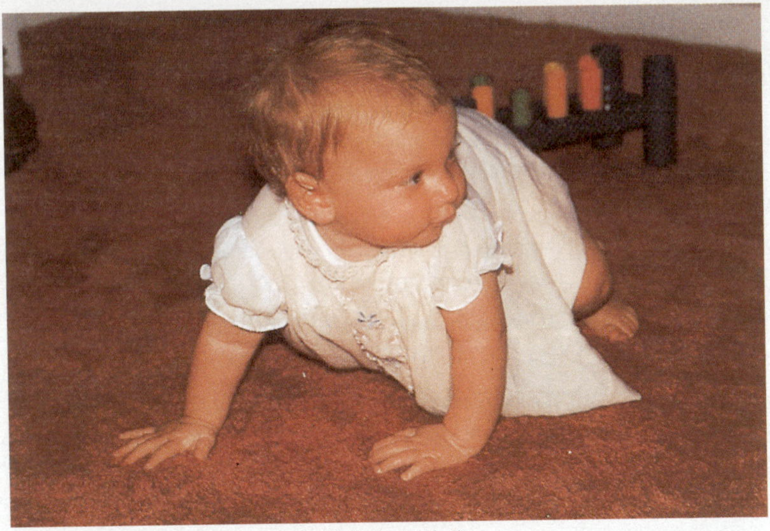

图 32 用手臂和腿作为支撑做出爬行体位
Getting into a crawling position

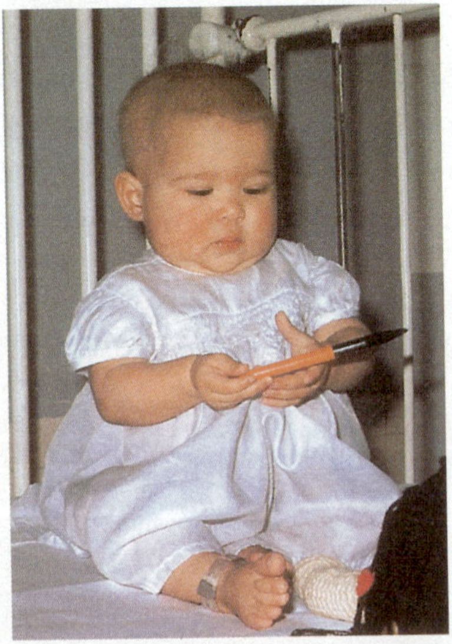

图 33 将物体从一只手转移到另一只手
Transferring objects

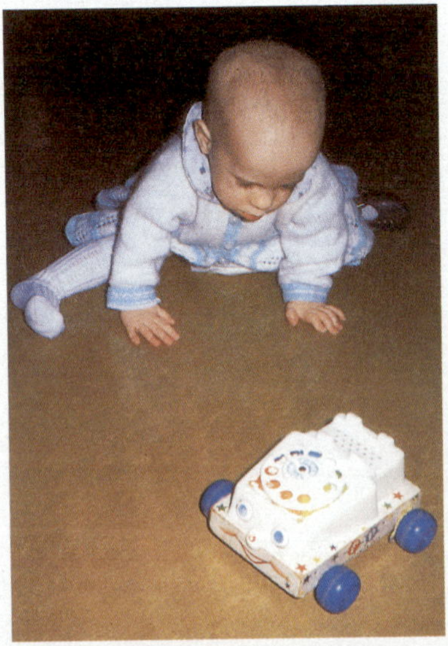

图 34 正常爬行运动的变异
Normal variant of getting around

12 ~ 18 个月

大运动

到12个月时，孩子通常可以握住大人的手行走（图35），并开始独自站立。

精细运动和视觉

用食指和拇指钳抓物体的动作更加精确，并且可以灵巧地捡起很小的物体（图36）。孩子可以用食指指向物体（图37）。他们会反复的投掷物体，通过劝说能按照要求把物体交给另一个人。他们可以用2 ~ 3块积木垒成塔形。

听觉和说话

他们已经有数个单词的词汇量，并且能重复自己的名字。在这个年龄段，理解能力要好于语言能力。他们喜欢看书中的图片，并且一边看，一边用手指和自言自语。

社交行为

到12个月时，孩子会用手指指向自己想要的东西。他们会自己从水杯中喝水，还能自己进食。他们开始试着自己穿衣。他们学会将物体抛掷给他人，也可以与你玩简单的游戏，如“躲猫猫”（图38）。

18 ~ 24 个月

大运动

可以很自信、很独立的走路。仅有3%的孩子到18个月时还不会走路。他们可以自己爬上椅子和楼梯，并且可以拿着玩具行走。

精细运动和视觉

开始用铅笔或蜡笔涂鸦。他们可以用3 ~ 4块积木垒成塔形。

表达能力和语言

他们至少有10 ~ 12个单词的词汇量，到24个月时，孩子可以用2 ~ 3个单词连成简单的句子。

社交行为

他们会用勺子和手指进食。他们也会坚持独立进食、穿衣和游戏，并且会对那些想要帮助他们的人的干扰表示抗议。

12-18 months

Gross motor

By 12 months, a child can usually walk with hands held (Fig. 35), and begins to stand alone.

Fine motor and vision

The pincer grip becomes more refined and tiny objects can be picked up delicately (Fig. 36). The child also points at objects with the index finger (Fig. 37). They cast objects down repeatedly and can be persuaded to give objects to another person on request. They build a tower with 2-3 bricks.

Hearing and speech

There is a vocabulary of several words and the child usually also repeats their own name. Comprehension is more advanced than speech at this age. They enjoy looking at pictures in a book and often point and babble while doing this.

Social behaviour

By 12 months, children indicate their wants, usually by pointing. They drink from a cup and help to feed themselves. They also begin to help with dressing. The child learns to throw and enjoys simple games such as peek-a-boo (Fig. 38).

18-24 months

Gross motor

Walks confidently and independently. Only 3% have not begun to walk by 18 months of age. The child will be able to climb onto chairs and up stairs, and will also hold onto toys while walking.

Fine motor and vision

Scribbles with a pencil or crayon. Builds a tower of 3-4 bricks.

Speech and language

There will be a vocabulary of at least ten to twelve words and, by 24 months, the child will link several words together in a short 2-3 word sentence.

Social behaviour

The child will spoon and finger feed. They will begin to assert more independence in feeding, dressing and play and will resist the intervention of others who try to assist.

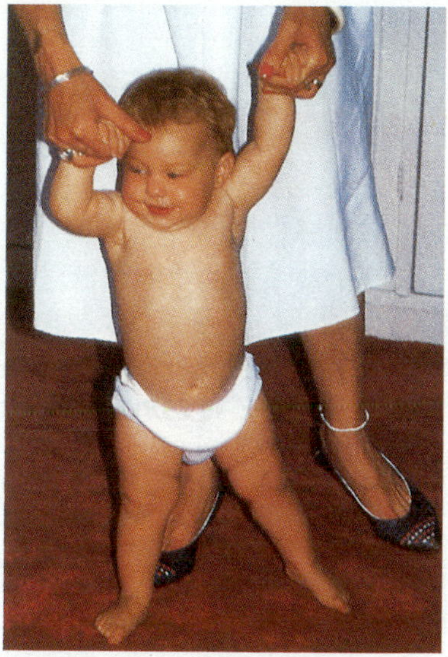

图 35　在他人帮助下行走
Walking with help

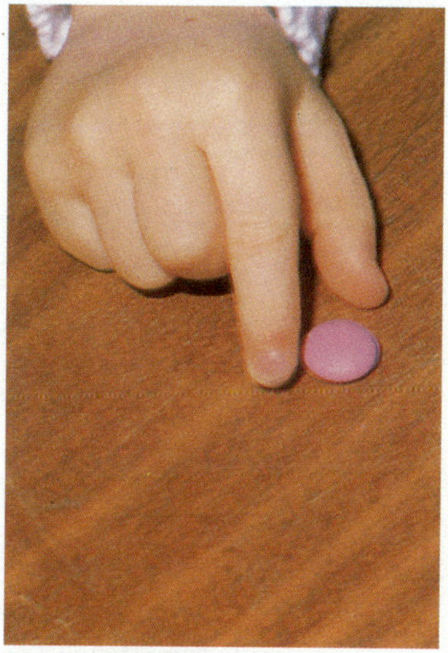

图 36　钳抓物体
Pincer grip

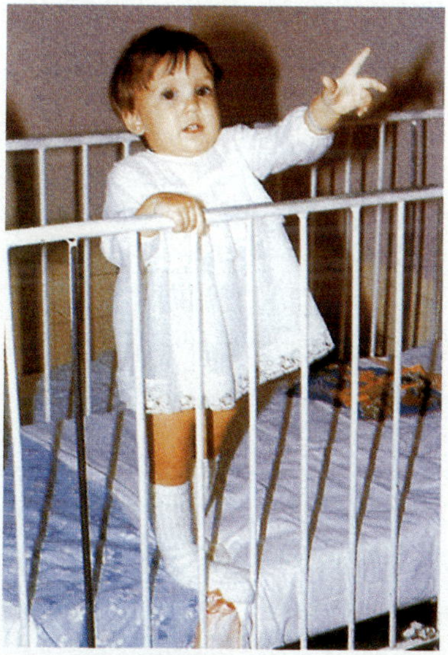

图 37　指向物体
Pointing

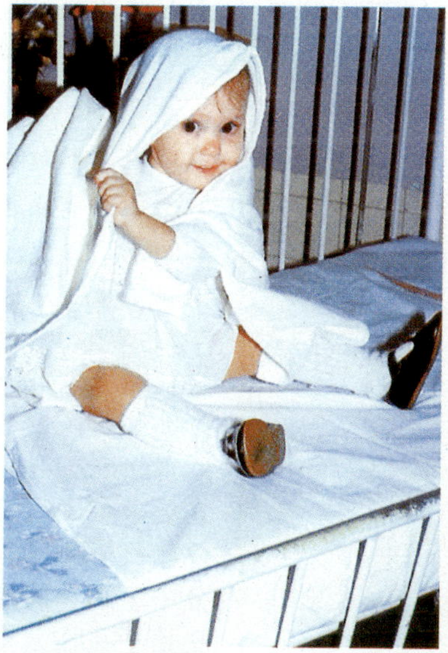

图 38　躲猫猫
Peek-a-boo

视力

在足月时，孩子的视觉神经髓鞘还未完全形成。先天性白内障和严重的先天性上睑下垂的早期纠治对于正常的视力发育很重要。出生时，孩子会将视线集中在母亲的脸上，到6～8周时，其视线可以在直线水平跟随物体移动。从 9 个月开始，可以用白色小球（Stycar测试球）测试其视敏度。3岁以后，孩子可以用分级字母卡来进行字母搭配（图 39）。

听力

新生儿可以被平和的声音所安抚，在生后几周后会对吵闹的声音做出惊跳、哭吵的反应。目前，在英国提倡对所有新生儿进行常规的听力筛查。一个最普通的新生儿筛查试验包括从中耳探测耳声发射（oto-acoustic emission，OAE）。到 7 ～ 9 个月时，婴儿会把他的头或视线转向声音刺激的方向，如响亮的碰撞声或在耳边的铃声（牵拉试验，distraction test）。正常语言的理解和模仿能力表示不可能有严重的听力缺失。

表达能力和语言

大多数孩子到 24 个月时都会将 2 ～ 3 个单词连成一个短句，到3岁时，就能说出较丰富的句子，并能够不间断地与人交谈，还会问许多重复的问题。如果孩子到3岁左右，其语言能力没有进步，或者发音不清晰，那么我们建议进行表达能力和语言的治疗。

绘画

在要求孩子所画的图中可提供有用的临床信息。可以让孩子画一个“人”，你可从他所画人体包含的部分中了解和探知孩子发育的阶段。一些图画可以反映孩子在临床交流中无法被了解到的情感问题（图40和41）。有时绘画可揭示隐藏的临床特征，比如一个偏盲的孩子只在纸的一边画图。

Vision

Myelination of the optic pathways is incomplete at term. Early correction of congenital cataracts or severe congenital ptosis is important for normal visual development. At birth, the child will fix on the mother's face, and by 6-8 weeks, follows objects in the direct line of vision. From 9 months, small graded white balls (Stycar test balls) can be used to test visual acuity. After 3 years of age, the child can usually match letters with graded letter cards (Fig. 39).

Hearing

The newborn infant will quieten with soothing noises and within a few weeks of birth reacts to loud noises by startling, or crying. In the UK, routine audiological screening of all newborn infants is now recommended. One commonly used neonatal screening test involves the detection of oto-acoustic emissions (OAEs) from the middle ear. By 7-9 months of age, infants will turn their heads or move their eyes towards a sound stimulus such as a high pitched rattle or bell at ear level (distraction test). Comprehension and imitation of normal speech indicates that severe hearing loss is unlikely.

Speech and language

Most children will be linking 2-3 words into short sentences by 24 months of age, and will have developed full sentences by 3 years of age. By 3 years, the child will talk incessantly and ask many repetitive questions. Referral to a speech and language therapist is indicated if there is not this progression or if the child's speech is not clearly articulated by around 3 years of age.

Drawings

The pictures a child is asked to draw can provide useful clinical information. A child can be asked to 'draw a man' and the parts of the body included in the picture are a good indication of the stage of development. Some pictures may indicate emotional problems that cannot otherwise be communicated to the clinician (Figs 40 and 41). Sometimes the drawing may reveal an undiscovered clinical feature such as hemianopia in a child who only draws on one side of the paper.

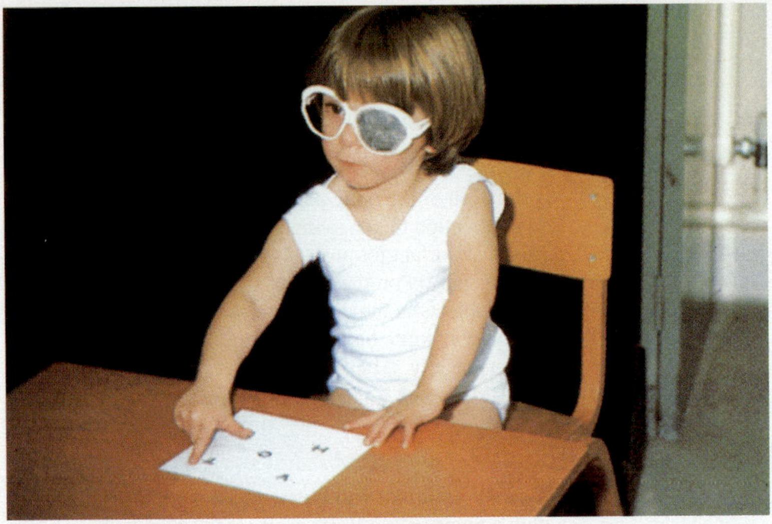

图 39　对 3 岁的孩子用分级字母卡测试视力
Testing vision with graded letter cards in a 3-year-old child

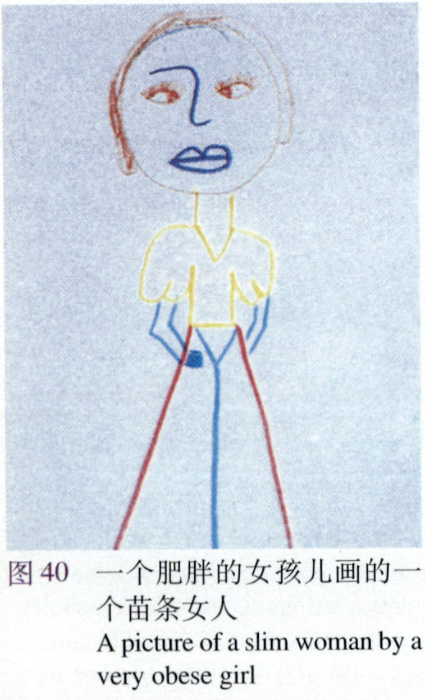

图 40　一个肥胖的女孩儿画的一个苗条女人
A picture of a slim woman by a very obese girl

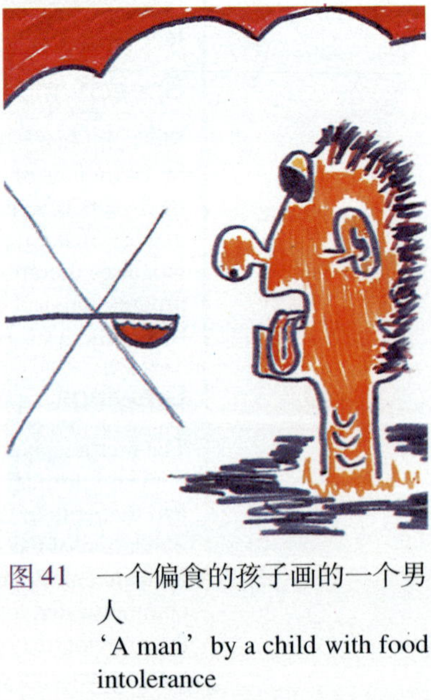

图 41　一个偏食的孩子画的一个男人
'A man' by a child with food intolerance

母乳喂养的优点是明确的（图42），并且应该从孩子一出生就开始。人工喂养不应鼓励，尤其是如果有家族性的过敏病史。母乳喂养优于人工喂养的主要方面在于前者有抗感染的特点，并且能够改善孩子的耐受力，尤其对于早产儿。从心理学方面来看，母乳喂养可以增进母婴之间的关系。许多早产儿由于发育不成熟或呼吸窘迫而不会吮吸，但是可以通过间歇性的鼻导管喂养法（鼻饲）喂食。低出生体重儿需要高蛋白和充分的液体摄入，并且通常需要补充钠、铁、维生素、钙、磷酸盐和叶酸。大部分儿童的生长发育情况与他们出生时所处的百分位点有关。那些由于在子宫内营养不良而造成出生时较小的新生儿很可能在出生后的前几年赶上正常生长发育。那些出生时相对于胎龄较大的新生儿（如糖尿病母亲所生的孩子），很可能越过其原来的百分位点，而处于相对较低的百分位点。

营养不良

临床特征

严重的全身性营养不良（消瘦）（图43）通常是由于无法进行母乳喂养和/或摄入食物不足所造成。它有时发生于一些慢性疾病中。极度消瘦以及对胃肠炎和其他感染的易患性增加是很常见的，蛋白质营养不良 (Kwashiorkor)是由于蛋白质摄入不足造成，可导致水肿、唇干裂、色素脱失和鳞状皮肤，以及稀疏、易折的淡红色头发（图44）。这些婴儿通常食欲较差，倦怠且易激惹。肝脏的脂肪浸润会造成肝大。

预防

社区的健康教育旨在预防营养摄入不足的情况发生。母乳喂养应该被鼓励，尤其是在发展中国家，因为在那里人工喂养是比较昂贵的。较廉价的地方性营养辅食应该在孩子4～6个月时加入他的饮食中。应早期识别营养不良，并早期逐步地添加地方性辅食。此外，应及时治疗感染，并且通常有必要添加维生素。

Breast-feeding has definite advantages (Fig. 42) and should begin in the delivery suite. Formula milk should be discouraged, especially if there is a family history of allergy. The major advantages of breast milk over formula milk are the anti-infective properties, and improved tolerance especially by preterm infants. Breast-feeding is also psychologically important to the maternal-infant relationship. Many preterm infants are unable to suck because of immaturity or respiratory distress, but they can be fed by intermittent gavage feeding through a nasogastric tube. Low birth weight infants require high protein and water intake, and supplements of sodium, iron, vitamins, calcium, phosphate and folic acid are usually necessary. Most children grow similar to their birth centile. Those who are small at birth because of intra-uterine undernutrition are more likely to achieve catch up growth in the early years after birth. Those who are large for gestational age at birth, (e.g. infants of diabetic mothers), are more likely to cross centiles to a lower centile.

Malnutrition

Clinical features

Severe generalized undernutrition (marasmus) (Fig. 43) is usually due to failure to breast-feed and/or inadequate dietary intake. It sometimes occurs in chronic illness. Extreme emaciation and increased susceptibility to gastroenteritis and infection are common. Protein energy malnutrition (kwashiorkor) results from inadequate dietary protein intake and results in oedema, cheilosis, depigmented and scaly skin, and sparse friable reddish hair (Fig. 44). The infant usually has a poor appetite and is listless and irritable. Fatty infiltration of the liver causes hepatomegaly.

Prevention

Community health education should aim to prevent nutritional deficiency states. Breast-feeding should be encouraged, particularly in developing countries where formula milks are often expensive. Cheap nutritious local foods should be introduced into the infant's diet from 4-6 months of age. Early recognition of deficiency states and gradual re-introduction of an adequate local diet. Associated infections may require treatment, and vitamin supplementation is usually necessary.

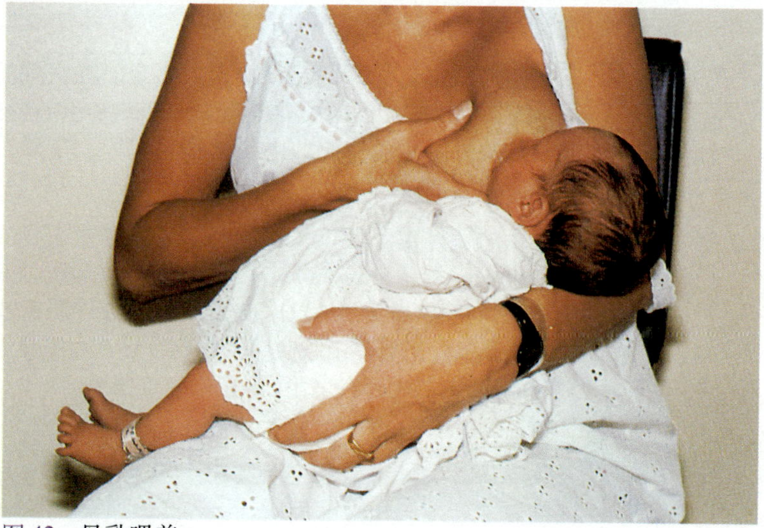

图 42　母乳喂养
Breast-feeding

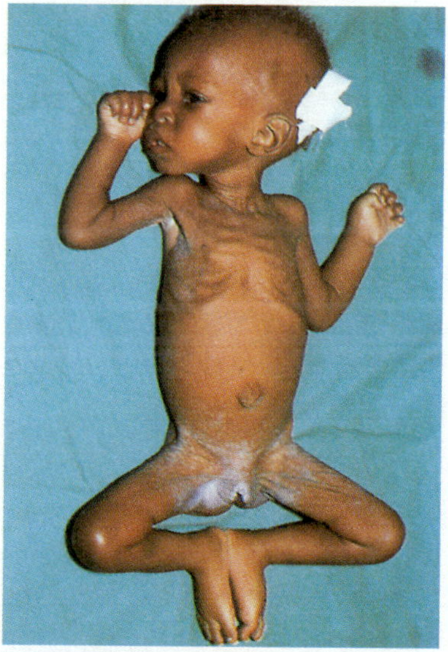

图 43　消瘦
Marasmus

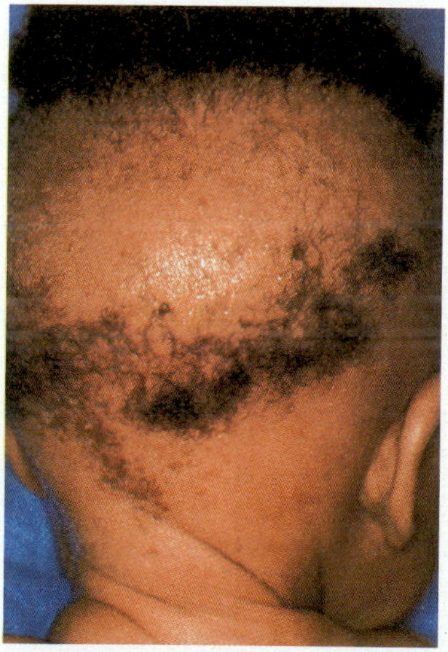

图 44　蛋白质营养不良造成的稀疏、易折的头发
Sparse friable hair in protein malnutrition (PEM)

发育停滞

病因学

发育停滞最常见的原因是食物摄入不足。在常规的体格检查中，先天性畸形、染色体疾病和特定综合征都应该被怀疑。儿童吸收不良的最常见原因是囊性纤维病和腹部疾病。

临床特征

在儿童早期体重不能以正常水平增长。体重表将显示距出生时的百分位点呈进行性偏离。臀部瘦且有肌肉废用性萎缩（图 45）。皮下脂肪丢失伴肌肉瘦弱。如果发育停滞是由吸收障碍引起，那么腹胀是最常见的表现（图 46），并且可能发生佝偻病。

检查

必须要评估饮食摄入。贫血和脂肪痢都提示有肠道吸收障碍。发汗试验和空肠活组织检查都可以分别证实囊性纤维病和腹部疾病。

佝偻病

病因学

维生素 D 缺乏通常是因为饮食中摄入不足引起。佝偻病也可由肠道吸收障碍、肝脏疾病、肾小管功能障碍和长期服用抗惊厥药引起。

临床特征

长骨干骺端隆起，尤其是腕关节（图47），此外还有弓形腿、胸廓畸形、串珠肋。在小婴儿可能会有颅骨软化和囟门闭合延迟。儿童通常易激惹和较烦躁，并且有骨压痛和肌无力。

诊断

经典的生化指标异常是低钙血症、低磷酸盐血症、维生素 D 缺乏和碱性磷酸酶升高。X 线片表现包括由于长骨骨骺骨化延迟而使干骺端呈杯口状张开。同时也可出现病理性骨折和负重长骨的畸形。

治疗

补充维生素 D 和改善饮食摄入。应用大剂量维生素 D 对于肾性佝偻病和遗传性低磷酸盐血症性佝偻病是有必要的。

Failure to thrive

Aetiology

The most common cause of failure to thrive is inadequate dietary intake. Congenital malformations, chromosomal disorders and specific syndromes can usually be suspected on routine physical examination. The most common causes of malabsorption in childhood are cystic fibrosis and coeliac disease.

Clinical features

Failure to gain weight at normal rate in early childhood. Weight chart will show progressive deviation from birth centile. Buttocks are thin and wasted (Fig. 45). There is loss of subcutaneous fat with poor muscle bulk. If failure to thrive is caused by malabsorption, abdominal distension (Fig. 46) is common and rickets may occur.

Investigation

Dietary intake must be assessed. Anaemia and steatorrhoea suggest malabsorption. Sweat test and jejunal biopsy will confirm cystic fibrosis and coeliac disease respectively.

Rickets

Aetiology

Vitamin D deficiency is usually due to inadequate dietary intake. Rickets is also caused by malabsorption, liver disease, renal failure, renal tubular dysfunction and long-term anticonvulsants.

Clinical features

Swelling of long bone metaphyses, particularly wrist (Fig. 47), bowing of legs, chest deformity, and rachitic rosary. Craniotabes and delayed closure of fontanelle may occur in young infants. The child is often irritable and fretful, and has bone tenderness and muscle weakness.

Diagnosis

Classic biochemical disturbances are hypocalcaemia, hypophosphataemia, vitamin D deficiency, and raised alkaline phosphatase. Radiological signs include splaying of metaphyses of long bones with delayed ossification of epiphyses. Pathological fractures and deformity of weight-bearing long bones may occur.

Management

Vitamin D supplementation and improved dietary intake. High dosage may be necessary in renal rickets or hereditary hypophosphataemic rickets.

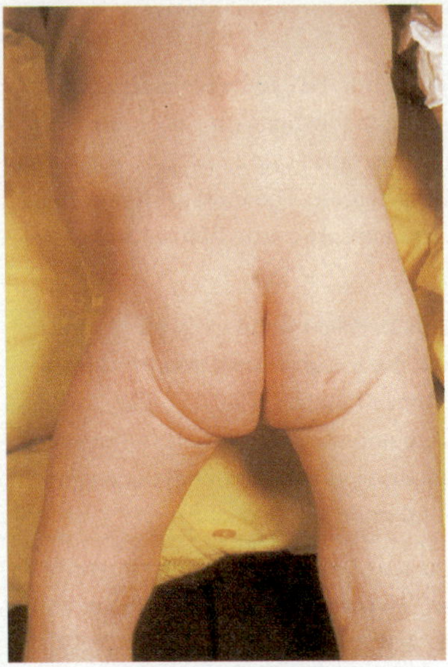

图 45　腹部疾病中臀部肌肉萎缩
Wasted buttocks in coeliac disease

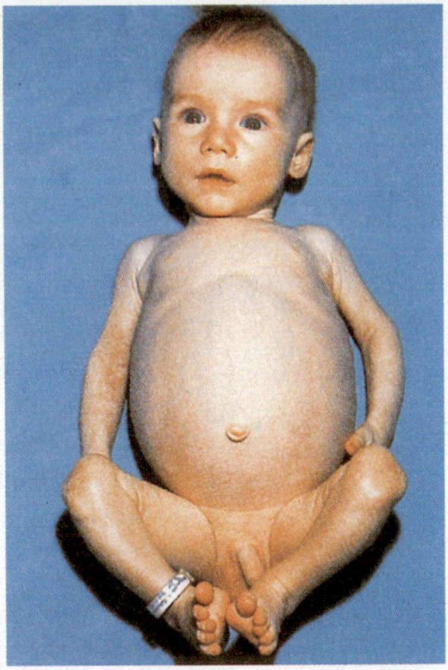

图 46　发育停滞伴腹胀和四肢废用性萎缩
Failure to thrive with distended abdomen and wasted limbs

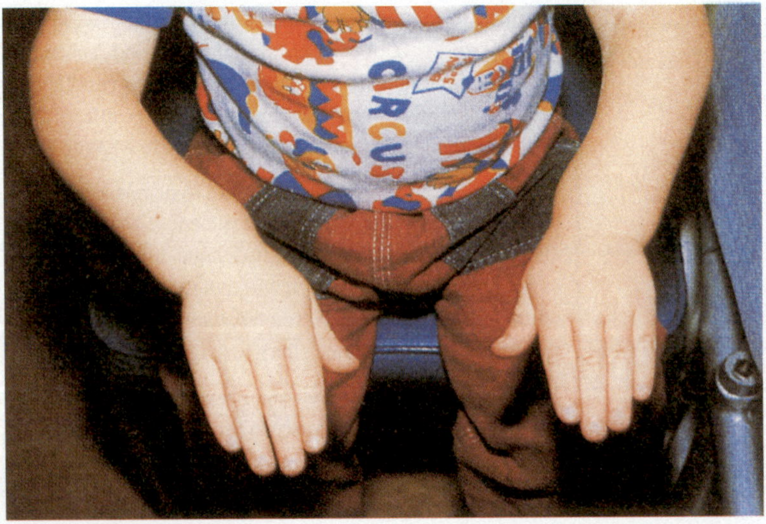

图 47　腕关节干骺端隆起
Swelling of metaphyses at wrists

正常生长

生长受到遗传、营养、情感因素以及疾病和激素分泌不足的影响。婴儿期的生长是迅速的，然后到儿童期逐渐变得缓慢而平稳，一直到青春期再次进入生长高峰，最后骨骺端融合达到最终生长高度。准确的身高、体重和头围的测量都应在生长百分位图表上绘成曲线。大多数儿童的生长在生长百分位图表上的进程都相似。有3%的正常健康儿童身高小于第三个百分位点。了解父母身高将有利于评定孩子身材矮小是遗传因素还是生长障碍。大部分早产婴儿都会通过生长而最终达到正常人群的身材，除非有严重的宫内生长受限。大脑发育和头围增长主要是在生后前三年内。在婴儿时期常见的颅骨和脸部不对称（斜头畸形）（图 48）是由于胎位关系或继发于宫内发育不完善（图 49）而造成的，但会随着年龄的增长而改善。由于颅骨骨缝过早地融合（颅缝早闭）而引起的头部的不对称是十分罕见的。

身材矮小

病因学

大多数身材矮小的孩子，其父母身材也都矮小。少部分是由于染色体异常（如 Turner 综合征、垂体功能减退、甲状腺功能减退、生长激素分泌不足、软骨发育不全），或医源性因素，包括长期使用类固醇治疗等。

临床特征和检查

体格检查常可发现一些染色体异常患儿的异形特征。软骨发育不全患儿通常有不成比例的短小四肢或躯干（图50），以及异常骨骼X线片表现。青少年期的甲状腺功能减退会导致进行性生长停滞（图 51）、严重的骨龄延迟、面容粗糙和智力发育迟缓。单一性生长激素缺乏症患儿有着与身高不相称的体重超重。连续性身高测量显示生长速率降低，脑垂体刺激试验证实生长激素缺乏。多发性垂体激素缺乏通常继发于肿瘤形成（如颅咽管瘤）、放疗或外伤。

治疗

激素缺乏需要特定的激素替代治疗。孩子是否今后能有一个正常的身材依赖于诊断的年龄、病程以及疾病的严重程度。

Normal growth

Growth is influenced by genetic, nutritional and emotional factors as well as by disease and hormonal deficiencies. Growth in infancy is rapid. There is then slow steady growth in childhood until the adolescent growth spurt, after which final height is reached and epiphyseal fusion takes place. Accurate measurements of height, weight and head circumference should be plotted on centile charts. In most children, growth follows a similar course to centile charts. Height <3rd centile occurs in 3% of normal healthy children. Parental height will help to assess whether short stature is genetic or a disorder of growth. Most preterm infants achieve normal adult size, unless there is severe intrauterine growth restriction. Major postnatal growth in brain and head circumference occurs in the first 3 years of life. Asymmetry of skull (plagiocephaly) and face (Fig. 48) caused by intrauterine posture, or secondary to immaturity (Fig. 49) is common in infancy and improves with age. Premature fusion of skull sutures (craniosynostosis) causing asymmetry is extremely rare.

Short stature

Aetiology

Most short children have short parents. A few have chromosomal abnormalities (e.g. Turner syndrome, hypopituitarism, hypothyroidism, growth hormone deficiency, chondrodysplasia), or iatrogenic causes, including long-term steroid therapy.

Clinical features and investigation

Physical examination usually reveals dysmorphic features in chromosomal abnormalities. In chondrodysplasia, there are usually disproportionately short limbs or trunk (Fig. 50), and abnormal skeletal X-rays. Juvenile hypothyroidism results in progressive growth failure (Fig. 51), severe retardation of bone age, coarse facies and intellectual retardation. In isolated growth hormone deficiency, the child is usually overweight for height. Serial height measurements show reduced growth velocity and pituitary stimulation tests demonstrate lack of growth hormone. Multiple pituitary hormone failure is usually secondary to neoplasia (e.g. craniopharyngioma), radiotherapy or trauma.

Management

Hormonal deficiency requires specific replacement therapy. Catch-up growth and ultimate height depend on age at diagnosis, duration and severity of underlying disorder.

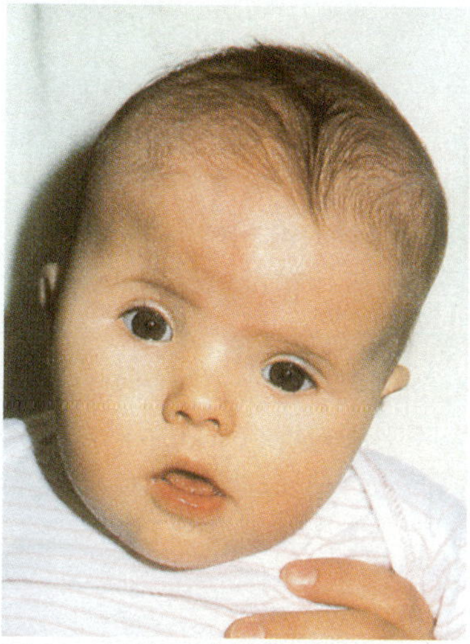

图 48 颅骨和脸部不对称
Asymmetry of face and skull

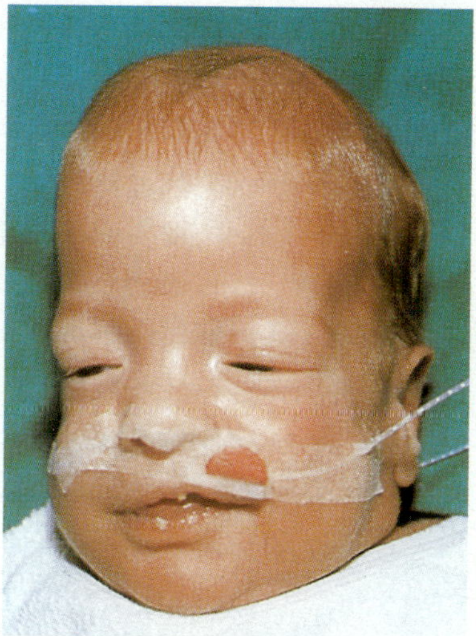

图 49 早产儿的狭长头形
Preterm infant with narrow, elongated head

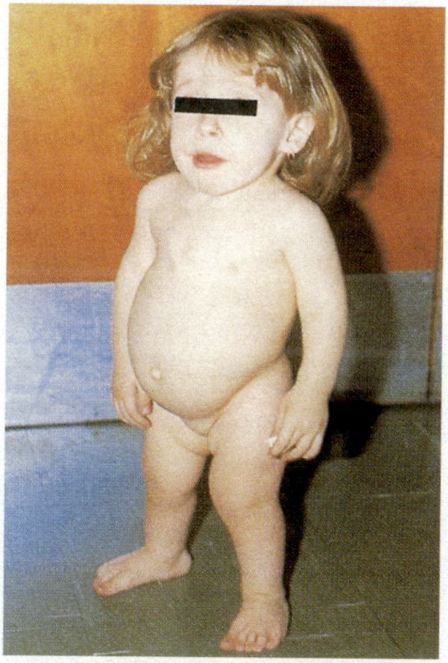

图 50 软骨发育不全的短小四肢
(经Dr G. Supramanian的许可)
Short-limbed chondrodysplasia
(courtesy of Dr G. Supramanian)

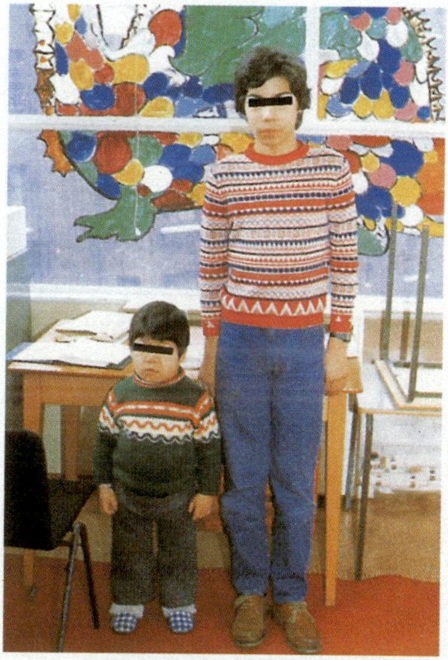

图 51 由于甲状腺功能减退而患有身材矮小症的 16 岁男孩与正常的 16 岁男孩
16-year-old boy with short stature due to hypothyroidism with a normal 16-year-old boy

糖尿病母亲的婴儿

发病率 在妊娠期较好的控制母亲的糖尿病能减轻糖尿病母亲所生婴儿的体征和症状，但是不能减少先天性畸形的高危险率。糖尿病母亲所生婴儿的先天性畸形的发生率（5%）要高于一般人群的危险率（3%）。目前还不知是否在怀孕前进行精细的糖尿病控制治疗可以减少这一高危险率。

临床特征 巨大肥胖婴儿（图 52 和 53），经常由于肺表面活性物质生成延迟而发生呼吸窘迫综合征。生后由于胰岛细胞增生、红细胞增多而有低血糖的危险。糖尿病母亲的婴儿在出生后前几个小时需要细心地观察，并规律地监测血糖。低血糖发生时需要多次喂奶，或者静脉输注葡萄糖。

病程和预后 如果对低血糖症有充分的认识，并予以正确处理，低血糖可在数天内缓解，而没有后遗症的危险。

贝克威思综合征

病因学 不明，多为散发。

临床特征 巨大出生体重婴儿，伴有舌下垂（图54）和脐膨出。低血糖是由于胰腺过度增生和红细胞增多症。

预后 在新生儿期有较高的死亡率。

肥胖症

病因学 肥胖在西方社会是一个常见的健康问题，但是由于内分泌紊乱而造成的肥胖很少见，而遗传因素则是常见原因。

临床特征 体重要高于身高的百分位点，即使这个孩子本来就很高。皮褶厚度极为丰满。

治疗 对于已有的肥胖很难治疗，因此在儿童早期进行预防很重要。

Infant of diabetic mother

Incidence

Good control of maternal diabetes throughout pregnancy reduces signs and symptoms in infants of diabetic mothers, but not the increased risk of congenital abnormalities. The frequency of congenital abnormalities (5%) is higher than the general population risk (3%). It is not yet known whether meticulous diabetic control before conception will reduce this high risk.

Clinical features

Large obese infants (Figs 52 and 53) who often develop respiratory distress syndrome due to delayed surfactant production. After birth, there is a risk of hypoglycaemia due to islet cell hyperplasia, and polycythaemia. Infants of diabetic mothers require careful observation in the first few hours after birth, with regular monitoring of blood sugar. Hypoglycaemia usually responds to frequent milk feeds or an intravenous infusion of dextrose.

Course and prognosis

Hypoglycaemia settles within a few days and, provided it has been recognized and treated adequately, will not give rise to sequelae.

Beckwith syndrome

Aetiology

Unknown and usually sporadic occurrence.

Clinical features

Large birth weight infants with glossoptosis (Fig. 54) and omphalocele. Hypoglycaemia due to pancreatic hyperplasia and polycythaemia often occur.

Prognosis

High mortality in the neonatal period.

Obesity

Aetiology

Obesity is a common health problem in Western society, but is rarely due to endocrine disturbance. A genetic component is common.

Clinical features

Weight is greater than expected for height centile, even though the child is often quite tall. Skin fold thickness is excessive.

Management

Established obesity is very difficult to treat, so prevention in early childhood is important.

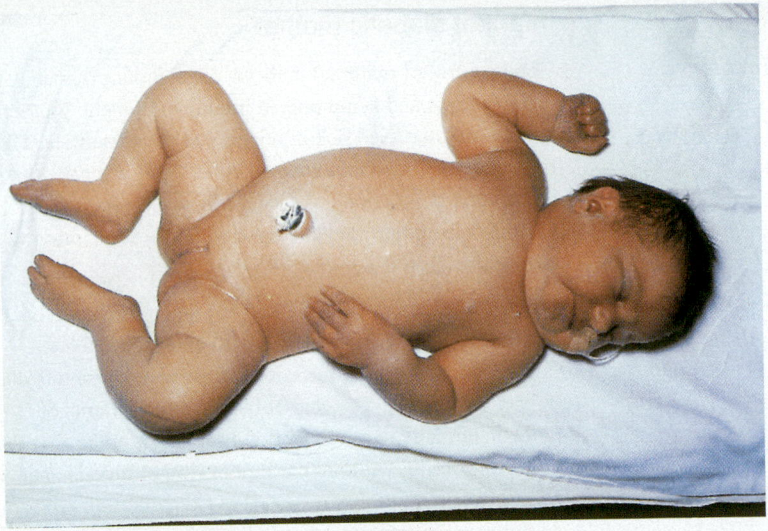

图 52　糖尿病母亲所生的巨大肥胖婴儿
Large obese infant of diabetic mother

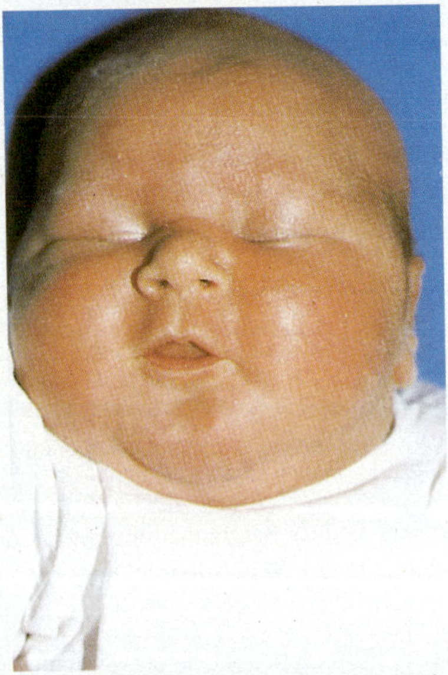

图 53　糖尿病母亲所生的具有“天使”般白胖面容的婴儿
Cherubic facies of infant of diabetic mother

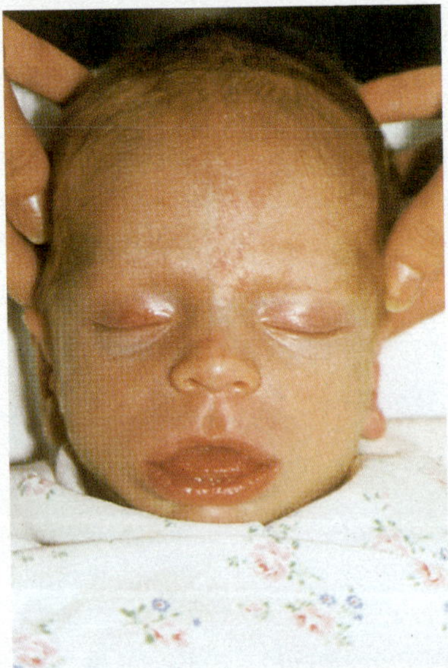

图 54　贝克威思综合征婴儿的舌下垂
Beckwith syndrome with glossoptosis

甲状腺功能减退

发病率 相对常见，每4000个出生存活新生儿中就有1个。

病因学 先天性甲状腺功能减退通常是由于甲状腺发育不全所造成。偶尔是由于遗传性激素合成途径发育不全所造成的。

临床特征 面容粗糙（图55），皮肤干燥，声音嘶哑干涩，缺少自发性活动。通常还有体温过低、肌张力减退以及体重增加缓慢。新生儿有时会出现脐疝（图56）、便秘和黄疸消退延迟。在婴儿期不能及早诊断对孩子今后造成的主要影响是智能迟钝。一些患儿还有小脑共济失调、近视和斜视。青少年的甲状腺功能减退出现较晚，患儿有生长不足，但如果在脑发育的关键阶段甲状腺功能正常，就很少有智力障碍。

治疗 进行终生的左旋甲状腺素替代治疗。剂量要调整到能达到正常的生长和骨龄，同时还要抑制促甲状腺激素。

甲状腺功能亢进

发病率 很少见。如果母亲有甲状腺毒症和因甲状腺刺激性免疫球蛋白引起Graves病的病史，那么其所生的婴儿有可能发生新生儿期甲状腺毒症。

临床特征 小婴儿有心动过速、呕吐、多汗、体重增长缓慢和易激惹的表现。大龄儿童也可能有快速生长、颤抖、眼球突出和甲状腺肿大的表现（图57）。

治疗 应用抗甲状腺药物，如卡比马唑，一直到症状缓解，通常需要数年。有些需要行甲状腺切除术。新生儿期的甲状腺毒症可以在数周内缓解，有时不需要治疗。

Hypothyroidism

Incidence
Relatively common, occurs in 1 in 4000 live births.

Aetiology
Congenital hypothyroidism is usually due to thyroid agenesis. Occasionally due to inherited dysgenesis of hormone synthesis.

Clinical features
Coarse facies (Fig. 55), dry skin, hoarse voice and cry, and paucity of spontaneous activity. Hypothermia, hypotonia and poor weight gain are common. Umbilical hernia (Fig. 56), constipation and prolonged jaundice sometimes occur in neonates. Intellectual retardation is the major long-term effect of delayed diagnosis in infancy. Some have cerebellar ataxia, myopia and squints. In juvenile hypothyroidism occurring in later childhood, there is growth failure, but very little intellectual impairment if thyroid function has been normal during the early critical period of brain growth.

Management
Lifelong replacement therapy with L-thyroxine. Dosage is adjusted to achieve normal growth and bone age as well as suppression of thyroid stimulating hormone.

Hyperthyroidism

Incidence
Uncommon. Neonatal thyrotoxicosis may occur in infants of mothers with a history of thyrotoxicosis and thyroid-stimulating immunoglobulins.

Clinical features
Young infants have tachycardia, vomiting, sweating, poor weight gain and irritability. Older children may also have rapid growth, tremor, and proptosis and goitre (Fig. 57).

Management
Antithyroid drugs such as carbimazole until spontaneous remission, usually within a few years. Some require thyroidectomy. Neonatal thyrotoxicosis resolves within a few weeks and sometimes no treatment is needed.

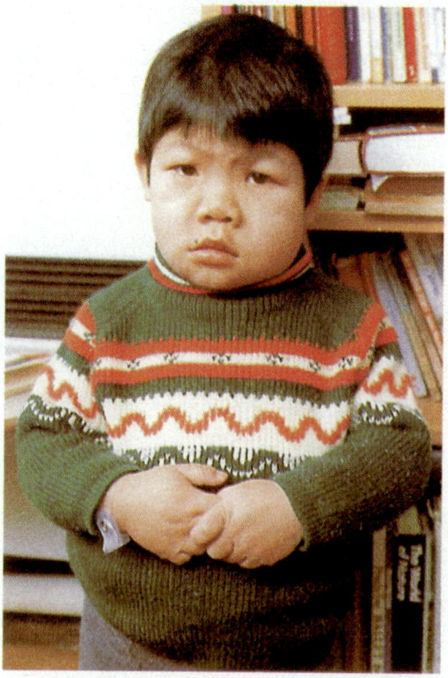

图 55　青少年甲状腺功能减退的粗糙面容
Coarse facies in juvenile hypothyroidism

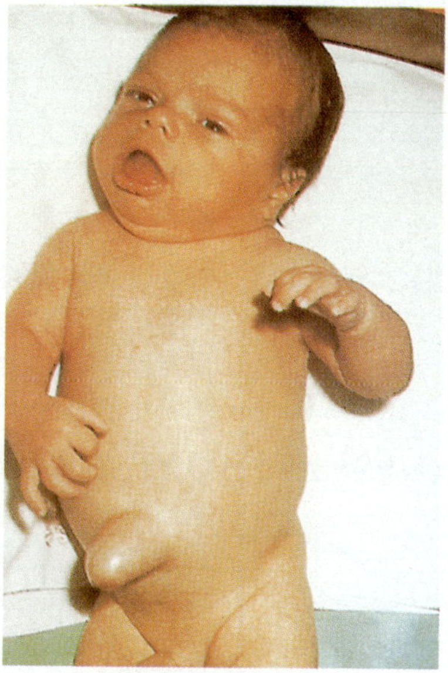

图 56　脐疝和大舌
Umbilical hernia and large tongue

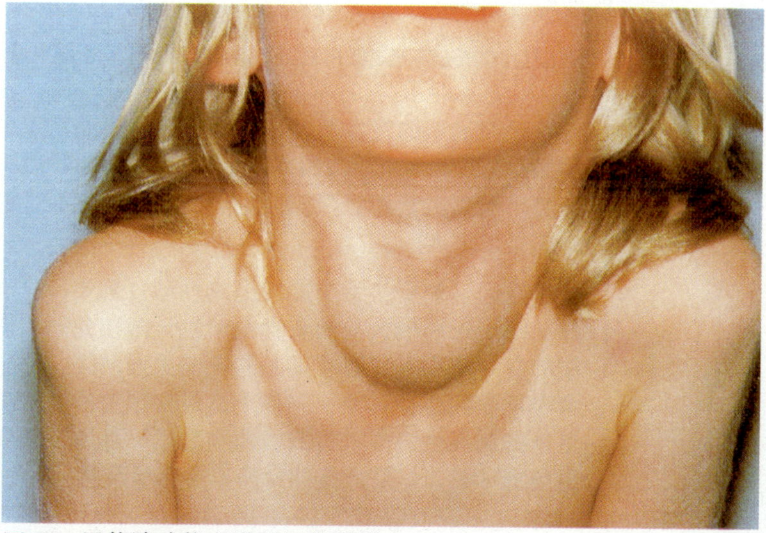

图 57　甲状腺功能亢进的甲状腺肿大
Goitre in hyperthyroidism

先天性肾上腺增生

病因学

是一种常染色体隐性遗传疾病，通常由于21-羟化酶缺乏导致皮质醇和醛固酮减少，睾酮生成过多。每5000个出生存活儿中就有1个患此病。进行产前诊断有可能发现。

临床特征

有女性男性化的表现（图58），女孩可能被误认为有严重尿道下裂和隐睾的男孩。如果“男性化”没有被早期认识到，婴儿可能在出生后第二周因危及生命的肾上腺危象而变得虚脱。

诊断和治疗

血浆17-羟黄体酮水平、血浆促肾上腺皮质激素和尿类固醇升高。失盐危象需要通过静脉输注盐溶液来进行复苏。需要进行长时间的氢化可的松替代治疗和应用保钠的甾类氟氢可的松。

性早熟

病因学

是下丘脑－垂体－性腺轴过早激活而造成。女孩青春期早熟的发生率高于男孩。孤立的乳房发育（青春期乳房过早发育）（图60）相对多见。脑肿瘤（如松果体瘤）和外源性类固醇用药也会引起早期第二性征发育（图59）。

临床特征

通过仔细的体格检查可以区分病理发育（男孩＜10岁，女孩＜8岁）与青春期开始早期的生理发育。发育顺序与通常的青春期发育顺序有差异（如出现了阴毛，但是没有乳房发育），则不可能是正常的生理发育。腹部触诊和超声扫描对于发现肾上腺和性腺肿瘤是很重要的。

治疗

病理原因（如甲状腺功能减退或肿瘤）需要特殊治疗。由于骨骺闭合前的青春期前生长时期变短而造成的身材矮小是青春期早熟的主要生理缺陷。同时青春期早熟还会对家长和孩子造成心理上的不安。用于抑制促性腺激素释放的药物治疗一直要持续到适当的年龄，但是最终的身高不会有所改善。

Congenital adrenal hyperplasia

Aetiology

Autosomal recessive disorder most commonly due to 21-hydroxylase enzyme deficiency resulting in reduced cortisol and aldosterone, and excessive testosterone production. Occurs 1 in 5000 live births. Prenatal diagnosis is possible.

Clinical features

Affected females are virilized (Fig. 58) and may be mistaken for males with severe hypospadias and cryptorchidism. If virilization is not recognized early, infants may collapse with a life-threatening adrenal crisis in the second week of life.

Diagnosis and management

Elevated plasma 17-hydroxyprogesterone level, plasma ACTH and urinary steroid excretion. Salt-losing crises require resuscitation with intravenous saline. Long term replacement hydrocortisone and a salt-retaining steroid fludrocortisone are required.

Precocious puberty

Aetiology

Premature activation of hypothalamo-pituitary-gonadal axis. Early puberty is more common in girls than boys. Isolated breast development (premature thelarche) (Fig. 60) is relatively common. Cerebral tumours, e.g. pineal tumours and exogenous steroid administration also cause early development of secondary sex characteristics (Fig. 59).

Clinical features

Careful physical examination may help to distinguish between physiological but early onset of puberty, and pathological development (<8 years of age in girls and <10 years of age in boys). Discrepancies from the usual sequence of puberty , (e.g. pubic hair but no breast development, are unlikely to be physiological). Abdominal palpation and ultrasound scanning are important in the detection of adrenal or gonadal tumours.

Management

Pathological causes (e.g. hypothyroidism or tumours) require specific treatment. Short stature is the major long-term physical disadvantage of early puberty because of the shorter period of prepubertal growth before epiphyseal fusion. Early puberty is also psychologically upsetting to both child and parents. Drug therapy may be used to suppress gonadotrophin release until the child reaches an appropriate age, but final height will not improve.

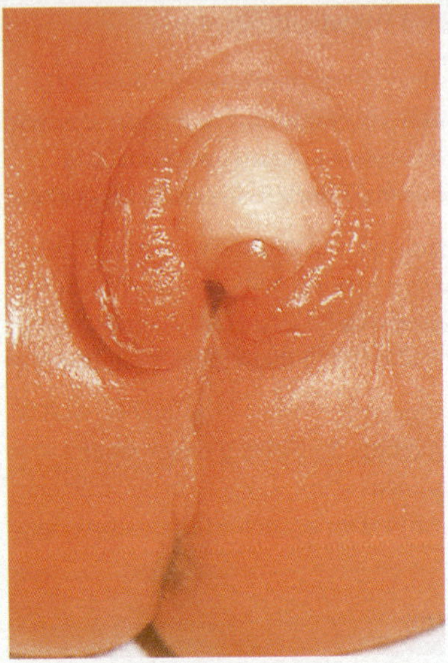

图 58 先天性肾上腺增生的肥大阴蒂
Enlarged clitoris in congenital adrenal hyperplasia

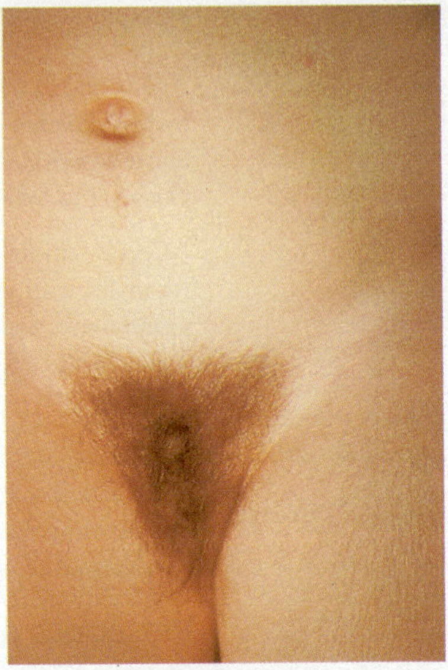

图 59 5 岁儿童的性早熟（肾上腺肿瘤）
Sexual precocity at 5 years of age (adrenal tumour)

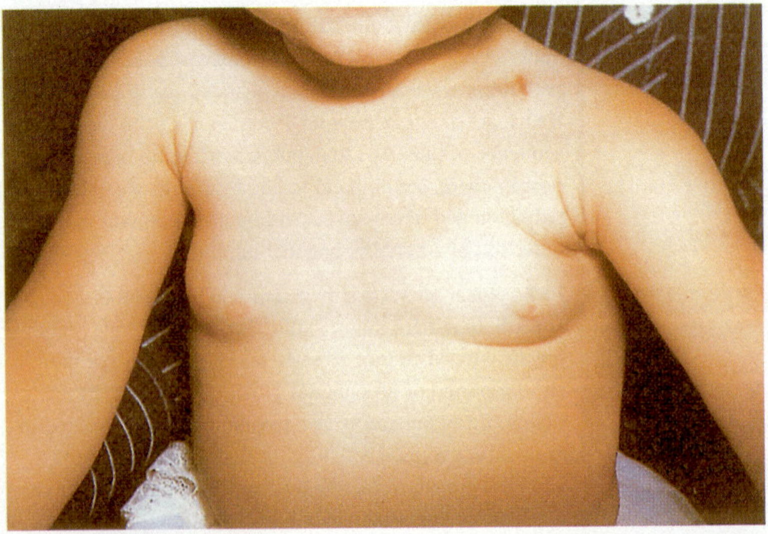

图 60 乳房的过早发育
Premature breast development

早产

发病率

在英国，将近6%～7%的出生存活儿是体重<2500g的低出生体重儿（Low birth weight infant, LBW）。其中，大约2/3的婴儿是胎龄<37周的早产儿。出生体重<1500g的新生儿占到出生婴儿的1%，但是有近50%在围产期死亡。

病因学

还不明确。绒毛膜羊膜炎和细菌性阴道病都与早产有关。有时早产可由母亲妊娠时的并发症引起（如先兆子痫、胎盘前置、宫颈机能不全、多胎妊娠和胎膜早破等）。

临床特征

肌张力差，呈蛙样体位（图61）。头相对较大，腹部隆起。由于颅骨较软和骨化不全，早产儿的头部经常呈狭长形，但是头形会随着年龄而改善。皮肤皱褶发育较差，尤其是足底部（图62）。30～36周胎龄的新生儿通常有较多胎毛，但是很少见于过早早产儿和过度成熟儿。耳廓弹性较差（图63）。皮肤透明发亮，皮下血管易见（图64），而且易被微小的外伤损伤。乳头直到28周胎龄后才会出现，乳腺组织需大于34周胎龄后才会形成。由于大阴唇较突出使得阴蒂相对较大，并伴有外阴裂隙。阴囊还未发育完善，并且有睾丸未降。

合并症

- 呼吸窘迫综合征
- 脑室周围出血
- 体温调节不良
- 易感染
- 喂养困难，不能吮吸
- 体液和电解质失衡

病程和预后

一般胎龄<24周新生儿存活率不高，胎龄≥30周新生儿存活率可以达95%。通过理想的护理，90%的存活早产儿不会有严重的神经系统残障。脑室周围白质软化，伴随有脑室周边的囊肿，会有较高神经系统残障的发生率。

Low birth weight infants (LBW)

Preterm

Incidence

In the UK, approximately 6-7% of live births are of LBW <2500 g. About two-thirds are preterm <37 weeks' gestation. Infants <1500 g comprise about 1% of births, but nearly 50% of perinatal deaths.

Aetiology

Often unknown. Chorioamnionitis and bacterial vaginosis are associated with preterm labour. Sometimes preterm birth occurs because of maternal complications (e.g. pre-eclampsia, placenta praevia, cervical incompetence, multiple pregnancy, premature rupture of membranes).

Clinical features

Poor muscle tone and tendency to lie in a frog-like position (Fig. 61). Relatively large head and prominent abdomen. Because the skull bones are soft and poorly mineralized, the head of the preterm infant often becomes narrow and elongated, but the shape improves with age. Skin creases are poorly developed, particularly on the soles of the feet (Fig. 62). Lanugo hair is often profuse in babies of 30-36 weeks' gestation, but is less common in very preterm or more mature infants. The pinna is poorly developed with little elastic recoil (Fig. 63). The skin is shiny and transparent with subcutaneous blood vessels readily visible (Fig. 64) and is easily damaged by even minor trauma. Nipples do not appear until 28 weeks' and breast tissue >34 weeks' gestation. The clitoris is relatively large with gaping of the vulva due to prominent labia majora. The scrotum is underdeveloped, and testes may be undescended.

Associations

- Respiratory distress syndrome.
- Periventricular haemorrhage.
- Poor temperature control.
- Increased susceptibility to infection.
- Feeding difficulties and inability to suck.
- Fluid and electrolyte imbalance.

Course and prognosis

Survival is uncommon <24 weeks, but 95% at 30 or >30 weeks' gestation. With optimal care, >90% of preterm infants who survive have no serious neurological handicap. Periventricular leucomalacia, with cysts alongside the ventricles is associated with a high incidence of neurological disability.

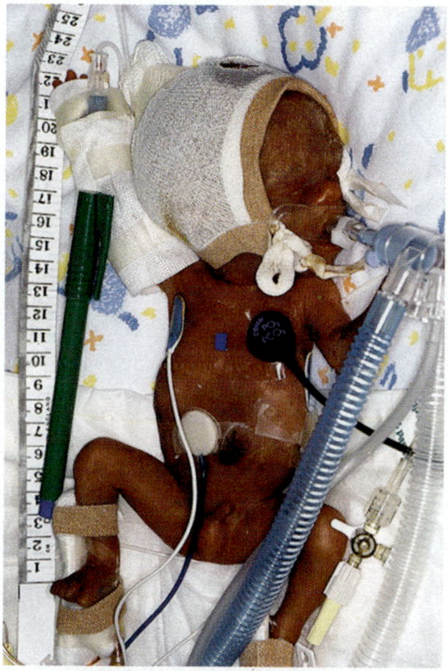

图 61　极低出生体重儿
Extremely low birth weight infant

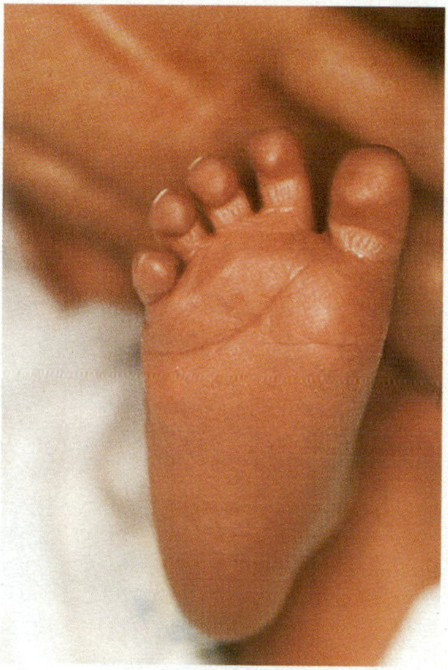

图 62　足底部皮肤皱褶发育较差
Poorly developed skin creases on feet

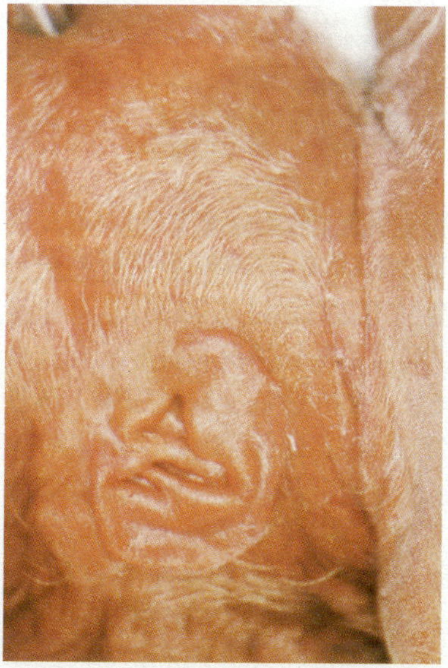

图 63　大量胎毛和原始耳发育
Profuse lanugo and primitive ear development

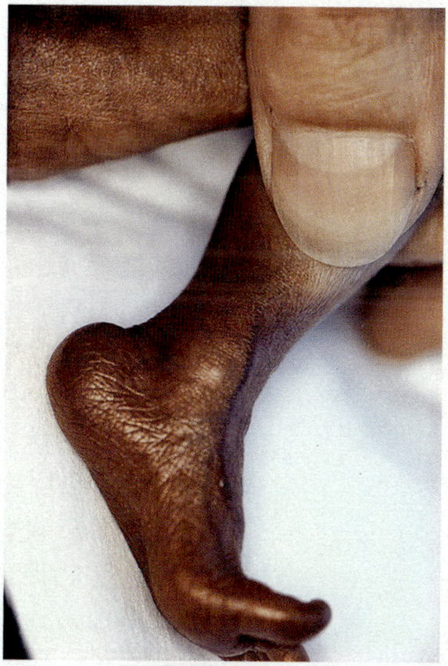

图 64　皮肤菲薄和静脉突出
Thin skin and prominent veins

小于胎龄儿（SGA）

同义词 足月小样儿（small for date）；宫内生长限制。

定义 相对于同一胎龄而言，出生体重＜第 10 个百分位点。

发病率 每 100 个出生存活儿中就有 2 个是 SGA，并且出生体重＜ 2500g。

病因学 可能与胎盘功能不全、母亲的先兆子痫、妊娠高血压、吸烟以及宫内病毒感染（如风疹病毒、巨细胞病毒、弓形虫病）有关。

临床特征 最常见的SGA婴儿通常是瘦长，皮肤干燥、脱屑（图65），并且指甲较长。除了出生体重外，他们的体貌外观和行为都与胎龄相适合。一些SGA婴儿均匀瘦小；有围产期窒息的危险，并且经常会有胎便污染皮肤（图66）、指甲和脐带的现象。除非他们生病或早产，否则SGA婴儿的喂养非常好，并且需要增加热量摄入。他们的生理体重丢失通常无关紧要，只要出生后有充分的营养补充，他们的体重增加十分迅速。他们在出生后前几天内有低血糖的危险。体温过低也可能发生。双胞胎在出生前的生长上可能有明显的差异（图67），尤其是存在慢性胎儿-胎儿输血的时候。

病程和预后 在没有宫内感染或新生儿低血糖的情况下，SGA 婴儿通常有着正常的智力和发育。LBW婴儿若头围和身长都与胎龄相适合（不对称的生长限制），只要生后给与充分的营养，其体重增长情况均良好，尤其是在生后第一年中。并且，在今后的生长过程中，其各方面都能够达到正常生长百分位点。如果出生时头围、体重和身长都低，表明有长期的宫内生长限制或遗传因素影响生长（对称的生长限制），其生后的生长可能总是低于正常百分位点。双胞胎间由于胎儿-胎儿输血造成的生长差异其预后很不确定，有较高的神经发育不良的危险。

Small for gestational age (SGA)

Synonyms Small for dates; intrauterine growth restriction.

Definition Birth weight <10th centile for gestational age.

Incidence Two in 100 live births are SGA and <2500 g.

Aetiology May be associated with placental insufficiency, maternal pre-eclampsia, hypertension or smoking, and intrauterine viral infection such as rubella , CMV or toxoplasmosis.

Clinical features The most common SGA infants are usually long and thin, with dry peeling skin (Fig. 65) and long nails. Their physical appearance and behaviour are appropriate for gestational age, not birth weight. Some SGA infants are uniformly small; they are at risk of perinatal asphyxia and often have meconium staining of the skin (Fig. 66), nails and umbilical cord. Unless they are ill or preterm, SGA infants feed very well and require increased caloric intake. Their physiological weight loss is usually insignificant and they gain weight rapidly with adequate postnatal nutrition. They are at risk of hypoglycaemia in the first few days after birth. Hypothermia may also occur. Twins may have a marked difference in prenatal growth (Fig. 67), particularly when there has been chronic feto-fetal transfusion.

Course and prognosis In the absence of intrauterine infection or neonatal hypoglycaemia, SGA infants are usually of normal intelligence and development. Infants of LBW but appropriate head circumference and length for gestation (asymmetric growth restriction) demonstrate good weight gain providing they receive adequate postnatal nutrition, particularly in the first year of life, and usually achieve normal centiles for all aspects of growth later. If the head circumference, weight and length are all low at birth indicating long-standing intrauterine growth restriction or a genetic influence on growth (symmetric growth restriction), postnatal growth may always remain below the normal centiles. The prognosis for twins with growth discrepancy due to feto-fetal transfusion is much more uncertain and there is a higher risk of poor neurodevelopmental outcome in these infants.

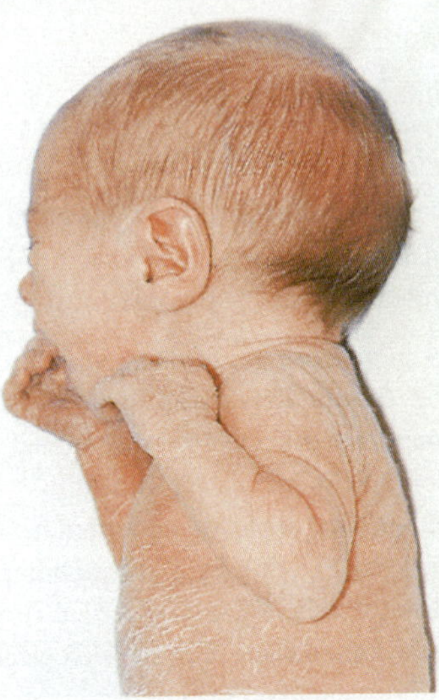

图 65　皮肤干燥、脱屑的 SGA 婴儿
Dry peeling skin of SGA infant

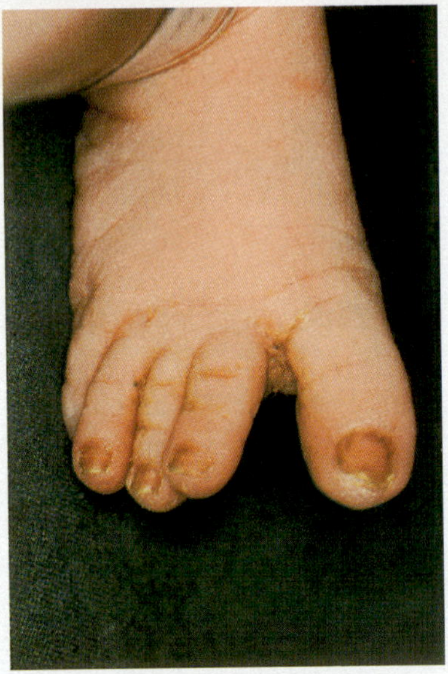

图 66　胎便污染皮肤和趾甲
Meconium staining of skin and nails

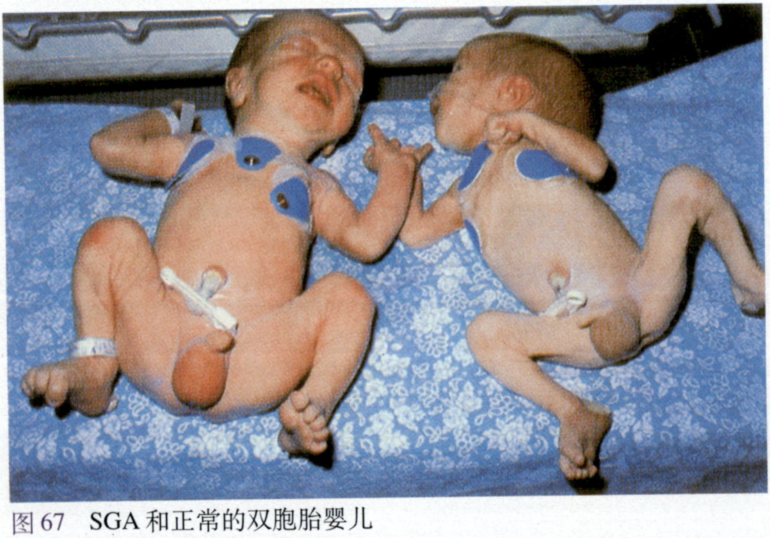

图 67　SGA 和正常的双胞胎婴儿
SGA and normal twins

呼吸窘迫综合征（肺透明膜病，HMD）

发病率

HMD是早产儿最常见的呼吸系统疾病。其原因是肺表面活性物质缺乏和肺组织结构不成熟。多见于有围产期窒息的婴儿和糖尿病母亲的婴儿。胎龄是HMD的主要决定因素，但是可以通过产前应用类固醇来减少发生危险。

临床特征

在出生后 4 小时内出现呼吸急促＞ 60 次 / 分钟，呼气时呻吟，发绀，肋间和肋下吸凹（图68）。HMD通常需与因肺间质水分延迟吸收而引起的暂时性呼吸急促相区别，前者生后 4 小时的 X 光片具有特征性肺不张的弥漫网状–粒状结构和支气管含气显影（图69）。随着婴儿的疲劳，HMD会逐渐恶化。如果病情不复杂，出生48小时后随着天然的表面活性物质生成，HMD会平稳的改善。早期应用外源性表面活性物质和机械通气，临床病程会得到改善。

并发症

在将近 10% 的 HMD 患儿中会出现气胸，尤其是应用机械通气时。偶尔会有间质性肺气肿、纵隔积气（图 70）或心包积气发生。大约有 20% ~ 30% 极低出生体重儿需要长时间应用氧疗（慢性肺病），一些甚至于在出院回家后仍继续氧疗。脑室周围出血(periventricular haemorrhage, PVH)、侧脑室胚层大血管出血是死亡的主要原因。胚层出血或脑室内出血很常见，不会造成严重后果。出血扩散到脑组织或引起脑积水都可致死，或引起神经系统后遗症。

治疗

在出生后即经由气管给予外源性表面活性物质，可以减少死亡率和减轻HMD的严重程度。通常需要机械通气，并且保持循环系统稳定性很重要，尤其是在发生 PVH 的前几天内。

预后

存活率和长期预后依赖于胎龄和并发症的发生。在过去10年间，随着机械通气技术的改善，PVH现在是生存率和神经系统残障的主要决定因素。通过理想的护理，只有＜ 10% 的早产儿会发生神经系统发育残障。

Respiratory distress syndrome (hyaline membrane disease, HMD)

Incidence

HMD is the most common respiratory disorder in preterm infants. It is due to surfactant deficiency and structural immaturity of the lungs. It is more common in infants with perinatal asphyxia and infants of diabetic mothers. Gestational age is the main determinant of HMD, but the risk can be reduced by antenatal steroids.

Clinical features

Tachypnoea >60/min, expiratory grunt, cyanosis, intercostal and subcostal recession (Fig. 68) within 4 h of birth. HMD can usually be distinguished from transient tachypnoea due to delayed lung liquid resorption by a characteristic diffuse reticulo-granular pattern due to atelectasis, and an air-bronchogram on chest X-ray (Fig. 69) after 4 h of age. HMD gradually worsens as the infant tires and if uncomplicated, steadily improves from 48 h as natural surfactant is produced. The clinical course is ameliorated by early administration of exogenous surfactant and mechanical ventilation.

Complications

Pneumothoraces develop in approximately 10% of infants with HMD, particularly if ventilation is required. Occasionally, pulmonary interstitial emphysema, pneumomediastinum (Fig. 70), or pneumopericardium occur. About 20-30% extremely LBW infants need prolonged oxygen therapy (chronic lung disease), some even at home after discharge from hospital. Periventricular haemorrhage (PVH), bleeding from the extremely vascular germinal layer of the lateral ventricles is the major cause of morbidity. Germinal layer haemorrhage or intraventricular haemorrhge is common and of no serious significance. Haemorrhage which extends into brain tissue or causes hydrocephalus may be fatal or cause long-term neurological sequelae.

Management

Exogenous surfactant, given into the trachea soon after birth, reduces mortality and severity of HMD. Mechanical ventilation is often required and maintainence of cardiovascular stability is important, particularly in the first few days when PVH may occur.

Prognosis

Survival and long-term prognosis depend on gestation and the occurrence of complications. With improvement in ventilatory techniques in the past decade, PVH is now the main determinant of survival and neurological handicap. With optimal care, <10% of preterm infants suffer major neurodevelopmental disability.

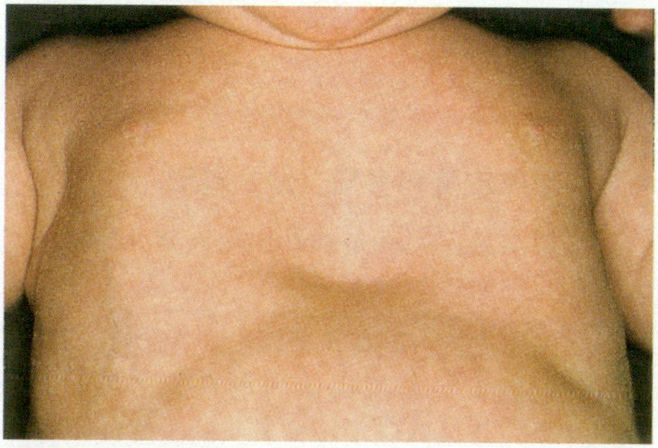

图 68 肋下吸凹
Subcostal recession

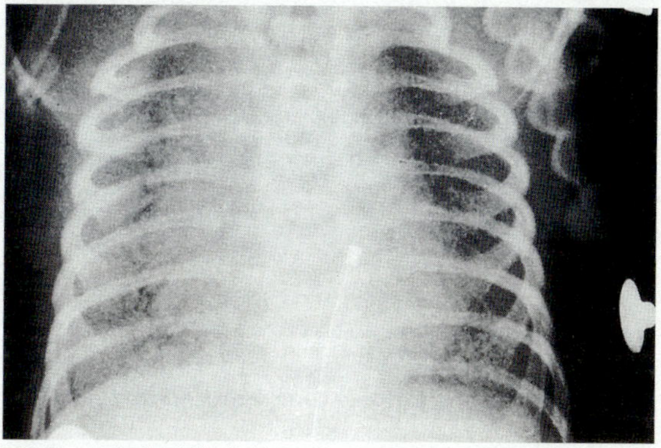

图 69 肺透明膜病的 X 光片表现
X-ray appearance of hyaline membrane disease

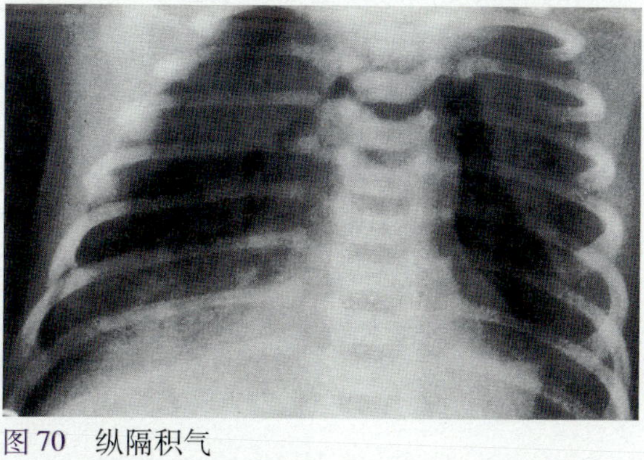

图 70 纵隔积气
Pneumonediastinum

附属皮赘和多指（趾）畸形

发病率和遗传特性

很常见，尤其是加勒比黑人婴儿。通常是常染色体显性遗传。

临床特征

附属皮赘（副耳）经常出现在脸部、耳前部（图71）。副乳头经常被误认为色素痣，可能是单个或是多个，并且多位于正常乳头的垂直线下方（图72）。从疏松的附属皮赘到完全成形的手指或脚趾，额外的指（趾）[多指（趾）] 形态多变。偶尔可能伴有两裂的掌骨或跖骨。通常只有外观上的畸形，但是额外的脚趾可能引起足前段增宽而造成今后穿鞋的困难。

治疗

如果皮赘的蒂和基底部非常狭窄，并且不包含软骨组织，可以对带蒂的皮赘进行结扎。皮赘会逐渐缺血坏死，没有疼痛，并且坏死的皮赘会在数天之内脱落，留下一个干燥的小伤痕。如果皮赘基底部很宽，或者皮赘内含有软骨组织，那么就需要进行整形外科手术。

羊膜索、截肢术和肢体缺如畸形

病因学

被广泛接受的关于羊膜索的假说是，在妊娠期前三个月中发生的羊膜外伤性破裂使发育中的胚胎可能错误移位于在羊膜和绒毛膜之间的一个腔隙中。膜可能形成环形环绕于胎儿肢体上。另外一种假说是由于胎盘血管的血栓形成栓塞，继发血管闭塞。羊膜索可能与胎儿畸形有关，尤其是肢体（图 73）或颅面缺损。肢体缺如畸形（图 74）在 20 世纪 60 年代的多发是由于致畸剂“沙利度胺（反应停）”的结果。但是，许多病例的发生没有任何可知原因。

治疗

如果畸形很严重，尤其是当限制了肢体功能，那么将婴儿早期转入多学科的假肢装配中心是有帮助的。

Accessory skin tags and polydactyly

Incidence and inheritance

Common, particularly in Afro-Caribbean infants. Usually autosomal dominant.

Clinical features

Accessory skin tags (accessory auricles) often occur on the face, anterior to the ear (Fig. 71). Accessory nipples are often mistaken for pigmented naevi and may be single or multiple and usually occur in a direct line below the normally situated nipple (Fig. 72). Extra digits (polydactyly) vary from loosely attached skin tags to fully-formed fingers or toes. Occasionally there may be an associated bifid metacarpal or metatarsal bone. Usually only a cosmetic deformity, but extra toes may cause broadening of the forefoot with difficulty in fitting shoes later.

Management

Small pedunculated tags can be ligated if the pedicle and base is very narrow and does not contain cartilage. The tag will become ischaemic, but it is not painful and will usually separate within a few days leaving a small dry scar. If the base is broad, or if the tag has a cartilaginous attachment, plastic surgery will be required.

Amniotic bands, amputations and limb reduction deformities

Aetiology

The most widely accepted hypothesis for amniotic bands is that the developing embryo may lie in a false cavity between the amnion and chorion after traumatic rupture of the amnion in the first trimester. The membranes may then form encircling bands around the limbs. An alternative hypothesis is vascular occlusion secondary to embolization from thrombosed placental vessels. Amniotic bands may be associated with fetal malformations, particularly limb (Fig. 73) or craniofacial defects. An epidemic of limb reduction deformities (Fig. 74) in the early 1960s was due to the effects of a teratogen – thalidomide. Many cases occur without any known cause.

Management

If the deformity is severe and particularly if it will interfere with limb function, early referral to a multi-disciplinary limb-fitting centre will be helpful.

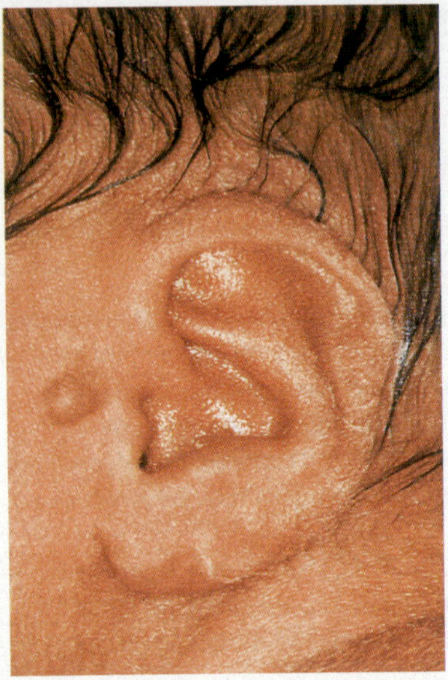

图 71　副耳
Accessory auricle

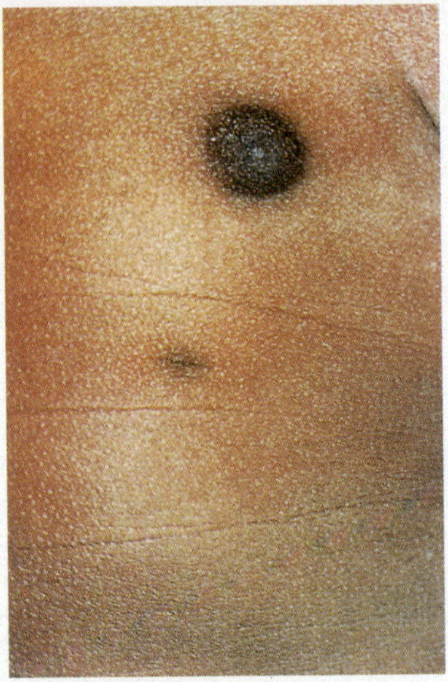

图 72　副乳头
Accessory nipple

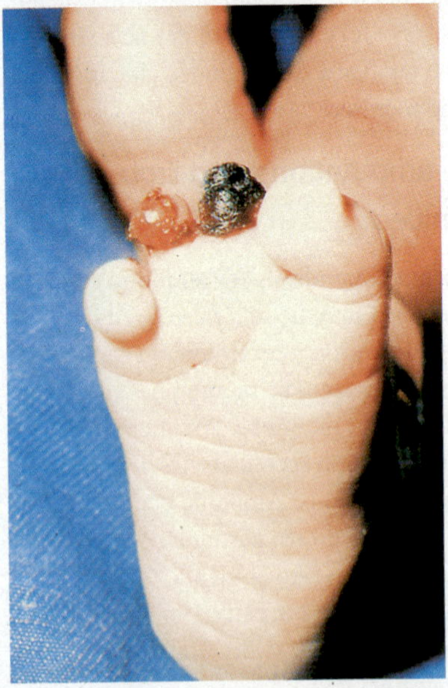

图 73　继发于羊膜索的脚趾坏疽
Gangrene of toes secondary to amniotic bands

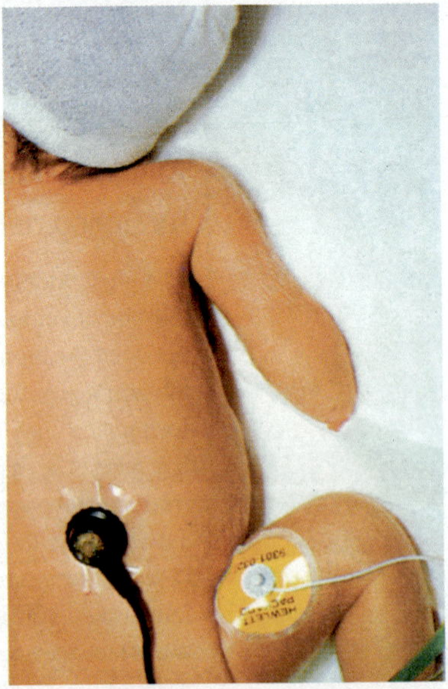

图 74　上臂缺如畸形，并残留手指遗痕
Arm reduction deformity with vestigial fingers

马蹄内翻足（畸形足）

发病率 每1000个出生存活儿中就有1个发生。这种疾病男孩的发病率是女孩的2倍。

病因学 尚未明确，可能是多基因遗传，子宫内受压也有一定的影响。

临床特征 患足被保持在一个固定的屈曲位（马蹄足）和内弯位（内翻）（图75）。它可以与位置性畸形足相区别，前者是真正的畸形足，不能进行被动的矫正。通常作为一个单独的畸形发生，但是也可与脊髓脊膜膨出、羊水过少和先天性髋关节脱位联合出现。

治疗 通常进行夹板疗法作为最初尝试矫正畸形的方法，但是如果矫形很困难，外科松解挛缩的腓肠肌和踝关节结构也许是必需的。

足和脚趾的畸形

发病率 常见，尤其是并趾畸形。

遗传特性 大多是常染色体显性遗传。

临床特征 并趾畸形多由于第2和第3趾的蹼化（图76）而出现。小趾重叠于第4趾上通常是双侧的。槌状趾(图77)通常发生于大脚趾，是由于先天性屈肌腱挛缩造成。当足前部由于内收而向内侧弯曲时，就形成了趾朝内畸形（内翻跖）。

治疗 并趾畸形不需要外科治疗。槌状趾或小趾重叠的足趾位置通常是不舒适的，可以进行外科矫正。尽管偶尔需要外科治疗，但是内翻跖会随着年龄增长和足的生长而改善。

Talipes equinovarus (club foot)

Incidence Occurs in 1 in 1000 live births. The condition is twice as common in males as in females.

Aetiology Uncertain, probably polygenic inheritance and intrauterine pressure play a part.

Clinical features The affected foot is held in a fixed flexion (equinus) and inturned (varus) position (Fig. 75). It can be differentiated from positional talipes because the deformity in true talipes cannot be passively corrected. Usually occurs as an isolated deformity but may occur in association with meningomyelocele, oligohydramnios and congenital dislocation of the hip.

Management Correction of the deformity is usually initially attempted by splinting, but if correction is difficult, surgical release of the contracted structures in the calf and ankle may be necessary.

Foot and toe deformities

Incidence Common – particularly syndactyly.

Inheritance Mostly autosomal dominant.

Clinical features Syndactyly usually occurs as webbing of the second and third toes (Fig. 76). Overlapping of the little toe over the fourth toe is usually bilateral. Hammer toe (Fig. 77) usually occurs in the big toe and results from a congenital contracture of the flexor tendons. In-toeing occurs when the feet tend to curve medially because of adduction of the forefoot (metatarsus varus).

Management Syndactyly of toes does not require surgery. The position of the toes in hammer toe or overlapping little toe is usually uncomfortable and surgical correction may be needed. Metatarsus varus improves with age and growth of the foot, although surgery is occasionally required.

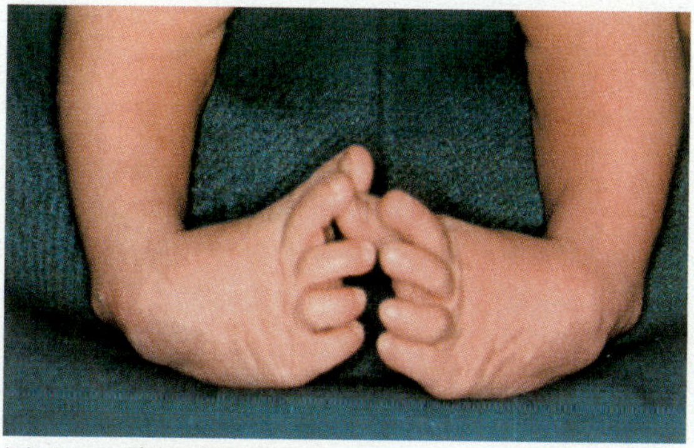

图 75　双侧马蹄内翻足
Bilateral talipes equinovarus

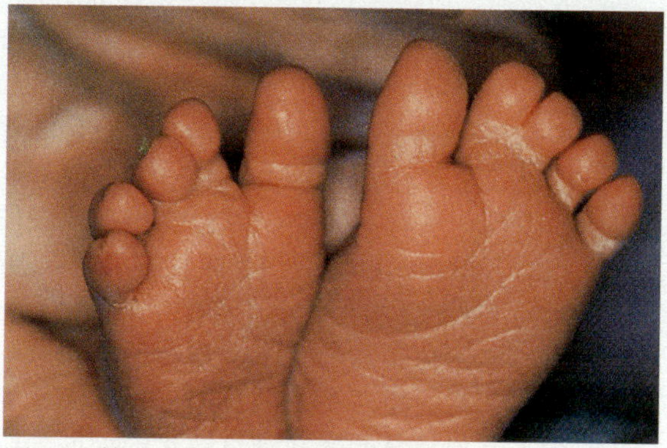

图 76　第 2 和第 3 趾的并趾畸形
Syndactyly of second and third toes

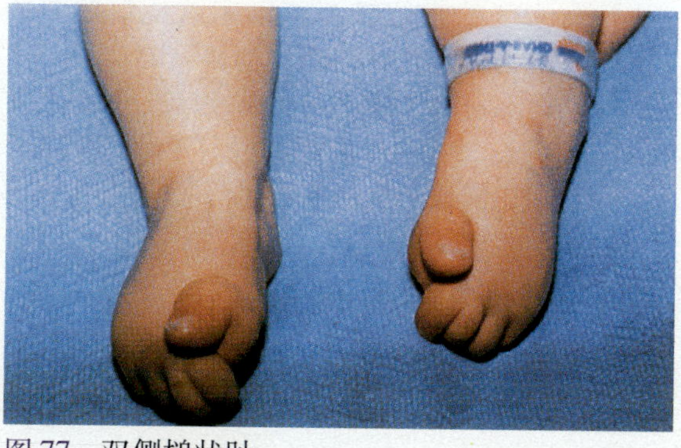

图 77　双侧槌状趾
Bilateral hammer toes

髋臼发育不良

同义词 先天性髋关节脱位。

发病率 很常见，每100个出生存活儿中就有1个发生髋关节脱位。通过早期诊断和治疗，髋关节脱位的流行病学显示在出生后第1年其发生率从1：1000下降到1：10 000。它多发生于臀先露的女孩中。

遗传特性 家族性。不是单纯的孟德尔式遗传。

临床特征 大多数都应该在新生儿期通过常规的筛查试验被发现。固定的脱位可以通过发现髋关节外展运动受限和有时患侧腿缩短而被诊断。检查可复位的髋关节脱位时，应将婴儿仰卧平放于坚硬的平面上。用拇指和其他手指握住大腿，将髋关节和膝关节屈曲（图78），每侧髋关节都应该从起始的中线位被慢慢地外展到90度（图79和80），当向后脱位的髋关节滑回到髋臼窝时，可触及到滑动感并伴随有响声。然后应再进行一次轻柔的尝试以诊断髋关节脱位。在腿内收时，拇指的压力施加于股骨的上部；然后腿外展，如同上面所述。超声对于诊断也是有用的。但是，这是一种劳动密集型技术，有着很高的假阳性率，因此，在英国超声主要被作为一种对高危婴儿或在临床上发现异常的婴儿进行筛查的辅助手段。超声作为一种主要筛查方法的作用尚未得到证实。

治疗 需要进行外展夹板疗法至少6周。对于有希望能够自行恢复的脱位髋关节也应该观察到孩子会走路为止。当对新生儿检查产生怀疑时，就应该在4～6个月对其进行全髋关节的X线片。诊断延迟可能会导致更长期的夹板治疗和外科手术。随着早期诊断和治疗，大部分髋关节发育不良婴儿应该不会有爬行和行走活动落后。

Developmental dysplasia of the hip

Synonym

Congenital dislocation of the hip.

Incidence

Dislocated or dislocatible hip at birth may be as common as 1 in 100 live births. With early detection and treatment, the prevalence of dislocated hip after the first year of life has been reduced from 1 : 1 000 to 1 : 10 000. It is more common in girls and after breech presentation.

Inheritance

Familial. There is no simple Mendelian pattern of inheritance.

Clinical features

The majority should be detected by routine screening tests in the neonatal period. Fixed dislocation can be diagnosed by finding restricted abduction of the hip and sometimes shortening of the affected leg. To examine for a reducible dislocation, the infant should be placed on its back on a firm surface. Holding the thighs between finger and thumb with the hips and knees both flexed (Fig. 78), each hip should be slowly abducted through 90 degrees starting from the midline (Figs 79 and 80). A palpable 'Clunk' will be felt as a posteriorly dislocated hip slips back into the acetabulum. A gentle attempt should then be made to diagnose a dislocatible hip. With the leg adducted, pressure is applied with the thumb on the upper part of the femur; the leg is then abducted, as above. Ultrasound is useful in diagnosis, but is labour-intensive, has a high false-positive rate and in the UK is therefore used mainly as an adjunct in screening high risk babies or where a clinical abnormality has been detected. The role of ultrasound as a primary screening test is unproven.

Management

Abduction splinting is required for at least 6 weeks. Even a dislocatible hip which resolves spontaneously should be observed until the child is walking. X-ray all hips at 4-6 months of age when neonatal examinations have aroused suspicion. Delay in diagnosis may involve more prolonged splinting or surgery. With early diagnosis and treatment, the majority of infants with developmental dysplasia of the hip should have no delay in crawling or walking.

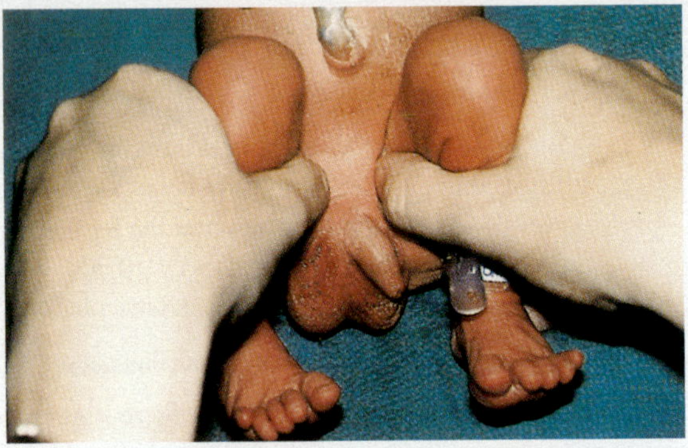

图 78 髋关节检查起始于中线位，使髋关节和膝关节都屈曲
Examination of the hips starting in the midline with hips and knees flexed

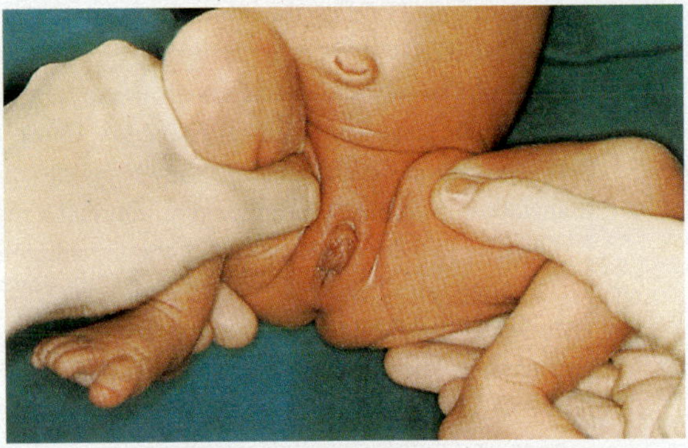

图 79 用拇指和其他手指握住大腿，将髋关节外展
Abduction of the hip holding the thigh between fingers and thumb

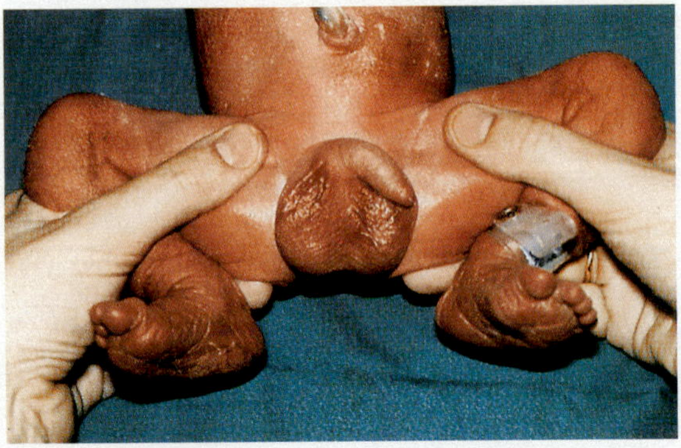

图 80 两侧的髋关节完全外展到 90 度
Full abduction of both hips through 90°

唇裂和腭裂

发病率 很常见，大约每600个出生存活儿中就有1个发生。

遗传特性 家族性，可能是多因素的，不是单纯的孟德尔式遗传。

临床特征 单独的腭裂经常发生于中线位。最不明显的一型是伴随有悬雍垂裂的黏膜下裂。唇裂和腭裂可以是单侧或双侧的（图81）。

合并症 喂养困难和牙列畸形都很常见。在腭裂患儿中，尤其是治疗较晚的患儿，可能出现语言问题。鼻咽部反流或出现脓毒血症时，可能继发耳聋。

治疗 一些婴儿可以进行母乳喂养，大部分婴儿可用较大奶嘴进行很好的喂养。导管或用勺喂养偶尔可能也需要。可以在不同的阶段实施外科手术治疗。用于外观畸形纠正的唇裂修补术的时间选择需要考虑到早期关闭的近期和远期好处。实施腭裂修补术需要稍晚些，但是也应该在生后第一年中就进行，因为这样可以达到较好的整形效果，并且可以避免或减少晚期修补带来的语言困难问题。如果初期的畸形很严重，就需要在稍晚些时候进行二期的唇和鼻部修补或咽成形术（图82）。

水囊状淋巴管瘤

病因学 颈淋巴管错构瘤，很少见。

临床特征 在颈外侧部柔软、多囊、边界不清、有波动感的淋巴肿胀瘤样组织（图83）。水囊状淋巴管瘤有透照性，并且在生后前几个月或前几年中增大缓慢。对患儿的影响取决于其大小和位置。偶尔会引起吞咽困难或呼吸障碍，尤其是在瘤体迅速增大的情况下。偶尔增大可能是由于感染和出血造成。

治疗 由于淋巴管侵入性和边界不清的特性给外科切除带来了困难，但是外科治疗通常是必要的。

Cleft lip and palate

Incidence Common; approximately 1 in 600 live births.

Inheritance Familial; probably polygenic, there is no simple Mendelian pattern.

Clinical features Isolated clefts of the palate always occur in the midline. The least obvious type is the submucous cleft which is often associated with a bifid uvula. Cleft lip and palate may be unilateral or bilateral (Fig. 81).

Associations Feeding difficulties and orthodontic deformities are common. Speech problems may occur with cleft palate, particularly after late closure. Deafness may arise secondary to regurgitation and sepsis in the nasopharynx.

Management Some infants can breast-feed; most infants feed well through a large teat. Tube or spoon feeding may occasionally be needed. Surgery is performed in several stages. Timing of repair of cleft lip to correct the cosmetic deformity requires consideration of short- and long-term benefits of early closure. Palatal repair is done later, but always within the first year of life when an excellent cosmetic result is usually achieved and speech difficulties of late closure are minimized. If initial deformity is severe, secondary repair of the lip or nose, or pharyngoplasty may be required later (Fig. 82).

Cystic hygroma

Aetiology Uncommon hamartoma of jugular lymphatic vessels.

Clinical features Soft, multicystic and ill-defined fluctuant lymphatic swelling in the lateral part of the neck (Fig. 83). Cystic hygromas transilluminate and enlarge slowly during the first few months or years of life. The effect on the child depends on size and site of the abnormality, but can occasionally cause dysphagia or respiratory obstruction, particularly if it enlarges rapidly. Occasionally enlargement may be due to infection or haemorrhage.

Management Surgical excision is difficult because of the invasive, ill-defined nature of the lymphatic channels, but it is usually necessary.

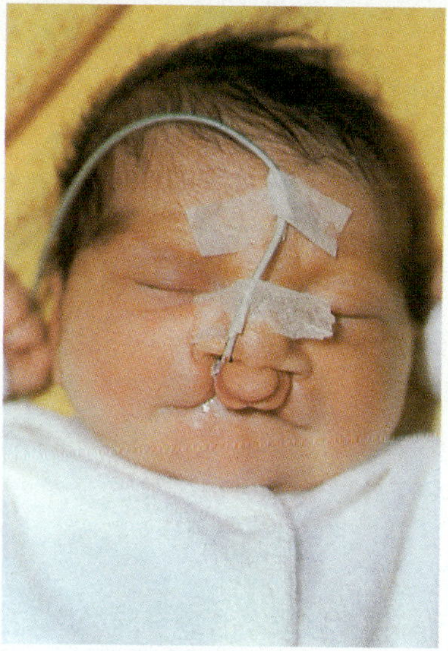

图 81　唇裂和腭裂
Cleft lip and palate

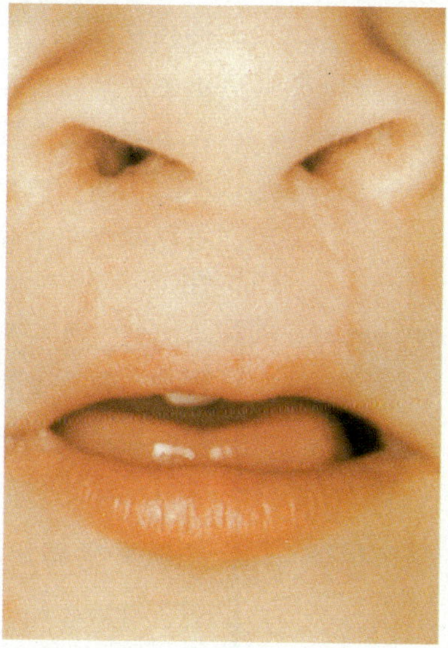

图 82　图 81 中的患儿手术后在 4 岁时
Same patient in Fig. 81 at 4 years of age, after surgery

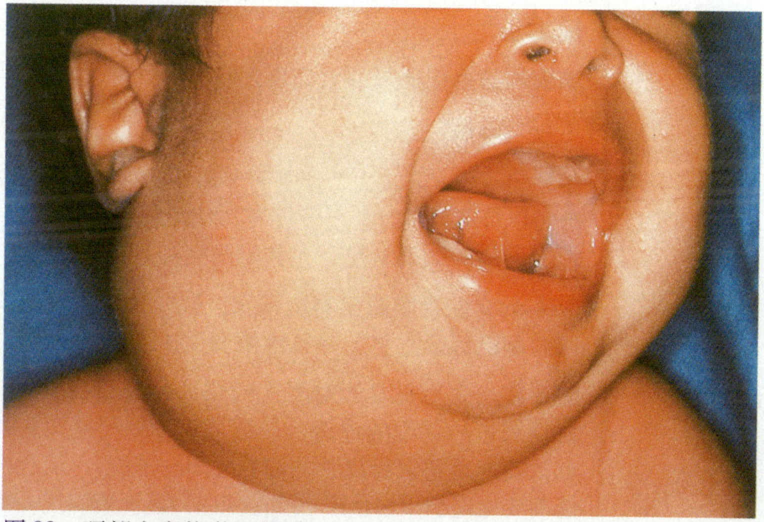

图 83　颈部水囊状淋巴管瘤
Cystic hygroma in the neck

神经管缺陷

发病率 由于产前筛查和母亲的营养状况改善，其患病率正在下降。隐性脊柱裂在人群中有约1%的发生率。

病因学 原因不明，但是普遍观念认为孕期母亲的叶酸补充可以减少对于高危家族人群神经管缺陷发生的危险性。

遗传特性 多因素。在一个孩子发生神经管缺陷后，再次妊娠过程中，就有1/20的再发危险率。

产前诊断 在妊娠中期三个月中羊水和母体血浆中甲胎蛋白浓度升高。该畸形通常在超声检查中很明显。

临床特征

脊髓脊膜膨出和脑（脊）膜膨出

包含有液体和/或神经组织的囊（脊髓脊膜膨出），有94%的病例伴随有潜在的腰骶区域脊髓弓缺损（图84）。残疾程度取决于缺损的严重程度和缺损的水平高度。有可能发生下肢弛缓性麻痹、感觉缺失、神经性膀胱功能障碍、尿失禁以及伴随有排便失禁的肛门扩展（图85）。脑（脊）膜膨出通常发生在胸髓（图86）或颈髓段。

脑膨出

脑膜和脑组织通过颅骨疝出。

无脑（畸形）

前脑和颅骨穹隆缺失，伴有面部和耳部畸变；虽然少数可以存活数小时甚至于数天，但最终不能存活。其他的伴随畸形很常见，尤其是腭裂和颈椎异常。

合并症 70%的脊髓脊膜膨出有脑积水。髋臼发育不良和马蹄内翻足都很常见，并且经常发生尿道感染。

治疗 需要在出生后前几天对婴儿的先天性畸形和神经系统情况进行仔细的评估，然后可对一些婴儿实施外科治疗。最初进行皮肤的修补关闭（图87），但是可能需要处理脑积水、矫形和泌尿的问题。胸髓或颈髓段的脑（脊）膜膨出通常有较好的预后，很少有神经系统后遗症。

Neural tube defects

Incidence

Prevalence is falling due to antenatal screening and improved maternal nutrition. Spina bifida occulta occurs in approximately 1% of people.

Aetiology

Unknown, but peri-conceptual maternal folic acid supplementation reduces the risk of neural tube defect in high risk families.

Inheritance

Polygenic. After one affected child, 1 in 20 risk of recurrence of neural tube defect in subsequent pregnancies.

Antenatal diagnosis

Elevated alpha fetoprotein concentrations in amniotic fluid and maternal plasma occur in second trimester of pregnancy. Defects are usually apparent on ultrasound examination.

Clinical features

Meningomyelocele and meningocele

Sac containing fluid and/or neural tissue (meningomyelocele), with underlying defect of spinal arch in lumbosacral region in 94% cases (Fig. 84). The degree of handicap depends on the level and severity of the defect. Flaccid paralysis of lower limbs, sensory loss, neurogenic bladder, urinary incontinence, and patulous anus (Fig. 85) with faecal incontinence may occur. Meningoceles often occur in thoracic (Fig. 86) or cervical spine.

Encephalocele

Herniation of meninges and brain through skull.

Anencephaly

Absence of forebrain and skull vault, with distortion of face and ears; incompatible with life although a few may survive for several hours or occasionally days. Other abnormalities are common, particularly cleft palate and abnormal cervical vertebrae.

Associations

Hydrocephaly occurs in 70% of meningomyeloceles. Developmental dysplasia of hip, and talipes equinovarus are common. Urinary tract infections often occur.

Management

Surgery may be indicated in some infants after careful assessment of congenital abnormalities and neurological state of infant in first few days of life. Skin closure initially (Fig. 87), but may require management of hydrocephaly, orthopaedic and urinary problems. Meningoceles in thoracic or cervical regions usually have excellent prognosis and fewer neurological sequelae.

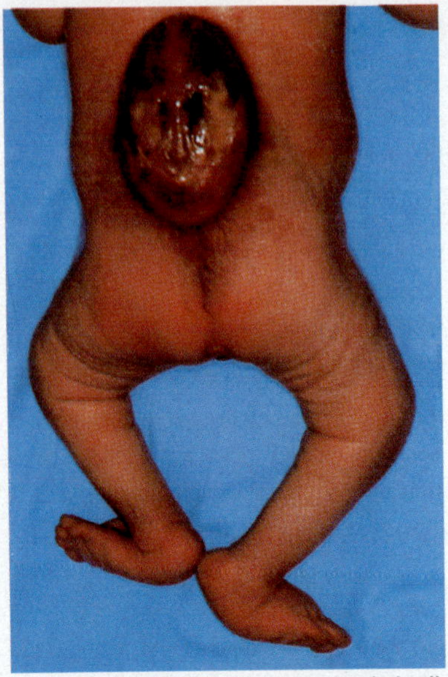

图 84　典型的腰骶区域脊髓脊膜膨出
Typical lumbosacral meningomyelocele

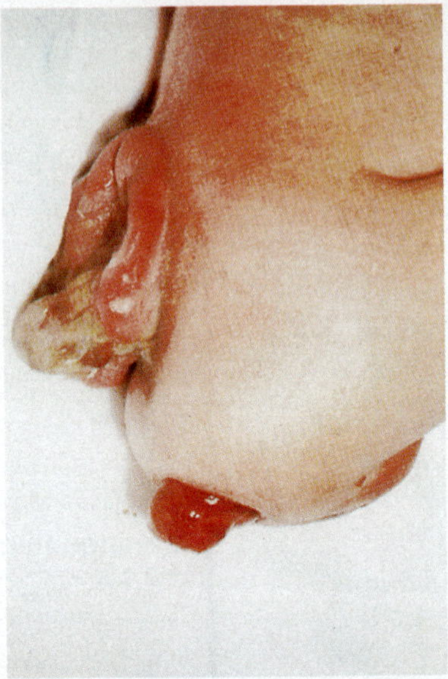

图 85　伴有肛门麻痹的脊髓脊膜膨出，有直肠脱垂
Meningomyelocele with paralysed anus. There is a rectal prolapse

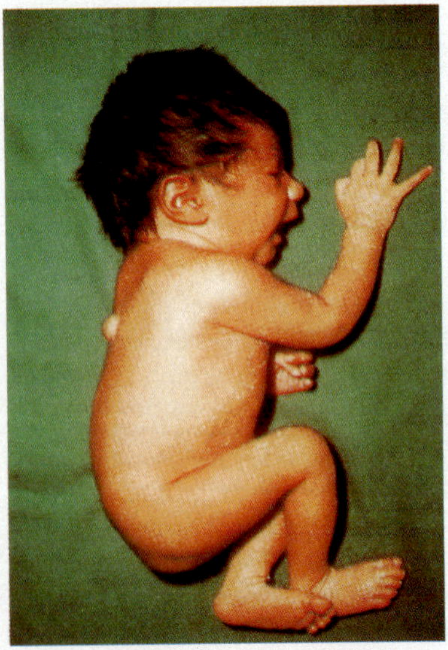

图 86　胸髓段脑（脊）膜膨出
Thoracic meningocele

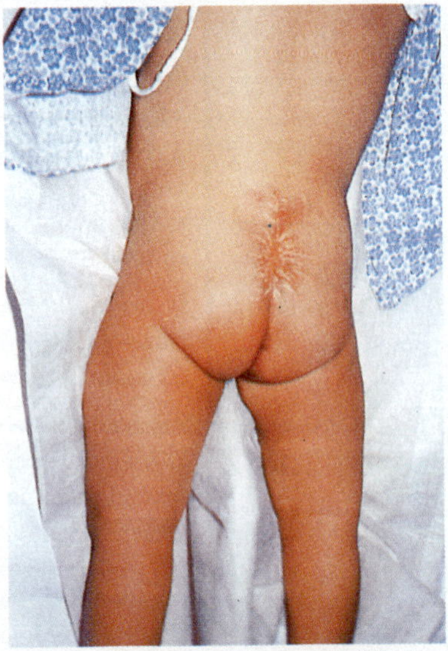

图 87　修补术后的脊髓脊膜膨出
Repaired meningomyelocele

脑积水

病因学

可作为先天性畸形而单独发生。这种疾病很常见，多是由于先天性脑导水管狭窄，或是继发于脑室周围出血或新生儿脑（脊）膜炎而形成。通常多伴发有神经管缺陷。

临床特征

颅骨的快速生长导致头围不成比例的增长（图 88），并且囟门和骨缝增宽。在对有出血后脑积水的早产儿进行常规头颅超声检查可以看到脑室指数增加。伴随有颅内压增高的症状（如嗜睡、呼吸暂停和呕吐）发生，但是在脑积水早期可能比较轻微。当情况很严重还未予以治疗时，脑积水会产生眼球的落日征、上运动神经元损害体征（尤其在腿部）以及神经系统发育问题。

治疗

取决于病因和病情严重程度。头颅超声和CT检查将会进一步证实诊断。如果有证据表明脑室和头围的生长持续偏离于正常的生长速率，那么就需要实行脑室腹膜分流术（图 89）或脑室心房分流术。

病程和预后

并不是所有的脑积水婴儿都需要进行脑外科手术。尤其是在脑室周围出血后，脑积水有可能是暂时性的，症状可通过分次腰椎穿刺来控制，一直到停止出现脑积水或脑室扩大消退为止。分流手术的预后取决于根本的病因、先前脑损害的程度以及分流术并发症的出现与否。

小头畸形

临床特征

头围小于同年龄和同胎龄的第3个百分位点，并且较小的头围与婴儿的身长和体重不相适应（图 90）。

病因学

一般不明确，通常伴随有智能迟钝。有些有较明确的产前因素（如先天性风疹病毒或巨细胞病毒感染）

Hydrocephaly

Aetiology

May occur as an isolated congenital abnormality. The condition is most commonly due to congenital aqueduct stenosis, or is secondary to peri-ventricular haemorrhage or neonatal meningitis. It is a common association of neural tube defects.

Clinical features

Accelerated rate of growth of the skull gives rise to a disproportinate increase in head circumference (Fig. 88), and widening of the fontanelles and sutures. Increasing ventricular index will be seen on routine cranial ultrasonography in preterm infants with post-haemorrhagic hydrocephaly. Associated symptoms of raised intra-cranial pressure (e.g. lethargy, apnoea, and vomiting) may occur but may be subtle in the early stages. When severe and untreated, hydrocephaly may give rise to a setting-sun appearance of the eyes, upper motor neurone signs particularly in the legs, and neurodevelopmental problems.

Management

Depends on aetiology and severity. Cranial ultrasonography and computed tomography scan will confirm the diagnosis. If there is evidence of continuing deviation from the normal rate of growth of the ventricles or skull circumference, a ventriculoperitoneal (Fig. 89) or ventriculoatrial shunt may be required.

Course and prognosis

Not all infants with hydrocephaly require neurosurgery. Particularly after peri-ventricular haemorrhage, hydrocephaly may be transient and symptoms may be conrolled by serial lumbar punctures until arrest or resolution of ventriculomegaly occurs. When shunt surgery is required, prognosis depends on the underlying aetiology, extent of preceding brain damage and occurrence of shunt complications.

Microcephaly

Clinical features

Head circumference <3rd centile for age and gestation, and which is inappropriately small for the length and weight of he infant (Fig. 90).

Aetiology

Usually unknown; often associated with intellectual retardation. Sometimes a clear prenatal cause is known (e.g. congenital rubella or cytomegalovirus infection).

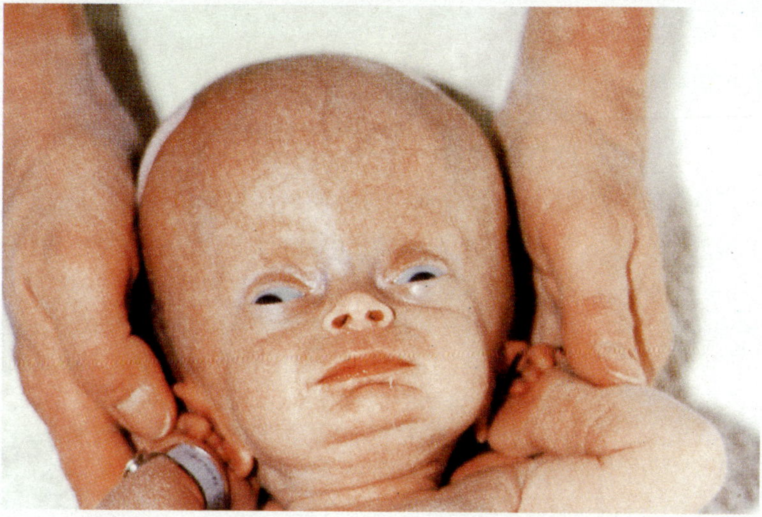

图 88　脑积水
Hydrocephalus

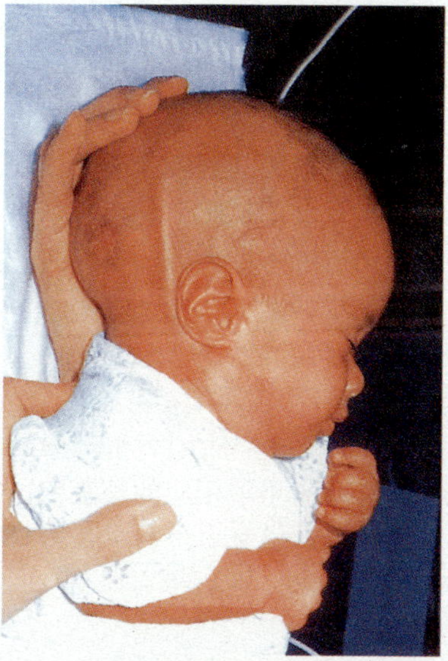

图 89　脑室腹膜分流术
Ventriculoperitoneal shunt

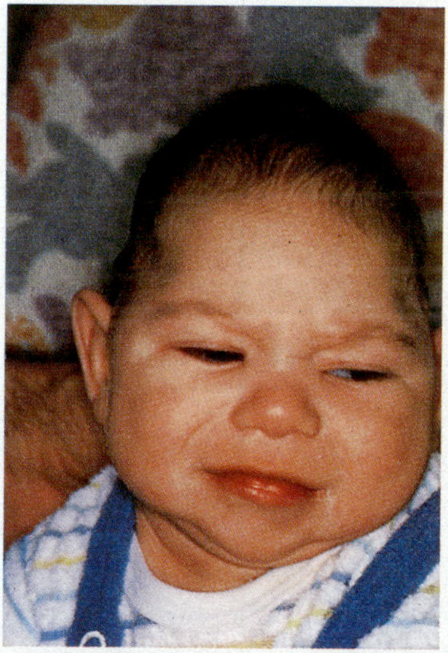

图 90　11 个月婴儿的小头畸形
Microcephaly at 11 months of age

唐氏综合征

同义词 21 三体综合征；过去常被称为先天愚型。

发病率 每600个出生存活儿中就有1个，是最常见的染色体异常疾病。

遗传特性 21 三体综合征在高龄产妇的孩子中有较高的发生率(母亲年龄为40岁时，每100个出生存活儿中就有1个发生；母亲年龄大于45岁时，每50个出生存活儿中就有1个发生)，但是大多数唐氏综合征婴儿的母亲都较年轻。一般再发危险率为1%，但是如果出现染色体易位，再发率可能会更高。

病因学 94% 的患儿有一条额外的 21 号染色体（21 三体），3% 的患儿有染色体易位，3% 的患儿为嵌合体型。

临床特征 低出生体重和生长限制很常见。通常会有扁平的满月脸和向上倾斜的眼睛（图 91），明显的内眦赘皮，全身肌张力减退，枕部扁平的短头畸形，第三囟门和单根掌横纹（通贯手）（图 92）。也可能有内弯、短小的第 5 指（指弯曲），第 2 和第 3 脚趾之间间隔宽阔（sandal gap），跖纹明显，有布拉什菲尔德点(Brushfield spots，即先天愚型婴儿虹膜表面的淡黄或白色斑点）（图 93）。30% 的唐氏综合征患儿会有先天性心脏病，最常见的是房室间隔缺损，应该常规进行超声心动检查。

合并症 呼吸道感染，急性髓性白血病，甲状腺功能减退，十二指肠闭锁，先天性巨结肠症和秃发症。

病程和预后 通常会有身材矮小和智力迟钝。平均IQ＜50，尽管社会行为能力经常超过其智能年龄相应的预期值。很多这些孩子现在在普通学校进行正常教育。男性常常不能生育，但是女性则不一定。其平均寿命是30～40岁。

产前诊断 高危母亲可以通过产前生化测试（三倍体测试）进行诊断。羊膜腔穿刺术或绒毛取样可为染色体分析或荧光原位杂交提供细胞标本。

Down syndrome

Synonyms

Trisomy 21; used to be called mongolism.

Incidence

Occurs in 1 in 600 live births. It is the most common chromosomal abnormality.

Inheritance

Increased incidence of trisomy 21 with older maternal age (1 in 100 live births after maternal age of 40 years and 1 in 50, over 45 years), but most infants with Down syndrome are born to young mothers. General risk of recurrence is 1%, but may be higher if there is translocation.

Aetiology

Trisomy 21 occurs in 94% infants, translocation in 3% and mosaicism in 3%.

Clinical features

Low birth weight and growth restriction are common. Flat moon-shaped facies with upward slanting eyes (Fig. 91), prominent epicanthic folds, generalized hypotonia, brachycephaly with a flattened occiput, a third fontanelle and single transverse palmar creases (simian crease (Fig. 92) are usually present. There may also be incurving of short fifth finger (clinodactyly), a wide gap between second and third toe (sandal gap), marked plantar crease, and Brushfield spots (Fig. 93). Congenital heart disease, most commonly atrio-ventriculo-septal defects, occur in 30% children with Down syndrome and routine echocardiogram should be performed.

Associations

Respiratory infection, acute myeloid leukaemia, hypothyroidism, duodenal atresia, Hirschsprung's disease and alopecia.

Course and prognosis

Short stature and intellectual retardation are always present. Average IQ is <50, although social performance is often beyond that expected for mental age. Many of these children are now educated in normal schools. Males are invariably infertile, but females are not necessarily so. Average life span is 30-40 years.

Antenatal diagnosis

Women at high risk can be identified by a combination of maternal biochemical tests (triple test) antenatally. Amniocentesis or chorionic villus sampling will provide cells for chromosomal analysis or fluorescence in situ hybridization.

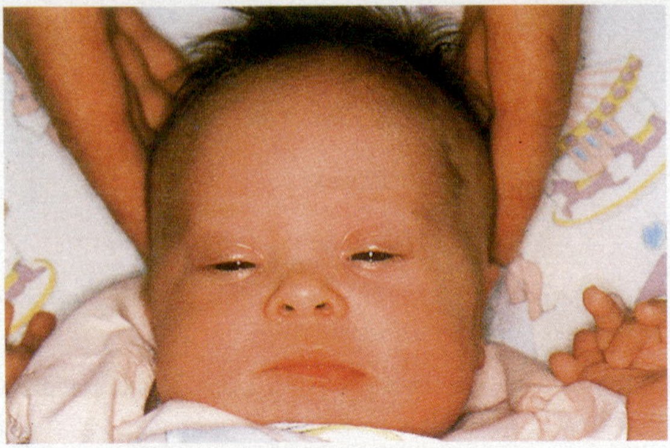

图 91　典型的唐氏综合征面容
Typical facies of Down syndrome

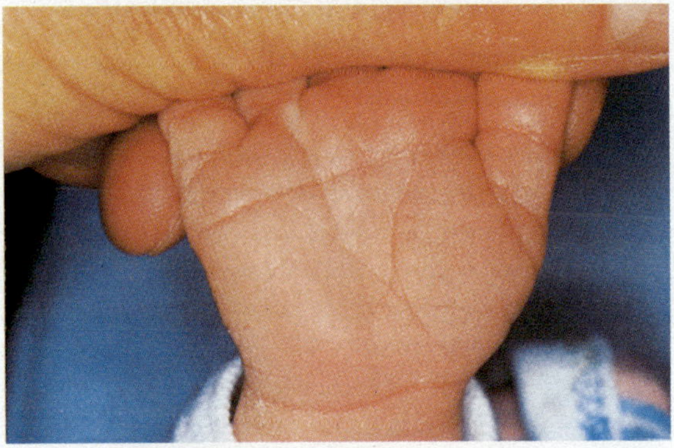

图 92　单根掌横纹（通贯手）
Single transverse palmar crease (Simian crease)

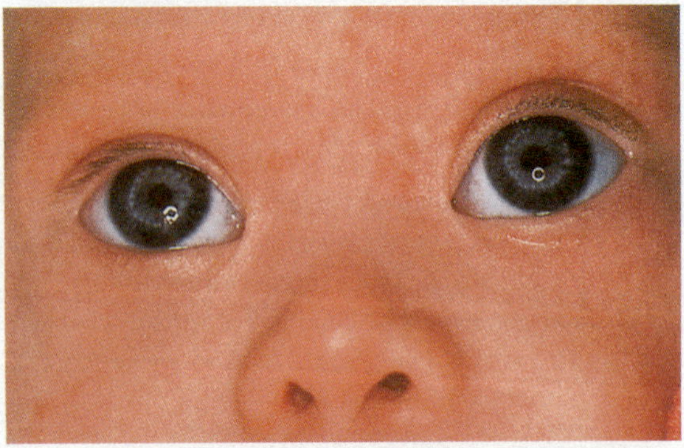

图 93　唐氏综合征明显的内眦赘皮，注意虹膜上的布拉什菲尔德点
Prominent epicanthic folds in Down syndrome. Note Brushfield spots on the iris

Edward 综合征（18 三体综合征）

发病率 每 3000 个出生存活儿中就有 1 个，是第二大常见染色体异常疾病。

临床特征 小于胎龄儿，小头畸形，严重智力迟钝，肺发育不全，先天性心脏病，臀部和四肢呈屈曲畸形样异常体位（图 94），钳夹样手，食指交叉于第 3 指上，第 5 指交叉于第 4 指上（图 95），摇篮样脚，肾脏异常，隐睾，以及枕部突出、小颌、多毛、睑裂短小、小口、面瘫和低位耳的颅面部异常。

病程和预后 大多数在生后前几周就死亡。仅有小于 10% 的婴儿存活超过 1 年。

帕塔综合征（13 三体综合征）

临床特征 脸部中线、眼睛和前脑缺陷，唇裂和腭裂，小头畸形，严重智力迟钝，耳聋，摇篮样脚，隐睾，先天性心脏病。

病程和预后 在出生后第一年中存活率$<$ 20%。

特纳综合征

发病率 每 5000 个出生存活儿中大约有 1 个，通常为散发。

病因学 卵巢功能不成熟。仅存在一个性染色体（XO 型）。

临床特征 低出生体重，手和脚短暂的先天性淋巴管性水肿（图 96），颈蹼，阔胸（乳头间距较宽），发际较低，短颈，臂外偏角较大（肘外翻）。约有10%患儿发生主动脉缩窄、耳聋和轻度智力缺陷。身材矮小和第二性征发育障碍会在以后的儿童期表现出来。

治疗 从青春期开始予以周期性的雌激素替代治疗将会诱导第二性征发育。永久性不育。重组生长激素将会改善最终的身高。

Edward syndrome (trisomy 18; E-trisomy)

Incidence

Occurs in 1 in 3000 live births; second most common chromosomal abnormality.

Clinical features

Small for gestational age, microcephaly, severe mental retardation, hypoplastic lungs, congenital heart disease, abnormal posture with flexion deformities of hips and limbs (Fig. 94), clenched hands with overlapping of index finger over third, and fifth finger over fourth finger (Fig. 95), rocker-bottom feet, renal abnormalities, cryptorchidism, craniofacial abnormalities with prominent occiput, micrognathia, hirsutism, short palpebral fissures, microstomia, facial palsy and low-set ears.

Course and prognosis

Most die within first few weeks. Fewer than 10% survive >1 year.

Patau syndrome (trisomy 13; D-trisomy)

Clinical features

Midline defects of face, eyes and forebrain, cleft lip and palate, microcephaly, severe mental retardation, deafness, rocker-bottom feet ,cryptorchidism, congenital heart defects.

Course and prognosis

Fewer than 20% survive the first year of life.

Turner syndrome

Incidence

Appoximately 1 in 5000 live births; usually sporadic occurrence.

Aetiology

Premature ovarian failure. Single X chromosome (XO).

Clinical features

Low birth weight, transient congenital lymphoedema of hands and feet (Fig. 96), webbing of the neck, broad chest with widely-spaced nipples, low hairline and short neck and a wide carrying angle (cubitus valgus). Coarctation of the aorta, deafness and mild mental deficiency occur in about 10%. Short stature and failure of secondary sexual development become apparent in later childhood.

Management

Cyclical oestrogen replacement therapy given from adolescence will induce secondary sexual development. Infertility is invariable. Recombinant growth hormone will improve final height.

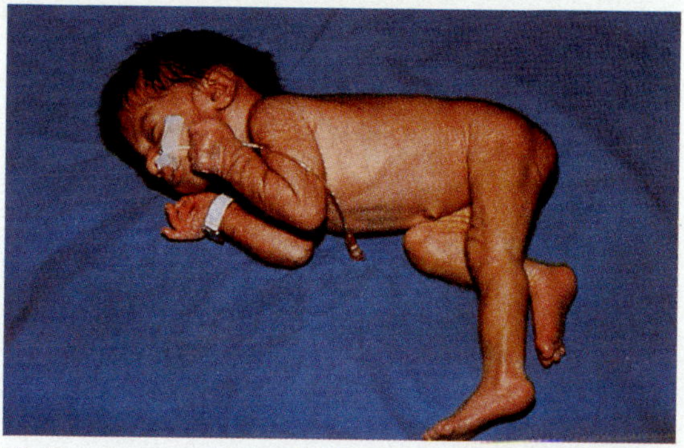

图 94 Edward 综合征臀部和四肢典型的异常屈曲体位
Edward syndrome with typical flexion deformities of hips and limbs

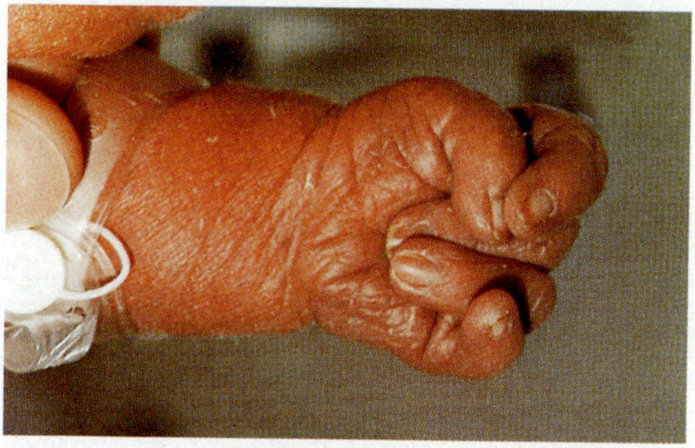

图 95 Edward 综合征钳夹样手，手指相互交叉
Clenched hands with overlapping of fingers in Edward syndrome

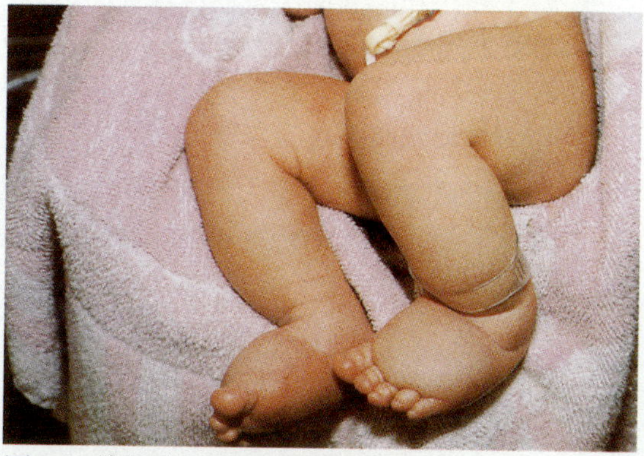

图 96 脚部先天性淋巴管性水肿
Congenital lymphoedema of feet

短肢侏儒

发病率 软骨发育不全，是最常见的软骨发育异常，每10 000个出生存活儿中就有1个。

遗传特性 常染色体显性遗传，但是约有90%是染色体的新生突变。软骨发育不全的致命形式（窒息性胸腔营养不良或致死性侏儒症）通常是常染色体隐性遗传（图97）。

临床特征 四肢短小（图98），大头（巨头畸形），前额突出，鼻梁较宽。

病程和预后 软骨发育不全性侏儒的智力一般正常，但早期运动发育比较慢。

成骨不全（脆骨病）

遗传特性 严重的先天性宽骨型成骨作用不全一般是常染色体隐性遗传。其他不太严重的类型可能常染色体显性遗传。

病因学 由于不明原因的胶原形成异常。

临床特征 颅骨和长骨骨化不良，伴有多发性骨折和骨痂形成。在一些严重类型中，患儿由于宫内骨折而在出生时有短小变形的四肢（图99）。在新近的骨折处可以有捻发感。有时会出现蓝色巩膜，但是仅凭这一点很难在新生儿期做出诊断。

预后 除了死产和因病情严重而早期死亡的婴儿，此病的自然发展史有较大变异性。过了婴儿期，生存情况会有所好转，但是孩子经常会因为外观畸形（图100）和因耳硬化而导致的耳聋形成残障。

治疗 必须予以谨慎地护理。外科矫形治疗骨折是唯一可提供的治疗方式，但是理想的治疗可以减少畸形。

Short-limbed dwarfism

Incidence

Achondroplasia, the most common chondrodysplasia, occurs in 1 in 10 000 live births.

Inheritance

Autosomal dominant inheritance but approximately 90% occur as a fresh mutation. The lethal forms of chondrodysplasia (asphyxiating thoracic dystrophy or thanatophoric dwarfism) are usually autosomal recessive (Fig. 97).

Clinical features

Short limbs (Fig. 98), large head (macrocephaly) and prominent forehead with broad nasal bridge.

Course and prognosis

Intelligence is usually normal in achondroplastic dwarfs, but early motor development may be slow.

Osteogenesis imperfecta (brittle bone disease)

Inheritance

The severe congenital broad-boned type of osteogenesis imperfecta is usually autosomal recessive. Other less severe forms may be autosomal dominant.

Aetiology

Abnormality of collagen formation of uncertain cause.

Clinical features

Poorly mineralized skull and long bones with multiple fractures and callus formation. In the severe form, they often have short, deformed limbs at birth due to intrauterine fractures (Fig. 99). Crepitus may be felt in bones with recent fractures. Blue sclerae are sometimes present, but may be difficult to diagnose in the neonatal period.

Prognosis

Wide variability in the natural history of this disorder, with stillbirth or early mortality among severely affected infants. Beyond infancy, the outlook for survival is good, but the child is often handicapped by orthopaedic deformity (Fig. 100) and deafness secondary to otosclerosis.

Management

Careful nursing is mandatory. Orthopaedic treatment of fractures is the only form of treatment that can be offered, but optimal management will limit deformity.

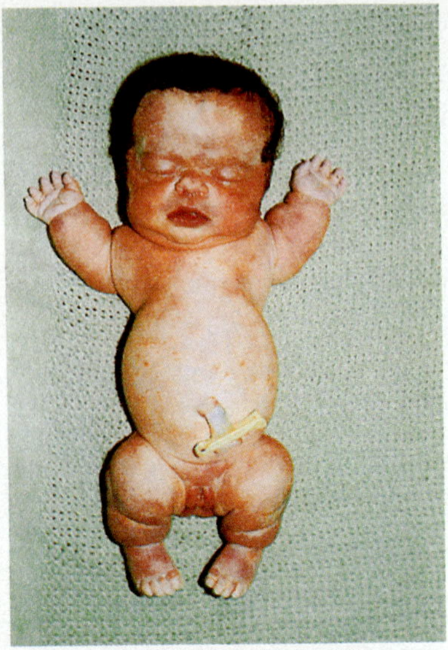

图 97　窒息性胸腔营养不良
Asphyxiating thoracic dystrophy

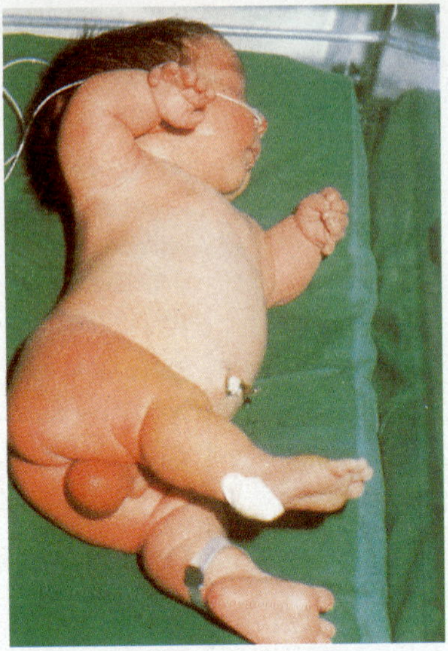

图 98　四肢短小的侏儒症
Short-limbed dwarfism

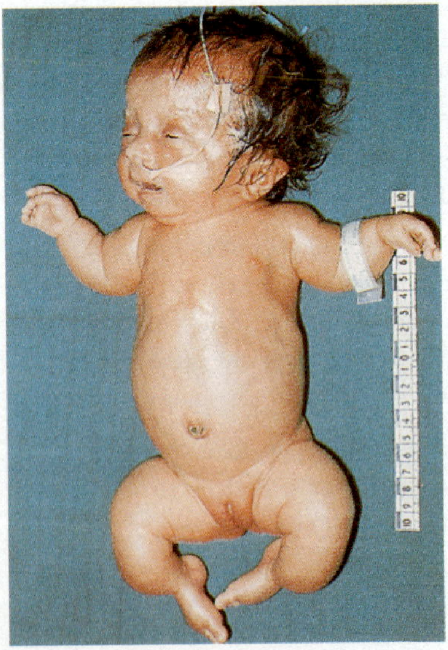

图 99　成骨不全
Osteogenesis imperfecta

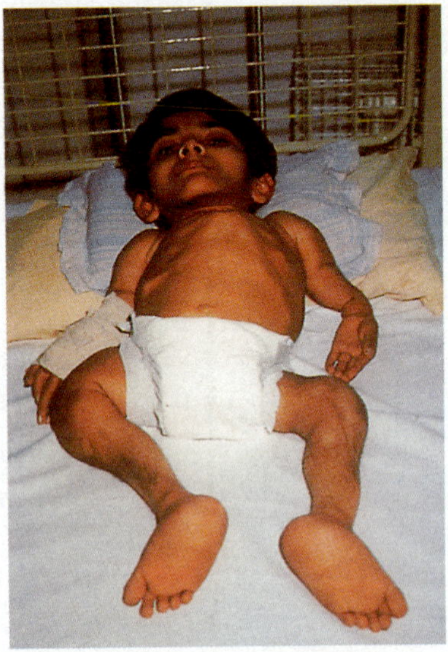

图 100　成骨不全伴骨畸形
Osteogenesis imperfecta with bony deformity

第一腮弓综合征

发病率 相对常见。

遗传特性 多为散发。

病因学 早期下颌骨发育不全导致畸形，舌后位，咽腭弓融合受损。

临床特征 严重小颌畸形和较广泛的正中线后位腭裂（图101和102）。

并发症 由于舌后坠进入腭裂而导致急性呼吸道阻塞；喂养困难。

治疗 需要精心的护理，俯卧位以避免呼吸道阻塞。关闭腭裂的外科手术应该在3个月大小以后实施。

病程和预后 由于急性呼吸道阻塞，在婴儿早期有着较高的死亡率。小颌和舌后坠在婴儿期会有所改善。

鳃弓综合征

同义词 面-耳-脊椎综合征。

发病率 相对常见。经常伴有眼睛和脊椎的异常，或眼球外层皮样囊肿（戈登哈综合征）。

临床特征 耳廓发育不良伴有外耳道缺失（图103），通常是单侧的。副耳也很常见。常有单侧的听力缺失，但是如果另一侧耳朵的听力正常，语言发育往往正常。颜面部发育不良，在颈前外侧常有鳃裂残留。

治疗 对听力的早期评估很重要。外科矫形手术效果通常是理想的，但也并不是都令人满意。

Pierre-Robin syndrome

Incidence Relatively common.

Inheritance Usually sporadic occurrence.

Aetiology Early developmental anomaly with mandibular hypoplasia, posterior location of the tongue and impaired closure of the posterior palate.

Clinical features Severe micrognathia and wide posterior midline cleft palate (Figs 101 and 102).

Complications Acute respiratory obstruction because of a tendency of the tongue to fall back into the cleft palate; feeding difficulties.

Management Expert nursing is required, often with the infant in the face-down posture to prevent respiratory obstruction. Surgical closure of the cleft palate should be performed after 3 months of age.

Course and prognosis High mortality in early infancy due to acute respiratory obstruction. Micrognathia and glossoptosis improve during infancy.

Branchial arch syndrome

Synonym Facio-auriculovertebral syndrome.

Incidence Relatively common. Often associated with ocular or vertebral anomalies or epibulbar dermoids (Goldenhar syndrome).

Clinical features Hypoplastic pinna with absent external auditory meatus (Fig. 103). Usually unilateral. Accessory pre-auricular tags are common. Unilateral hearing loss is common, but speech is usually normal if hearing is normal on the other side. Facial hypoplasia, and branchial cleft remnants in the anterolateral neck are common.

Management Early assessment of hearing is important. Cosmetic surgery is usually desirable, but not always satisfactory.

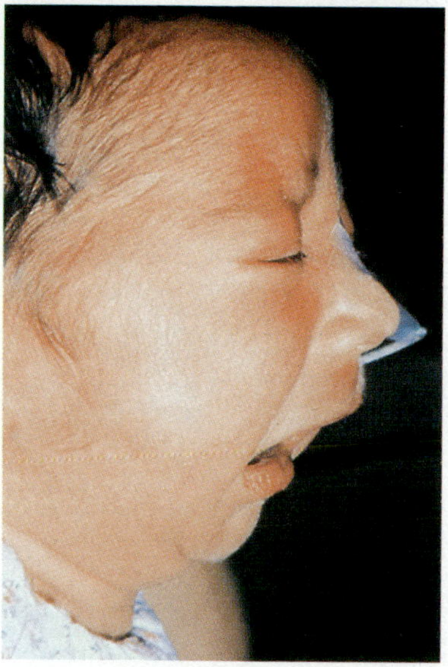

图 101 第一腮弓综合征的严重小颌畸形
Severe micrognathia of Pierre-Robin syndrome

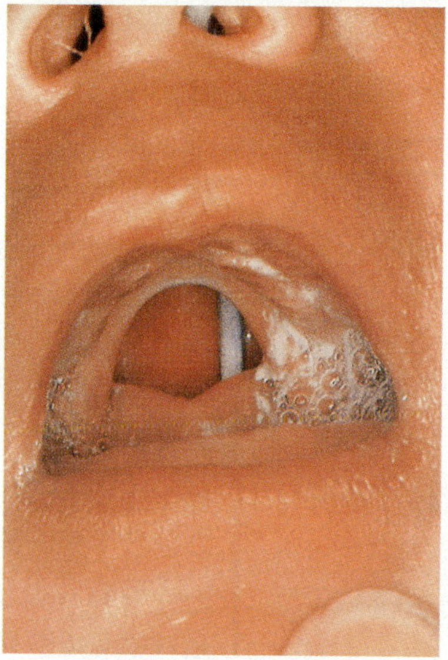

图 102 较广泛的正中线后位腭裂
Wide posterior midline cleft palate

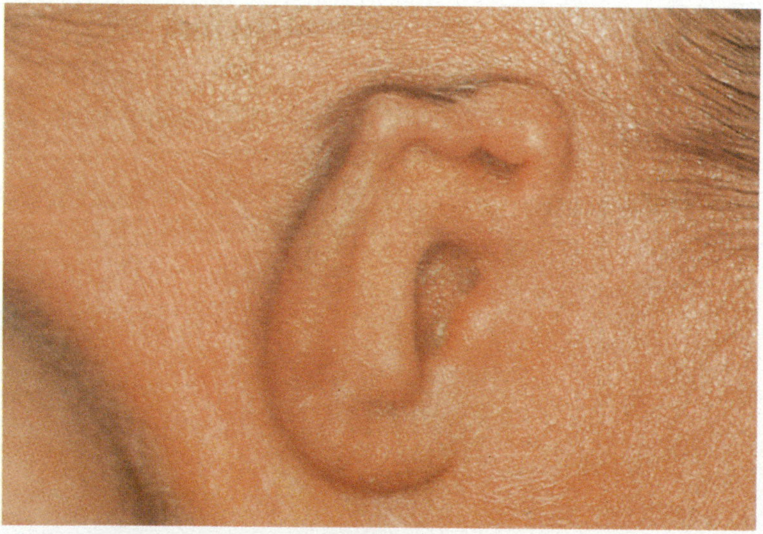

图 103 耳廓发育不良伴有外耳道缺失
Hypoplastic pinna with absent external auditory meatus

波特综合征

同义词 肾缺如。

发病率 每3000个出生存活儿中就有1个。常规产前超声会检查发现严重的羊水过少。

病因学 Potter描述的典型综合征是由于不明原因的肾缺如引起。其他肾缺陷（婴儿多囊肾或慢性尿道闭塞）或慢性羊水渗漏，也可能引起羊水过少和相似的临床表现（如四肢挛缩和肺发育不良）。

遗传特性 散发。

临床特征 低出生体重，低位耳（图104），主要异常情况有四肢屈曲挛缩、肺发育不良和肾衰竭。

病程和预后 会发生肾衰竭和进行性生化指标紊乱。通常由于生后呼吸衰竭而导致死亡。

干梅状腹综合征

发病率 不常见。

遗传特性 散发。

临床特征 腹壁肌肉组织缺损形成多皱纹的干梅状腹部外观（图105），睾丸未降和多发性肾异常，常常有尿路闭塞（图106）。

治疗 如果条件允许，可以对肾畸形进行外科手术治疗。在以后的阶段需进行腹壁重建手术。

预后 依赖于肾畸形的严重性和对肾功能的影响。通常会发生慢性肾功能不全。

Potter syndrome

Synonym
Renal agenesis.

Incidence
Occurs in 1 in 3000 live births. Routine antenatal ultrasonography will show severe oligohydramnios.

Aetiology
The classic syndrome described by Potter was due to renal agenesis of unknown aetiology. Other renal defects (infantile polycystic kidneys or chronic urinary tract obstruction) or chronic leakage of amniotic fluid, may also give rise to oligohydramnios and similar clinical manifestations (e.g. contractures of limbs and hypoplastic lungs).

Inheritance
Sporadic occurrence.

Clinical features
Low birth weight, low set ears (Fig. 104), compression abnormalities with flexion contractures of limbs, hypoplastic lungs, and renal failure.

Course and prognosis
Renal failure and progressive biochemical derangement occur. Death is normally due to respiratory failure soon after birth.

Prune-belly syndrome

Incidence
Uncommon.

Inheritance
Sporadic occurrence.

Clinical features
Deficient abdominal wall musculature giving a rugose, prune-belly appearance (Fig. 105), undescended testis and multiple renal anomalies, usually obstructive uropathopathies (Fig. 106).

Management
Surgical management of renal abnormalities if appropriate. Reconstitution of abdominal wall at a later stage.

Prognosis
Depends on the severity of the renal abnormalities and the effect on renal function. Chronic renal failure is common.

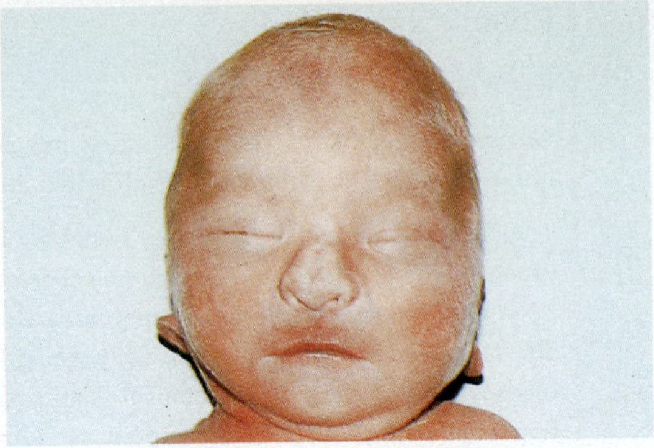

图 104 波特综合征（经 Dr G. Gau 许可）
Potter syndrome (courtesy of Dr G. Gau)

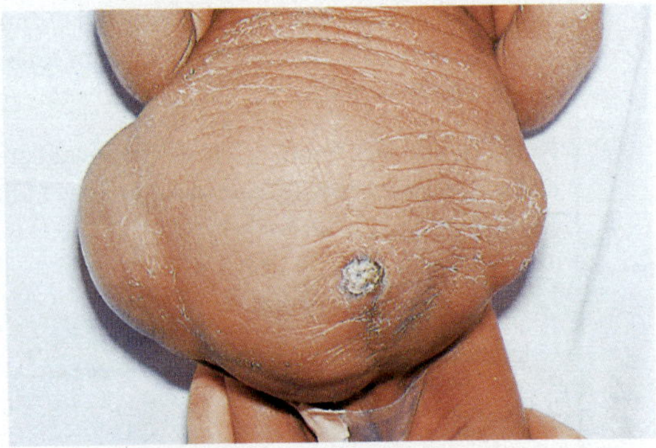

图 105 干梅状腹综合征松弛的腹壁肌肉组织
Prune-belly syndrome with lax abdominal wall musculature

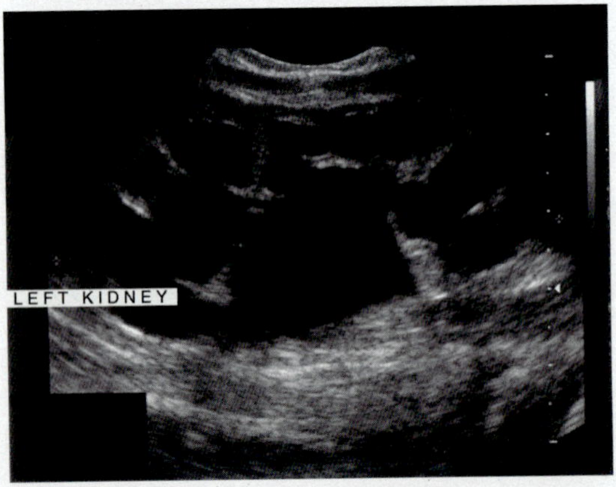

图 106 尿路闭塞引起的大量肾积水
Gross hydronephrosis in obstructive uropathy

外胚层发育不良

发病率和遗传特性 很罕见，X 连锁和常染色体显性遗传。

临床特征 指甲和牙齿发育不良或缺如。毛发通常较细且稀疏。在一些类型中会有汗腺和皮脂腺功能异常。

指甲-髌骨综合征

临床特征 指甲发育不良或缺如（图 107），髌骨缺如。到成年以后膝关节会出现骨关节炎。

门克斯综合征（门克斯卷发综合征）

遗传特性 很罕见，是 X 连锁隐性遗传。

病因学 可能是由于铜结合金属蛋白缺陷所致。

临床特征 特征性稀疏、卷曲纠结的毛发（图 108 和 109），其毛发在显微镜下呈现部分断裂和扭曲形态。有严重的进行性神经衰退，并且从婴儿早期开始就出现发育停滞。通常在出生后前几年死亡。

产前诊断 在培养羊膜细胞时发现铜摄入过多。

德朗热综合征

遗传特性 不明原因，散发存在。

临床特征 都会有身材矮小，发育停滞和多毛症。其特征性的面容（图110）为浓密的眉毛，长而卷的睫毛，小颌症，带有前倾鼻孔的小鼻子和下翻的嘴唇。

病程和预后 所有患儿都有严重的智能发育迟缓，并且经常在儿童早期死亡。

Ectodermal dysplasia

Incidence and inheritance — Rare; X-linked and autosomal dominant inheritance described.

Clinical features — Hypoplastic or absent nails and teeth. Hair is usually fine and sparse. Abnormalities of sweat and sebaceous glands also occur in some varieties.

Nail-patella syndrome

Clinical features — Hypoplastic or absent nails (Fig. 107) and absent patellae. Osteoarthritis of the knees develops in adult life.

Menkes syndrome (Menkes kinky hair syndrome)

Inheritance — Rare, X-linked recessive.

Aetiology — Probably a defect of copper-binding metalloprotein.

Clinical features — Characteristic sparse, twisted kinky hair (Figs 108 and 109) which has partial breakages and twists on microscopic examination. There is profound progressive neurological deterioration and failure to thrive from early infancy. Death is usual within the first few years.

Antenatal diagnosis — Excessive copper uptake in cultured amniotic cells has been demonstrated.

de Lange syndrome

Inheritance — Sporadic condition of unknown aetiology.

Clinical features — Short stature, failure to thrive, and hirsutism are invariable. Bushy eyebrows, long curling eyelashes, micrognathia, small nose with anteverted nostrils, and down-turned mouth give a characteristic facial appearance (Fig. 110).

Course and prognosis — All are severely mentally retarded and death usually occurs in early childhood.

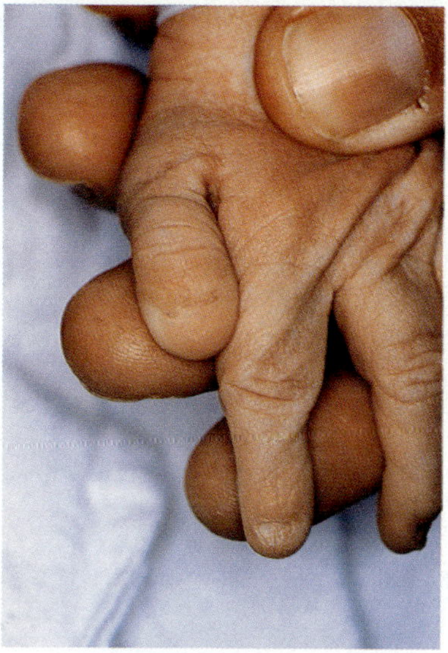

图 107 指甲发育不良
Hypoplastic fingernails

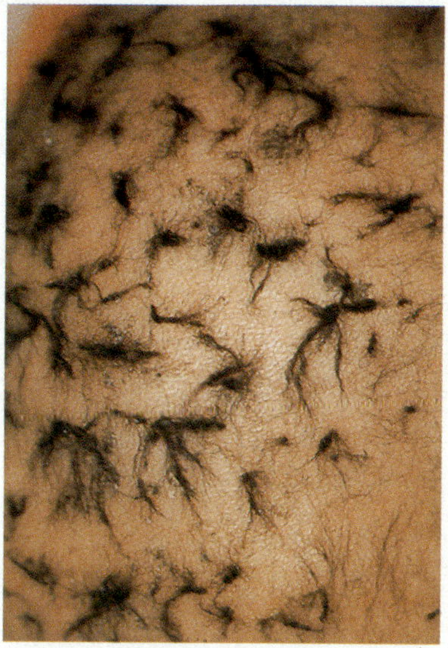

图 108 门克斯综合征卷曲纠结的毛发
Kinky hair in Menkes syndrome

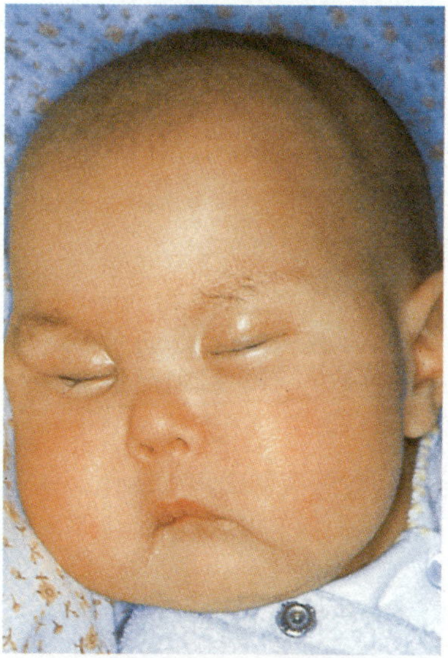

图 109 门克斯综合征颜面部：浮肿的脸颊和卷曲的眉毛
Facies of Menkes syndrome showing puffy cheeks and kinky eyebrows

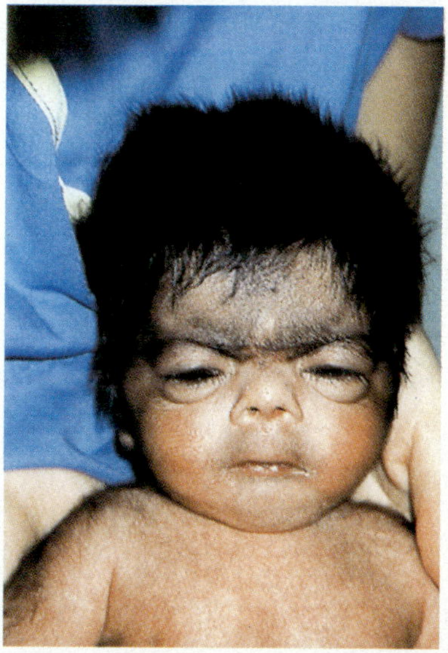

图 110 德朗热综合征特征性的多毛面容
Characteristic hirsuite facial appearance of de Lange syndrome

结节性脑硬化

发病率 不常见，但是有些较轻的类型可能没有做出诊断。

遗传特性 常染色体显性遗传，但是至少 80% 是由于染色体新的突变造成。

临床特征 综合征的严重程度和表现变化度很大，甚至于在一个家族中。通常会有癫痫，智能缺陷和一些皮肤表现。到孩子 7 ~ 8 岁时都会在 CT 检查中发现有脑组织肉芽肿损害（结节）。皮肤表现包括典型的皮脂腺腺瘤（图 111）、纤维瘤、鲨革斑、咖啡牛奶斑和色素脱失斑（图 112）。常见有内脏错构瘤和视网膜损害。

瓦尔登伯格综合征

发病率 不常见。

遗传特性 常染色体显性遗传。

临床特征 额发发白（图113）或部分性白化病和先天性耳聋比较常见。有时会有虹膜异色症和皮肤白癜风现象。

预后 耳聋是最严重的特征，通常是双侧的和严重的感觉神经性耳聋。

莱-尼综合征

发病率 很罕见。

遗传特性 X 连锁伴性遗传。

病因学 先天性酶缺陷导致尿酸生成过多。目前已经开始对高危家庭进行产前诊断。

临床特征 精神发育迟缓，手足徐动症样或舞蹈病样动作，发音困难，肌无力，腱反射活跃，跖伸肌反射。由于不能控制的攻击性冲动而导致特征性的自残（图 114），这似乎与感觉损伤和高尿酸血症无关。

治疗 可应用别嘌呤醇来控制高尿酸血症，但是临床病程不会被改变。

预后 很差，大多在儿童期死亡。

Tuberous sclerosis

Incidence Uncommon, but mild forms may be underdiagnosed.

Inheritance Autosomal dominant, but at least 80% are due to a new mutation.

Clinical features Severity and expression of the syndrome varies enormously, even within families. Usually epilepsy, mental deficiency and some skin manifestations occur. All have granulomatous, lesions (tubers) in the brain which become visible on CT scan by 7-8 years of age. Skin manifestations include the typical adenoma sebaceum (Fig. 111), fibromas, shagreen patch, café-au-lait spots, and depigmented patches (Fig. 112). Visceral hamartomas and retinal lesions are common.

Waardenburg syndrome

Incidence Uncommon.

Inheritance Autosomal dominant.

Clinical features White forelock (Fig. 113) or partial albinism and congenital deafness are usual. Sometimes there is heterochromia of the iris and vitiligo of the skin.

Prognosis Deafness is the most serious feature; usually bilateral and severe sensorineural deafness.

Lesch-Nyhan syndrome

Incidence Rare.

Inheritance X-linked.

Aetiology Enzyme deficiency resulting in excess production of uric acid. Antenatal diagnosis is now available for high-risk families.

Clinical features Mental retardation, athetoid or choreiform movements, dysarthria, muscle weakness, brisk tendon reflexes and extensor plantar responses. Characteristic self-mutilation (Fig. 114) due to uncontrollable aggressive impulses which appear to be unrelated to impaired sensation or hyperuricaemia.

Management Hyperuricaemia can be controlled with allopurinol, but clinical course remains unchanged.

Prognosis Poor. Most die in childhood.

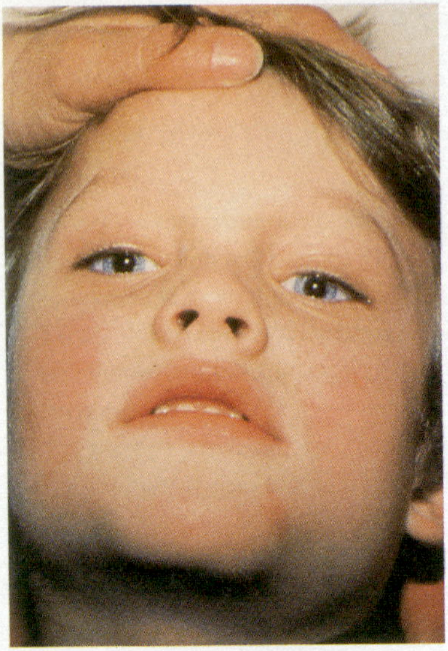

图 111　颏部的皮脂腺腺瘤
Adenoma sebaceum on the chin

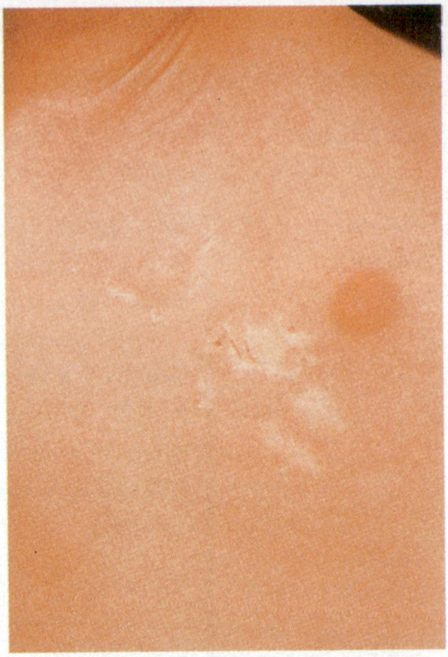

图 112　结节性脑硬化的色素脱失斑
Depigmented patches in tuberous sclerosis

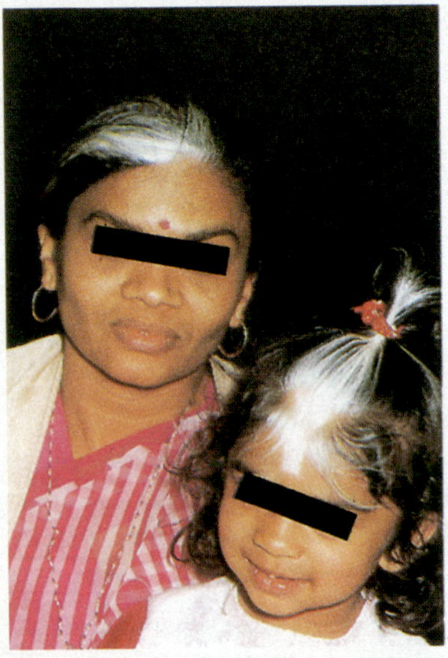

图 113　瓦尔登伯格综合征的额发发白
White forelock of Waardenburg syndrome

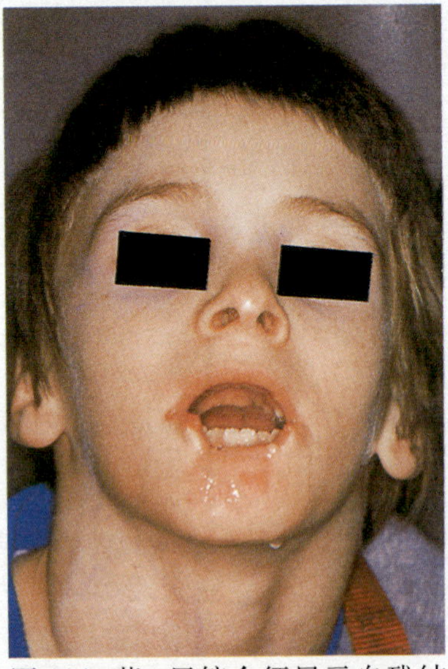

图 114　莱－尼综合征显示自残结果
Lesch-Nyhan syndrome showing effects of self-mutilation

黏多糖累积病

遗传特性和发病率 常染色体隐性遗传，不常见。

病因学 不同的特异性酶缺陷导致细胞质内黏多糖蓄积。最常见的类型是Ⅰ型黏多糖病（Hurler 综合征）（图115）、Ⅱ型黏多糖病（Hunter综合征）、Ⅳ型黏多糖病（Morquio综合征）和Ⅶ型黏多糖病（Sanfilippo综合征）。

临床特征 婴儿出生时表现正常。通常在出生后头两年逐渐发育出现面容粗糙、生长发育迟缓、精神发育迟缓、骨骼异常和肝脾大（图116）。角膜混浊见于Ⅰ型黏多糖病。在Ⅳ型黏多糖病中有严重的骨骼异常和生长发育迟缓，但是智力正常。

治疗 不能治愈，但是骨髓移植可能是阻止病程进展的有效治疗形式，并可能使疾病改善。

拉-西综合征

遗传特性和发病率 通常是散发的，不常见。

临床特征 是一种在胎内就存在的极度生长发育迟缓综合征（图117），四肢不对称，第5指短小内弯。颅面骨发育不全，具有小三角形脸和小的下翻嘴唇。

病程和预后 在以后的儿童期生长速率会逐渐改善，但是成年后的最终身高较矮。

科凯恩综合征

遗传特性和发病率 较罕见的常染色体隐性遗传，进行产前诊断有可能发现。

临床特征 身材矮小，从婴儿期就出现皮下脂肪丢失。会出现脊柱后凸（图118）、关节活动受限、灰色稀疏毛发和精神发育迟缓。视网膜色素沉着和皮肤光过敏也很常见。

Mucopolysaccharidoses

Inheritance and incidence
Autosomal recessive; uncommon.

Aetiology
Various specific enzyme deficiencies which result in accumulation of cytoplasmic mucopolysaccharides. Most common types are Hurler (type I) (Fig. 115), Hunter (type II), Morquio (type IV) and Sanfilippo (type VII) syndromes.

Clinical features
The infant appears normal at birth. Coarse facies, growth retardation, mental retardation, skeletal abnormalities and hepatosplenomegaly develop within the first 2 years of life (Fig. 116). Cloudy cornea is found in Hurler syndrome. In Morquio syndrome, there is severe skeletal deformity and growth retardation, but normal intelligence.

Management
There is no cure, but bone marrow transplantation may be a useful form of treatment to halt the progression of the condition, and may cause it to regress.

Russell-Silver syndrome

Inheritance and incidence
Usually sporadic; uncommon.

Clinical features
A syndrome of extreme growth retardation of prenatal onset (Fig. 117), asymmetry of the limbs and shortened incurved fifth finger. There is craniofacial dysostosis with small triangular facies and a small down-turned mouth.

Course and prognosis
Gradual improvement in growth rate may occur in later childhood, but final adult height remains small.

Cockayne syndrome

Inheritance and incidence
Rare autosomal recessive; antenatal diagnosis possible.

Clinical features
Short stature with loss of subcutaneous fat from infancy. Dorsal kyphosis (Fig. 118), limitation of joint movement, grey sparse hair and mental retardation are present. Retinal pigmentation and photosensitive skin are common.

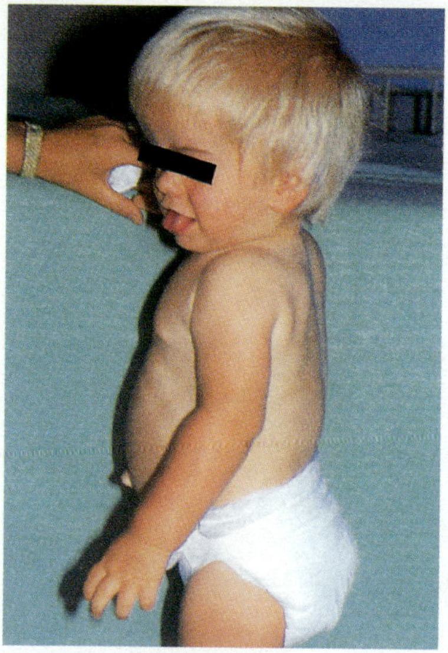

图 115　I 型黏多糖病
Hurler syndrome

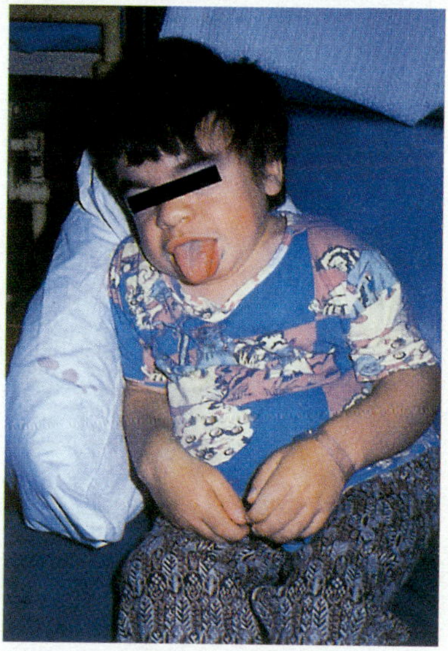

图 116　严重的黏多糖累积病
Advanced mucopolysaccharidosis

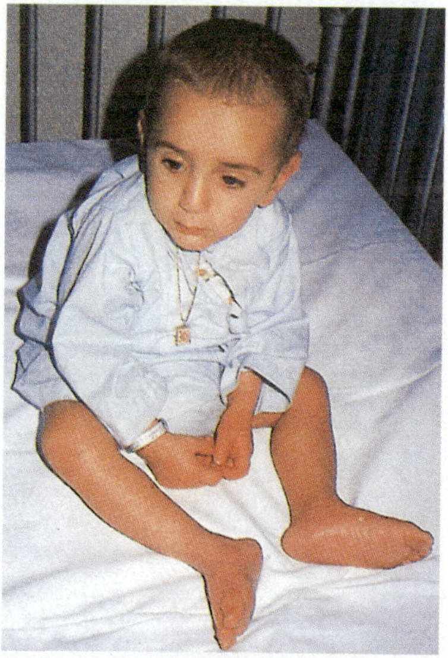

图 117　拉－西侏儒症
Russell-Silver dwarfism

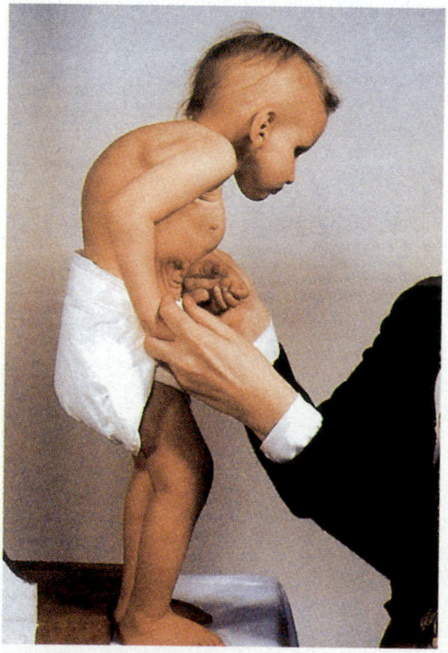

图 118　科凯恩综合征
Cockayne syndrome

克鲁宗综合征

发病率 不常见。

遗传特性 常染色体显性遗传，具有多种表现型。

临床特征 颅面骨发育不全，冠状缝、人字缝和矢状缝的颅缝早闭。由于眼眶较浅和眼距过远而引起眼球突出，形成一种特殊面容（图 119）。

治疗 对于严重的颅面骨发育不全可进行外科手术以使脑组织正常生长，或出于美容原因进行外科手术。

预后 如果早期进行外科手术治疗，预后良好。

早老综合征

发病率和遗传特性 是一种不明原因、极其罕见的综合征。大多数为散发。

临床特征 从婴儿期开始就出现早熟和快速老化（图 120）。有严重的生长发育迟缓、皮下脂肪丢失和全身性动脉粥样硬化。有时还会有秃发、指甲发育不良和屈曲畸形。

病程和预后 通常脑发育和智力发育正常。预期寿命严重缩短（平均 15 年），通常由于心肌梗死引起死亡。

洛氏综合征

同义词 眼-脑-肾综合征。

遗传特性和发病率 X 连锁；很罕见。

临床特征 精神发育迟缓、肌张力减退、关节活动过度、多动和生长发育迟缓很常见。通常会有白内障和失明（图 121）。也会有肾小管功能不全和隐睾。

预后 很差。

Crouzon syndrome

Incidence Uncommon.

Inheritance Autosomal dominant with variable expression.

Clinical features Cranial facial dysostosis with craniosynostosis of coronal, lambdoid and sagittal sutures. Ocular proptosis because of shallow orbits and hypertelorism give a characteristic facial appearance (Fig. 119).

Management Surgery to allow normal brain growth when craniosynostosis is severe, or for cosmetic reasons.

Prognosis Good if surgery is performed early.

Progeria

Incidence and inheritance Extremely rare syndrome of unknown aetiology. Most cases are sporadic.

Clinical features Premature and rapid ageing (Fig. 120) with onset in infancy. Severe growth retardation, loss of subcutaneous fat and generalized atherosclerosis. Alopecia, hypoplastic nails and flexion deformities sometimes occur.

Course and prognosis There is normal brain development and intelligence. Life expectancy is severely shortened (average 15 years) and death is usually due to myocardial infarction.

Lowe syndrome

Synonym Oculo-cerebro-renal syndrome

Inheritance and incidence X-linked; rare.

Clinical features Mental retardation, hypotonia, joint hypermobility, hyperactivity and growth retardation are common. Cataracts and blindness (Fig. 121) usually occur. Renal tubular dysfunction and cryptorchidism are also found.

Prognosis Poor.

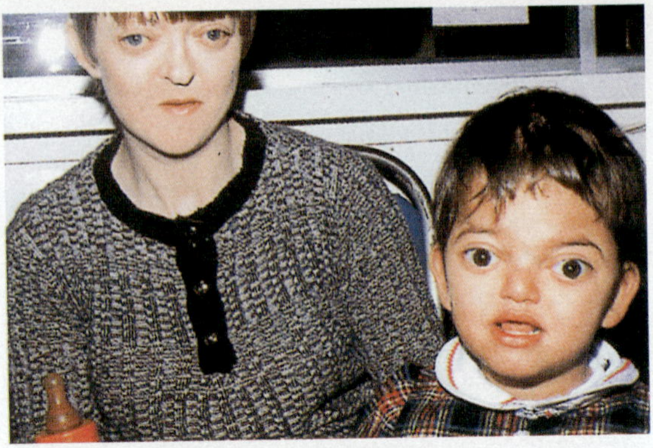

图 119 克鲁宗综合征（经由 Dr A. Kilby 许可）
Crouzon syndrome (courtesy of Dr A. Kilby)

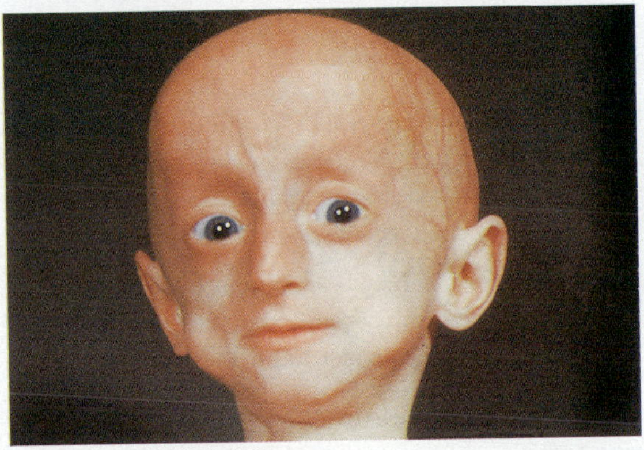

图 120 早老综合征
Progeria

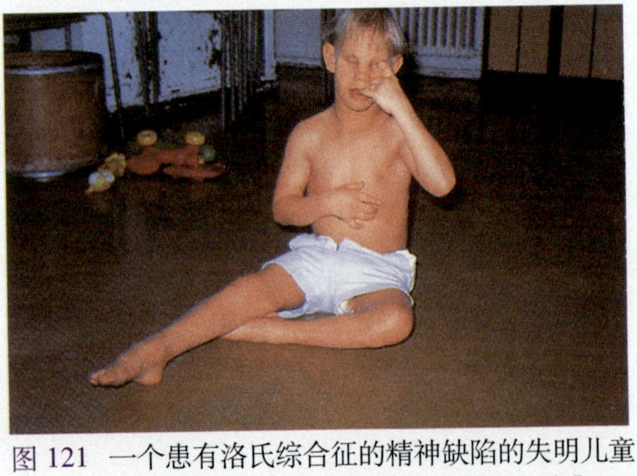

图 121 一个患有洛氏综合征的精神缺陷的失明儿童
A mentally handicapped blind child with Lowe syndrome

胎儿水肿

发病率 因为有可能在产前就予以 D 抗体以预防恒河猴溶血病的发生，因此胎儿水肿较为少见。

病因学
- 溶血性疾病，尤其是恒河猴溶血病的同族免疫作用
- α - 重型地中海贫血
- 宫内病毒感染，尤其是巨细胞病毒
- 先天性梅毒
- 伴有充血性心力衰竭的室上性心动过速
- 先天性肾病综合征
- 先天性细小病毒的感染
- 胎盘血管瘤

临床特征 苍白，全身性水肿（图 122 和 123），腹水，胸腔积液，充血性心力衰竭，以及由于肺水肿或肺发育不良而造成的严重呼吸窘迫。

治疗 取决于水肿的原因。如果水肿是继发于溶血性疾病，那么交换输血和机械通气是主要的治疗方法。如果存在继发于快速型心律失常的心力衰竭，那么就需用药物和除颤针对心律失常进行治疗，并针对心力衰竭予以支持性治疗。

预后 取决于原发病因；如果婴儿能度过新生儿期，一般预后良好。

克利佩尔-费尔综合征

遗传特性和发病率 不明原因，散发存在。每 40 000 个出生存活儿中就有 1 个，女性较多见。

临床特征 颈部短且固定，继发性颈蹼，发际较低（图 124），颈椎融合。有时会出现偏侧脊柱发育不全、肋骨缺损、脊柱侧凸和Sprengel肩（先天性肩胛翼状畸形，即先天性肩胛向上移位）。

合并症 大约 30% 的病例有耳聋。有可能是作为神经管发育过程中出现的很多严重缺陷的一部分而出现。

预后 多变，取决于潜在的骨骼异常情况。

Hydrops fetalis

Incidence
Less common since prevention of rhesus haemolytic disease has been possible with antenatal anti-D administration.

Aetiology
- Haemolytic disease, particularly rhesus isoimmunization.
- Alpha-thalassaemia major.
- Intrauterine viral infections, particularly cytomegalovirus.
- Congenital syphilis.
- Supraventricular tachycardia with congestive cardiac failure.
- Congenital nephrotic syndrome.
- Congenital parvovirus infection.
- Placental angioma.

Clinical features
Pallor, gross generalized oedema (Figs 122 and 123), ascites, pleural effusions, congestive heart failure, and severe respiratory distress due to pulmonary oedema or pulmonary hypoplasia.

Management
Depends on the cause of hydrops. If hydrops is secondary to haemolytic disease, exchange transfusions and ventilatory support are the mainstay of treatment. In the presence of cardiac failure secondary to a tachyarrhythmia, treatment is directed towards correcting the arrhythmia with drugs or defibrillation, and supportive treatment of cardiac failure.

Prognosis
Depends on underlying cause; usually good if infant survives neonatal period.

Klippel-Feil syndrome

Inheritance and incidence
Sporadic occurrence of unknown aetiology; occurs in 1 in 40 000 live births; female predominance.

Clinical features
Short immobile neck, secondary webbing of neck, low hairline (Fig. 124) and fusion of cervical vertebrae. Hemivertebrae, rib defects, scoliosis and Sprengel`s shoulder sometimes occur.

Associations
Deafness in approximately 30% of cases. May occur as part of a more serious defect of neural tube development.

Prognosis
Variable and dependant on the underlying skeletal abnormality.

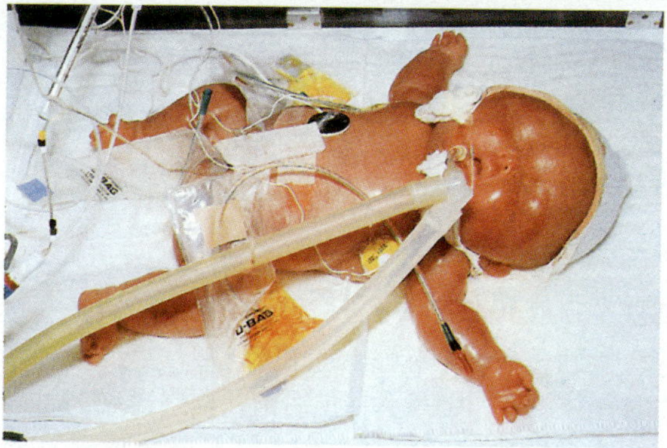

图 122
胎儿水肿疾病的全身性水肿
Gross generalized oedema of hydrops fetalis

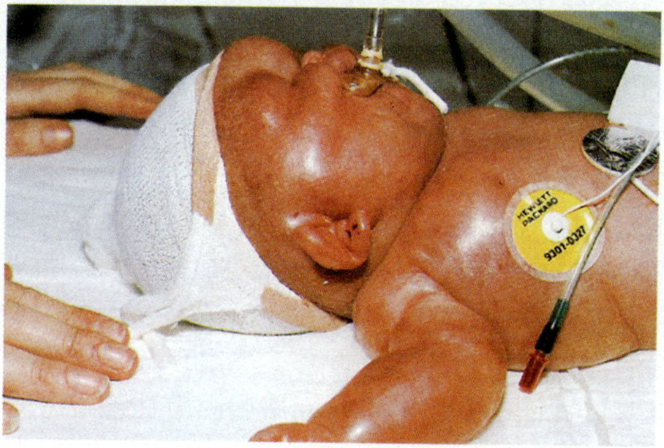

图 123
由于恒河猴溶血病引起的胎儿水肿的苍白和水肿
Pallor and oedema in hydrops fetalis due to rhesus haemolytic disease

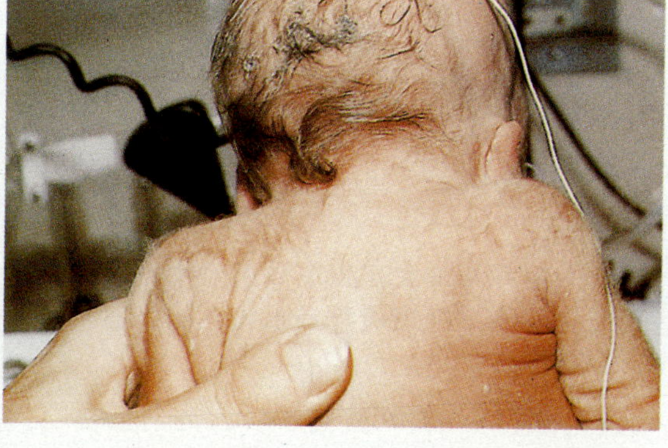

图 124
克利佩尔－费尔综合征的短颈和低发际
Short neck and low hairline in Klippel-Feil syndrome.

草莓样痣

发病率 常见，尤其在早产儿。

病理学 毛细血管扩张和/或内皮细胞增生。

临床特征 隆起、柔软、有凹痕的鲜红色血管瘤，边缘不连续。出生时往往没有，但是会在生后前几周内出现。通常先是小而微微隆起的鲜红色斑，逐渐变化成草莓样痣。它可以是单发，也可以是多发，可以出现在身体的任何部位。其大小多数会在生后第一年中迅速增加。在草莓样痣中心出现溃疡和由此继发的感染。经过数年，所有的草莓样痣都会慢慢消退。当草莓样痣中心出现浅灰色的纤维化区域（图125）时，说明它开始消退。它们最终会完全消失，仅留下一个扁平、苍白的脱色区域。

病程和预后 除非有出血、感染或影响到患处功能的严重美容畸形，否则不需要治疗。除了类固醇外，所有治疗方法都会留下一些皮肤瘢痕；在大多数草莓样痣中，让其自然消退是最理想的处理方法。当出现草莓样痣压迫重要器官或严重出血时，应用类固醇往往是有效的。

单纯痣（毛细血管扩张痣）

发病率 很常见，见于30% ~ 50%的婴儿。

病理学 毛细血管瘤。

临床特征 粉红色鲜亮的“斑点”样毛细血管瘤，可见于眼睑、鼻梁（图126）、上嘴唇和颈背部（图127）。在前额有时会有一个“V”字形的皮损，民间传说中认为是鹳喙的标记。单纯痣受压后不会变白。

病程和预后 所有脸上的单纯痣都会在出生后第一年自行消退。那些在颈背部的单纯痣通常是永久性的，但不需要治疗。

Strawberry naevi

Incidence

Common, particularly in preterm infants.

Pathology

Dilated capillaries +/- endothelial proliferation.

Clinical features

Raised, soft, pitted, bright red haemangiomata with a discrete edge. Not usually present at birth, but appear within the first few weeks of life. Often preceded by a small and slightly raised, bright red spot, which evolves into a strawberry naevus. May be single or multiple and occur anywhere on the body. Majority increase rapidly in size during the first year of life. Ulceration and subsequent infection may occur in the centre of the lesion. All strawberry naevi regress slowly over a few years. Involution has started when pale grey areas of fibrosis appear in the centre of the naevus (Fig. 125). They eventually disappear completely and leave only a flat, pale depigmented area.

Course and prognosis

No treatment is required, unless there is haemorrhage, infection or severe cosmetic deformity interfering with function of affected part. All forms of treatment except steroids will leave some scarring of skin; natural resolution is the optimal management in majority of strawberry naevi. When there is pressure on a vital organ or severe bleeding, steroids may sometimes be helpful.

Simple naevus (stork bite naevus)

Incidence

Very common; seen in 30-50% of infants.

Pathology

Capillary haemangioma.

Clinical features

Bright pink 'macular' capillary haemangiomata seen on eyelids, bridge of nose (Fig. 126), upper lip and nape of neck (Fig. 127). On the forehead, there is sometimes a V-shaped lesion said in folklore to be the mark of the stork`s beak. Simple naevi do not blanch on pressure.

Course and prognosis

All simple naevi on the face disappear spontaneously in the first year. Those on the nape of the neck are usually permanent, but never require treatment.

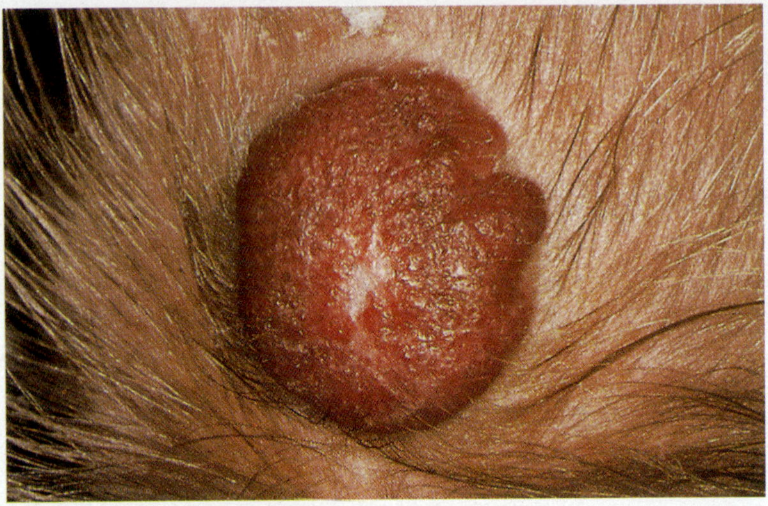

图 125 草莓样痣开始消退
Strawberry naevus beginning to regress

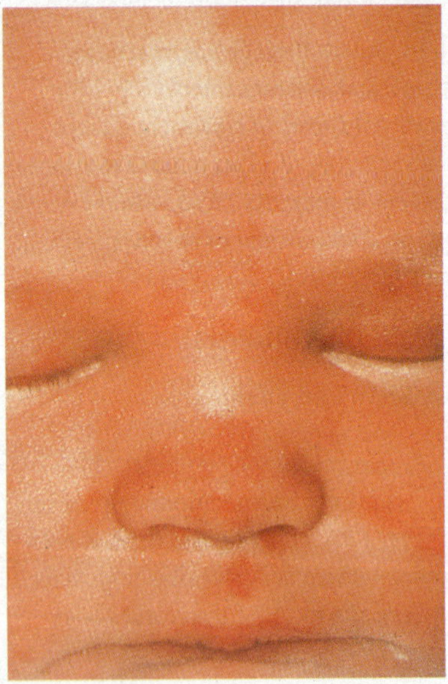

图 126 眼睑、鼻和上嘴唇的单纯痣
Simple naevus on eyelids, nose and upper lip

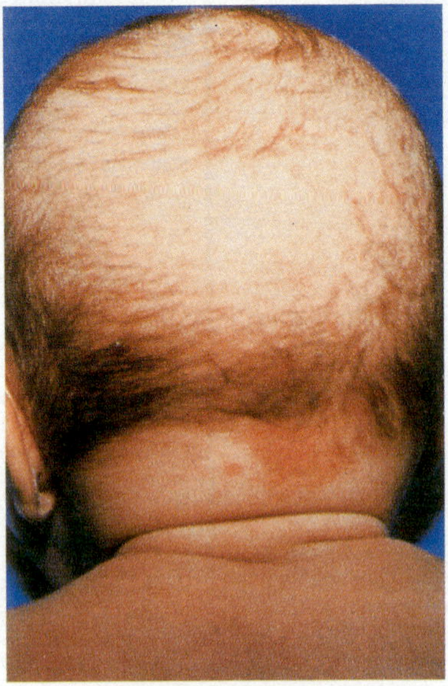

图 127 颈背部的单纯痣
Simple naevus on nape of the neck

海绵状血管瘤

临床特征 柔软的皮下兰红色团块（图 128），边缘不如草莓样痣清楚；扩大的静脉吻合性的含血腔隙，在其表面常常有毛细血管成分。

病程和预后 大多数海绵状血管瘤不会消退，其大小实际上可能会增加。有时会有出血和感染，偶尔在痣里会有血小板扣留现象从而导致血小板减少症。

治疗 外科切除通常比较困难，在局麻状态下进行硬化剂注射可以加速其纤维化。

葡萄酒色痣（鲜红斑痣）

临床特征 边界锐利、扁平的毛细血管瘤，其颜色多变，从淡粉红色到深紫色。它们在出生时即有，以后其大小不会增加。可以出现在身体任何部位（图 129），但是最常出现在脸上。

病程和预后 它们大多数是永久性的皮肤变色。

合并症 大多数葡萄酒色痣都是独立出现的，但有时会有部分皮肤呈现多孔状，累及其他脏器或形成可识别血管综合征的一部分（如斯特奇-韦伯综合征）。

治疗 外科整形并不令人满意。对于大龄儿童化妆掩饰可能有所帮助。激光治疗对于某些病人较为有用，推荐早期就诊于相关的专家。

斯特奇-韦伯综合征

遗传特性 多数为散发，偶见常染色体显性遗传。

临床特性 颜面部葡萄酒色痣（图 130），特征性地按照三叉神经区域分布，可有癫痫发作，有时会有精神发育迟缓。经常会出现同侧脑膜出血，并且会引起对侧偏瘫、脑萎缩、大脑钙化和大头畸形。

Cavernous haemangiomata

Clinical features

Soft, subcutaneous bluish-red mass (Fig. 128) with a less distinct edge than a strawberry naevus; dilated blood-filled cavities with venous anastamoses and often a surface capillary element.

Course and prognosis

The majority do not regress and may actually increase in size. Haemorrhage and infection sometimes occur, and occasionally sequestration of platelets within the naevus may cause thrombocytopenia.

Management

Surgical excision is often difficult. Injection of sclerosing agents under anaesthetic may promote fibrosis.

Port wine stains (naevus flammeus)

Clinical features

Sharply demarcated 'flat' capillary haemangiomata which may vary in colour from pale pink to deep purple. They are present at birth and do not increase in size after birth. May occur anywhere on the body (Fig. 129), but are most common on the face.

Course and prognosis

The majority remain as permanent discoloration of the skin.

Associations

Most port wine stains occur as an isolated defect but sometimes are partly cavernous, involve other organs or form part of a recognizable vascular syndrome, (e.g. Sturge-Weber syndrome).

Management

Surgery is cosmetically unsatisfactory. Cosmetic cover-up cream may be helpful in older children. Laser treatment is helpful for some and early referral to a specialist is recommended.

Sturge-Weber syndrome

Inheritance

Majority sporadic; occasionally autosomal dominant.

Clinical features

Facial port-wine stain (Fig. 130), characteristically in trigeminal distribution, seizures and sometimes mental retardation. Meningeal haemangioma often present on same side and may cause contralateral hemiplegia, cerebral atrophy, cerebral calcification and macrocephaly.

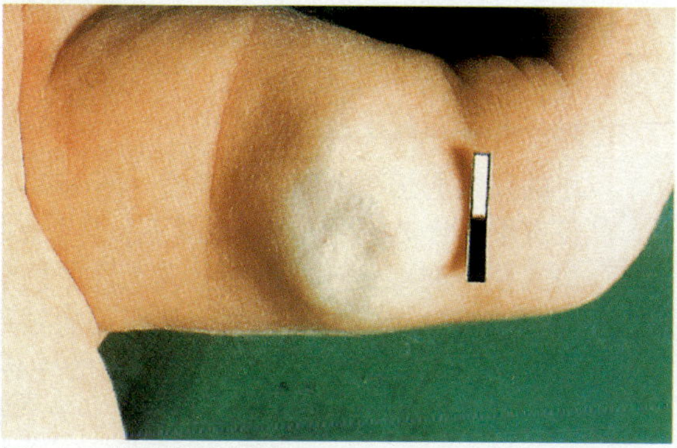

图 128 海绵状血管瘤
Cavernous haemangioma

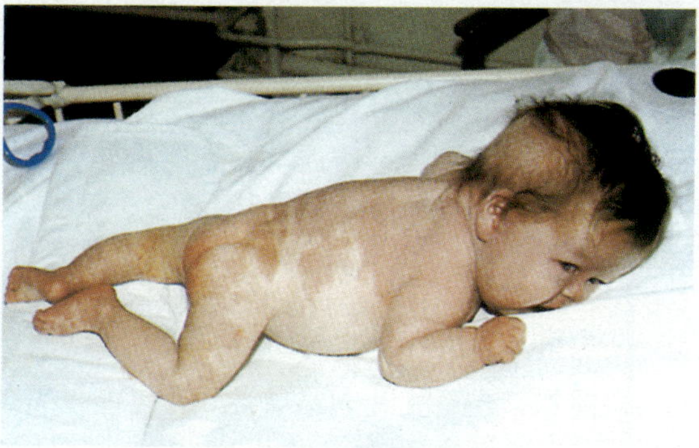

图 129 广泛的葡萄酒色痣
Extensive port wine stain

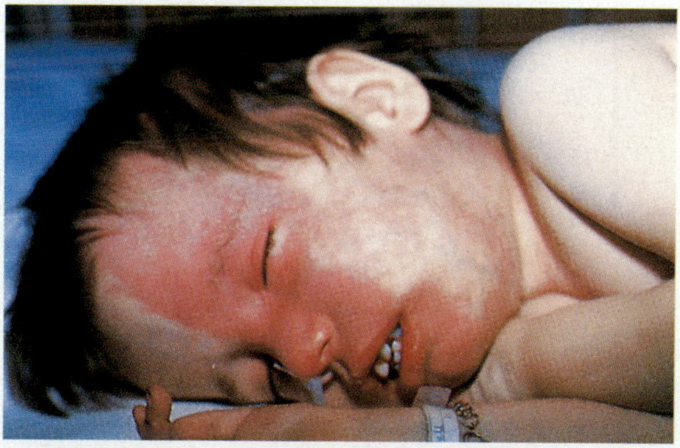

图 130 斯特奇－韦伯综合征的颜面部痣
Facial naevus of Sturge-Weber syndrome

色素痣

发病率 除了胎斑非常常见外，色素痣在新生儿期并不常见，尤其在深皮肤的婴儿中。

临床特征 小的局限的褐色或黑色色素痣（图 131），在临床上没有重要意义，通常在儿童期不会高于皮面，但是在成人期可能可触摸到。一些先天性的色素痣还含有毛囊。罕见而巨大的躯干下部痣可能导致严重的外观异常。色素失调症是一种罕见的性连锁遗传疾病，最初在新生儿期为炎性水疱，后来会发展为色素纹（图 132）。

合并症 大多数是无害的。在一些特殊综合征中可以看到多发性色素痣，如多发性神经纤维瘤。在成人，交界痣偶尔会发展成为恶性黑色素瘤，但是很少见。

治疗 主要是针对有外观异常和同时存在有相关疾病者。巨大的躯干下部痣通常会有严重外观毁损，可在生后数月通过擦皮法得到改善。

脱色素痣

发病率 不常见，可以作为单独的症状出现。

临床特征 偶尔，在新生儿期结节性硬化可能仅表现为皮肤或毛发区域色素脱失。

皮脂腺痣

临床特征 通常是位于新生儿发际或头皮处的蜡状、黄色、有凹痕但无毛发的斑块（图 133）。

病程和预后 持续存在的皮损部位有恶变可能，因此建议在青春期予以切除。

合并症 很少有，可能会合并有惊厥和神经发育问题。

Pigmented naevus

Incidence

Uncommon in neonatal period except for Mongolian blue spots which are very common, particularly in infants with dark skin.

Clinical features

Small localized brown or black pigmented naevi (Fig. 131) are of no clinical significance and are usually not elevated during childhood, but may become palpable during adult life. Some congenital pigmented naevi contain hair follicles. Severe cosmetic deformity may occur with the rare giant bathing trunk naevus. Incontinentia pigmenti, a rare sex-linked hereditary disorder, initially consists of inflammatory bullae in the neonatal period which progress to pigmented streaks (Fig. 132).

Associations

Majority are harmless. Multiple pigmented naevi are seen in certain syndromes such as neurofibromatosis. Junctional naevi occasionally develop into malignant melanoma in adults, but this is rare.

Management

Depends on the cosmetic deformity and co-existence of associated disorders. Giant bathing trunk naevi are often grossly disfiguring and may be improved by dermabrasion in the first few months.

Depigmented naevus

Incidence

Uncommon and may occur as an isolated finding.

Clinical features

Occasionally, areas of skin or hair depigmentation may be the only manifestation of tuberous sclerosis in the neonatal period.

Sebaceous naevus

Clinical features

Waxy, yellow, pitted but hairless plaque usually found around the hairline or scalp (Fig. 133) in newborn infants.

Course and prognosis

Malignant transformation may occur in lesions which persist, hence excision is advised in adolescence.

Associations

Rarely, may be associated with convulsions and neurodevelopmental problems.

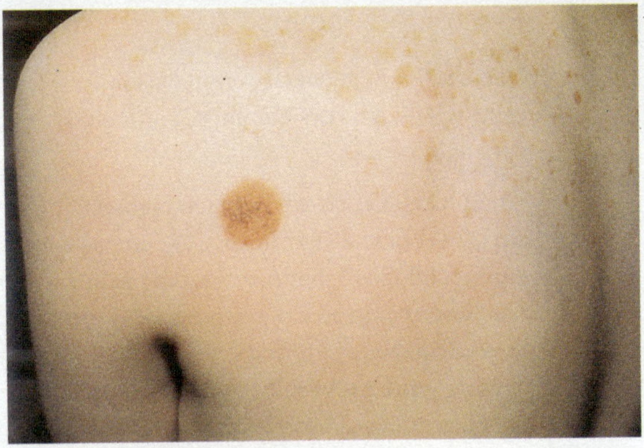

图 131 多发性色素痣
Multiple pigmented naevi

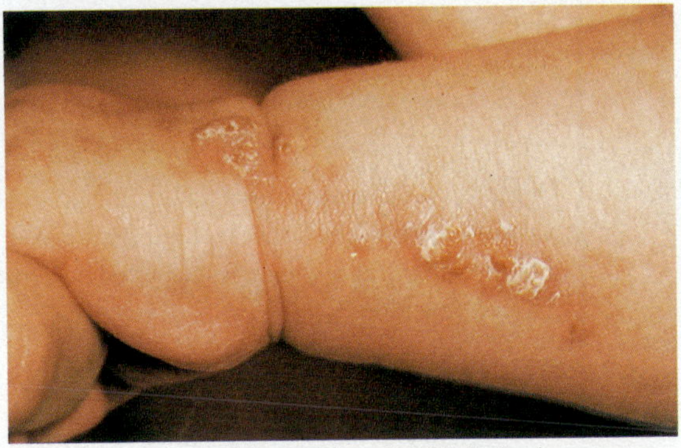

图 132 色素失调症的皮损呈线性分布
Lesions of incontinentia pigmenti in a linear distribution

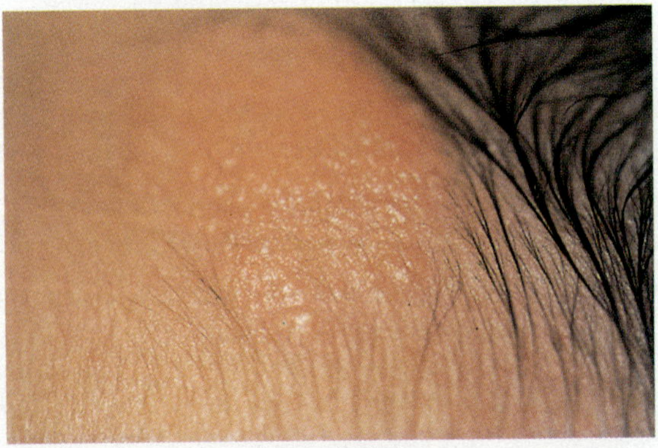

图 133 在发际附近的皮脂腺痣
Sebaceous naevus near the hairline

局限性脱发（斑秃）

发病率 不常见，全秃就更为罕见。在唐氏综合征中发病率则较高。

病因学 未知，有时会在精神紧张和压力较大时出现。

临床特征 局限性脱发常常会引起局限性头皮毛发脱落（图134）。它具有特征性明显的毛干边界，没有红斑和皮屑，因此可以与头癣相鉴别。

病程和预后 通常具有自限性；但是偶尔会发展为全秃，导致全身毛发脱落。没有有效治疗方法。

部分皮肤层缺失

发病率 罕见。

病因学 未知。

临床特征 通常是一种浅表的溃疡性损伤，多出现于头皮（图135）。头皮的部分皮肤层缺失有时发生于13三体综合征（帕塔综合征），但大多数是作为一种单独的先天性异常而出现。小面积头皮缺失有时被错误的归因于产科损伤（如胎儿头皮血采样和头皮电极）。产科操作通常只会引起较小的皮肤损伤（图136），只要小心的取下头皮夹，它会自行愈合，而没有瘢痕形成和脱发。

病程和预后 缺失是通过肉芽形成而愈合的。如果皮损不是浅表的，或如果发生继发性感染，愈合后可能会有瘢痕形成和收缩。可能会在头皮上留下永久性的脱发区域。

Alopecia areata

Incidence

Uncommon; alopecia areata totalis is very rare. There is an increased incidence in Down syndrome.

Aetiology

Unknown; sometimes occurs during periods of stress.

Clinical features

Alopecia areata commonly causes localized hair loss on the scalp (Fig. 134). It can usually be distinguished from tinea capitis by the characteristic margin of exclamation mark hair shafts, and the absence of erythema and scaling.

Course and prognosis

Usually self-limiting; but occasionally may progress to alopecia totalis which results in total body hair loss. No effective treatment.

Partial thickness skin defects

Incidence

Rare.

Aetiology

Unknown.

Clinical features

The lesion is usually a superficial area of ulceration, most commonly found on the scalp (Fig. 135). Partial thickness skin defects of the scalp sometimes occur in trisomy 13 (Patau syndrome), but most occur as an isolated congenital anomaly. Small scalp defects are sometimes mistakenly attributed to obstetric trauma (e.g. fetal scalp sampling or scalp electrodes). Obstetric manipulations usually only cause minor skin trauma (Fig. 136) which heal without scarring or hair loss providing care is taken when removing scalp clips.

Course and prognosis

The defect heals by granulation. If it is not superficial, or if secondary infection occurs, healing may result in scar formation and contraction. A permanent bald patch may be left on the scalp.

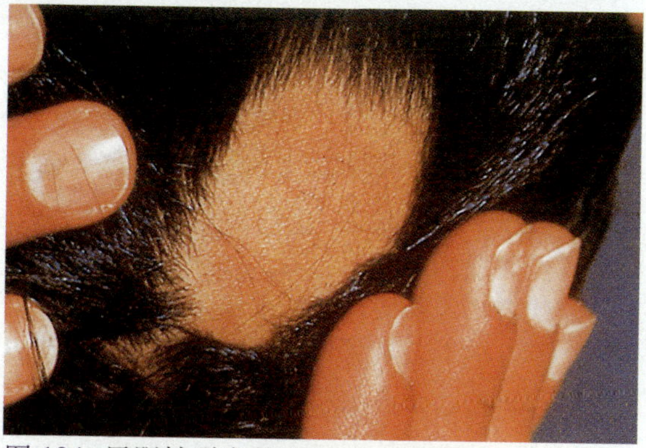

图 134 局限性脱发的头皮毛发脱落
Scalp hair loss in alopecia areata

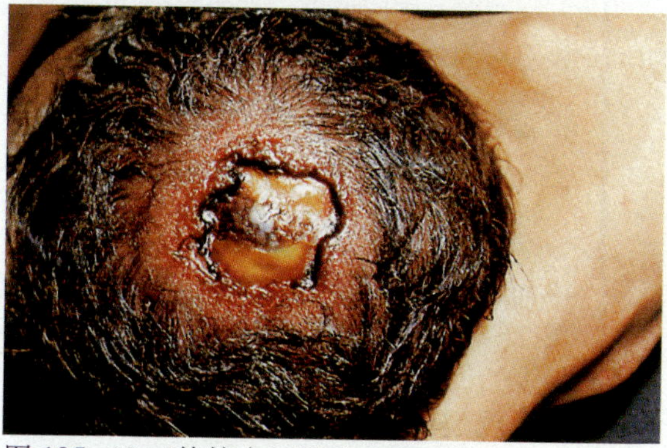

图 135 13 三体综合征的头皮皮肤缺失
Scalp skin defect in trisomy 13

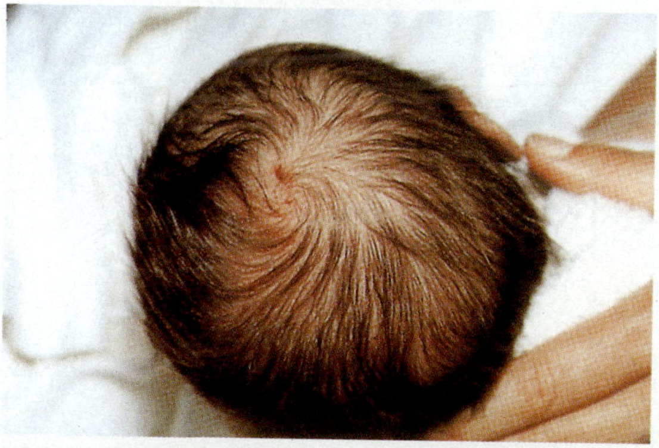

图 136 用于胎心监护的头皮夹所造成的损伤
Wound from a scalp clip used for fetal heart monitoring

尿布疹

病因学

通常是由于长时间的使用潮湿尿布刺激皮肤而造成，有时被称为"氨皮炎"。在尿布覆盖区域其他主要皮疹是念珠菌感染和脂溢性皮炎的皮疹。

临床特征

红斑，脐部脓疱，会阴和生殖器溃疡，但是通常不累及腹股沟区（图137)。如果呈现散发的卫星样皮损，或者累及腹股沟区，则提示有念珠菌感染（图138)。婴儿的粪便较稀薄，经常会有肛周红斑。

治疗

应该经常更换尿布。对于单纯尿布疹，应该暴露会阴部，并涂抹防护性软膏。念珠菌感染则应在局部涂抹制霉菌素或咪康唑软膏。如果用简单的治疗不能使皮疹消退，则应考虑念珠菌感染。脂溢性皮炎通常需要使用温和的类固醇软膏。

脂溢性皮炎

病因学

在小婴儿中很常见；病因未知。

临床特征

特殊的脂样渗出，鳞状皮屑，红斑样皮疹或斑块，通常会在出生后前几个月出现。眉毛（图 139)、耳后皮肤以及会阴都是好发部位。常会在头皮上发现较稠厚的油脂样皮屑，一般称之为"乳痂"。偶尔从尿布疹周围会有盘状皮损向上蔓延到躯干部位（尿布牛皮癣)。在较轻的类型中，脂溢性皮炎可能被误诊为特应性湿疹，特别是当皮疹影响到了肢体屈曲部位。不会引起全身性疾病，即使存在大面积的脂溢性皮炎（莱纳综合征炎)。但有时会有继发性感染。

治疗

温和的皮质类固醇软膏，如1%的氢化可的松。乳痂通常用角质溶解洗剂或软膏，但是经常会复发。

Napkin or diaper rash

Aetiology

Usually due to irritation from prolonged wearing of wet napkins; sometimes called 'ammonical dermatitis'. Monilial infection and seborrhoeic dermatitis are the other main rashes in the napkin area.

Clinical features

Erythema, umbilicated pustules, and ulceration of the perineum and sometimes the genitalia, but usually sparing the groin flexures (Fig. 137). The presence of discrete satellite lesions or involvement of the flexures is suggestive of monilial infection (Fig. 138). In babies with loose stools, there is often perianal erythema.

Management

Napkins should be changed frequently. In simple napkin rash, exposure of the perineum and a protective barrier cream is all that is required. Monilial infection responds to topical nystatin or miconazole cream. Monilia should always be considered when a rash does not respond to simple treatment. Seborrhoeic dermatitis often requires the application of a weak steroid cream.

Seborrhoeic dermatitis

Aetiology

Very common in young infants; aetiology unknown.

Clinical features

Distinctive greasy, scaly, erythematous rash or plaques, which usually appear within the first few months of life. The eyebrows (Fig. 139), skin behind the ears, and perineum are commonly affected. Thick greasy scales are often found on the scalp where the condition is commonly called 'cradle cap'. Occasionally, there may be discoid lesions on the trunk spreading up from a napkin rash (napkin psoriasis). In mild forms, seborrhoeic dermatitis may be mistakenly diagnosed as atopic eczema, particularly when the rash affects the flexures. There is never any systemic illness, even with widespread seborrhoeic dermatitis (Leiner syndrome), but secondary infection sometimes occurs.

Management

Mild corticosteroid cream such as 1% hydrocortisone. Cradle cap usually responds to a keratolytic shampoo or cream, but often recurs.

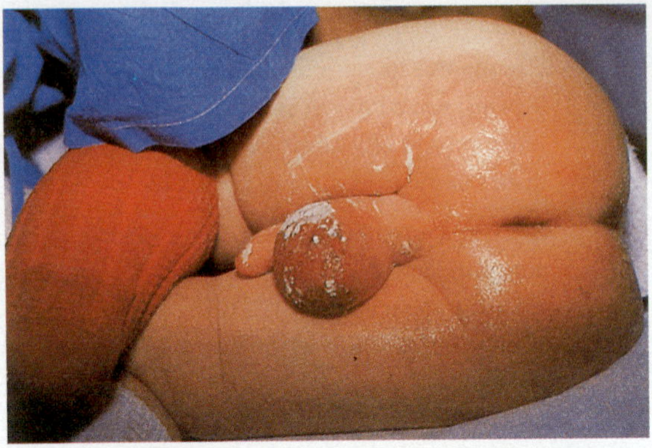

图 137 单纯尿布疹
Simple napkin rash

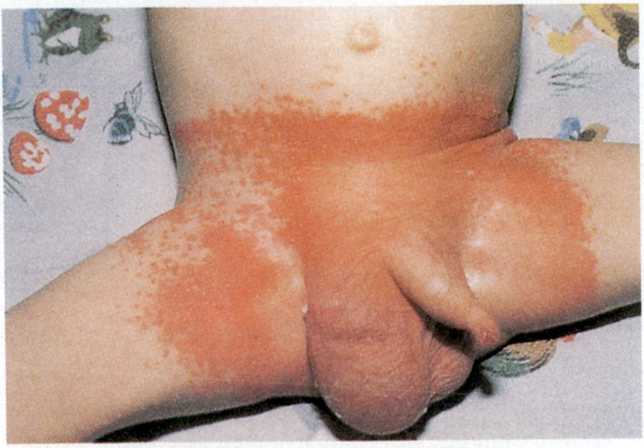

图 138 念珠菌感染散发的卫星样皮损
Monilial infection with discrete satellite lesions

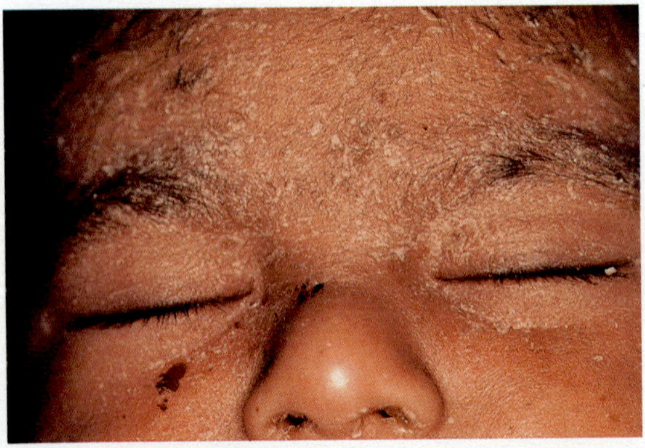

图 139 脂溢性皮炎
Seborrhoeic dermatitis

大疱性表皮松解症

发病率和遗传特性 很罕见，一般是常染色体隐性遗传。

病理学 是位于表皮的基底膜和真皮的结缔组织之间的表皮下大水疱。

临床特征 大水泡，常常是由小的损伤引起，在出生时或出生后不久既有，累及广泛（图 140）。在新生儿类型中死亡率较高。在婴儿期起病的通常是常染色体显性遗传，常有营养不良，而且会导致瘢痕形成。

鉴别诊断 大疱性表皮松解症的外表可能与广泛的葡萄球菌性皮肤感染相类似（新生儿天疱疮或毒性表皮坏死溶解）。

治疗 需要好的护理，尤其强调要尽量减少操作，因为皮肤上的小损伤会对病情有显著的影响。如果有继发性细菌感染，需要用抗生素。

产前诊断 如果有以前曾患此病的前一胎婴儿的DNA，就可能进行产前诊断。

火棉胶婴儿和先天性鱼鳞癣胎儿（斑色胎）

发病率 很罕见，病因不明。

临床特征 出生时，新生儿被包围在一个有光泽的、黄褐色的、玻璃纸样的膜内，可能有面部特征和四肢的扭曲(图141)。由于胸廓的伸展受到限制会出现呼吸窘迫。先天性鱼鳞癣胎儿是一种比较严重的通常可致命的疾病，有相似的皮肤外观，但是在鳞片状皮肤之间有深的裂隙，有时有睑外翻和嘴唇外翻(鱼口状)。

病程和预后 出生后出现皮肤膜样脱落。除了用大量的软膏来起到润滑作用（图142）外，没有特殊的治疗方法。继发感染应该及时治疗。大多数火棉胶婴儿在以后的儿童期有正常的皮肤，少数会在以后发展成为鱼鳞癣样皮肤。

Epidermolysis bullosa

Incidence and inheritance
Very rare; usually autosomal recessive.

Pathology
Subepidermal bullae with blisters between basement membrane of epidermis and connective tissue of dermis.

Clinical features
Bullae, often resulting from minor trauma, occur at or soon after birth and cover large areas of the body (Fig. 140). High mortality in the neonatal form. Later onset in infancy, is usually autosomal dominant and often dystrophic, resulting in scar formation.

Differential diagnosis
Epidermolysis bullosa may be similar in appearance to widespread staphylococcal skin infection (pemphigus neonatorum or toxic epidermal necrolysis).

Management
Good nursing care is required, with particular emphasis on minimal handling because of the dramatic effect of minor trauma on the skin. Antibiotics may be required if there is secondary bacterial infection.

Antenatal diagnosis
Possible when there is DNA from a previously affected infant.

Collodion baby and harlequin fetus

Incidence
Very rare; unknown aetiology.

Clinical features
At birth, the infant is encased in a shiny, brownish-yellow, cellophane-like membrane which may distort facial features and extremities (Fig. 141). Respiratory embarrassment may occur because of restriction of chest expansion. Harlequin fetus is a more serious condition which is usually fatal, with a similar appearance of the skin, but also deep fissures between scale-like areas of skin, and sometimes ectropion and everted lips (fish-mouth).

Course and prognosis
Desquamation of the membranous skin occurs after birth. No particular treatment apart from copious lubrication of skin with creams (Fig. 142). Secondary infection should be treated promptly. Most collodion babies have normal skin in later childhood, a few develop ichthyotic skin changes later.

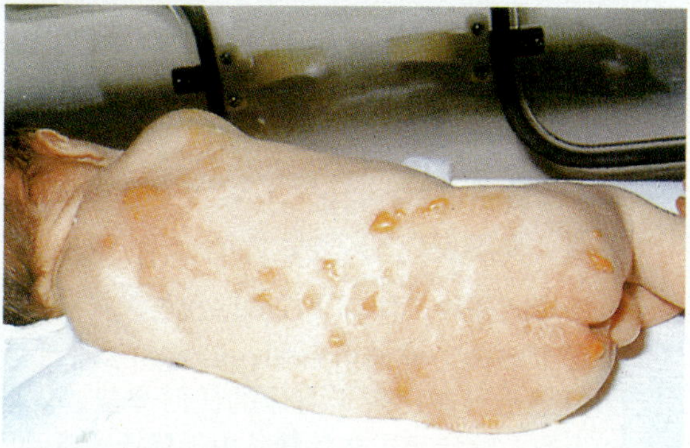

图 140　广泛的大水疱
Widespread bullae

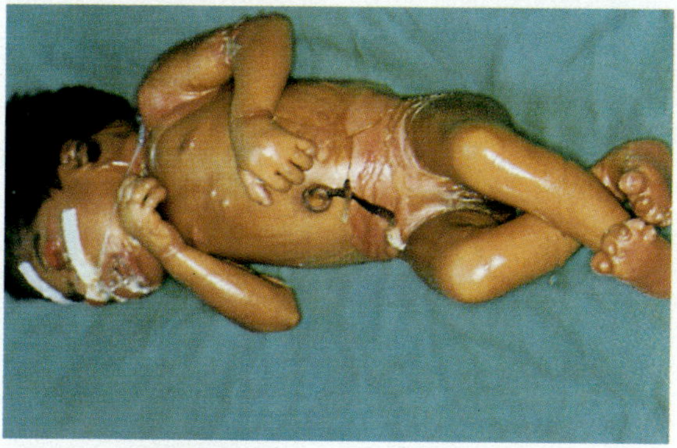

图 141　火棉胶婴儿
Collodion baby

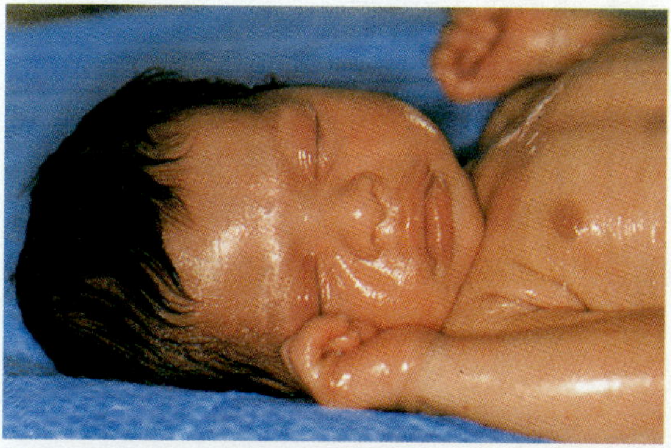

图 142　生后20天情况有所好转，注意油亮的皮肤。
Improvement is seen after 20 days. Note the oiled skin

湿疹

发病率 常见，儿童的发病率有3%。通常在出生后的前几年中出现。

遗传特性 常有其他遗传性过敏性疾病的家族史（如哮喘、枯草热、变态反应）。

临床特征 瘙痒的斑块，伴有表皮脱落和苔癣样变，特征性地出现于面部、膝关节背面、肘窝和手腕部（图 143），但是也可能出现于身体的任何部位。皮肤经常性地干燥，瘙痒是主要症状。由于搔抓通常会引起继发性的感染。

检查 嗜酸粒细胞增多、血清IgE增高或者皮试阳性常常对遗传性过敏症的一般诊断有帮助。但是在临床治疗中帮助不大，因为本病通常涉及多种因素。

治疗 避免使用肥皂，可以用润滑油或乳化软膏来替代。对于干燥的皮肤可以大量使用亲水乳膏。在病情急性加剧期间可以对严重的斑块少量使用温和的皮质甾类乳膏全身性抗组织胺类药对于控制瘙痒和搔抓，尤其在入睡时，常常有用。如果有明确的因食用某种食物而引起病情恶化的病史，那么避免食用该种食物会有所帮助。

病程和预后 病情易反复，到儿童后期常会有所改善。

银屑病（牛皮癣）

发病率 在儿童期不常见；通常发生于有很强家族史的群体中。病因不明。

临床特征 有鳞状皮屑的红色斑块样皮损（图 144），尤其出现于在肘部、膝部、发际周围和头皮（图 145）。

治疗和病程 银屑病通常有终生患病的趋势。治疗取决于皮损的严重程度。皮质类固醇、煤焦油和水杨酸软膏是治疗的一线药物。

Eczema

Incidence

Common; affects 3% of children. Onset usually within first few years of life.

Inheritance

Often family history of other atopic disorders (e.g. asthma, hay-fever, allergy).

Clinical features

Itchy plaques with excoriation and lichenification, characteristically occurring on the face, behind the knees, antecubital fossae and wrists (Fig. 143), but can occur anywhere. The skin is often dry, and itching is a prominent symptom. Secondary infection is common because of scratching.

Investigation

Eosinophilia, raised serum IgE or positive skin tests are sometimes helpful in the general diagnosis of atopy, but are rarely useful in clinical management, as multiple factors are usually involved.

Management

Soap should be avoided, and emollient oil or emulsifying ointment used instead. Aqueous cream can be used liberally on the dry skin. Weak corticosteroid cream may be applied sparingly to bad patches during acute flare-ups. Systemic antihistamines are sometimes useful to control itching and scratching, which occur particularly during sleep. When there is a clear history of aggravation by certain foods, an exclusion diet may help.

Course and prognosis

Fluctuating course; usually improves in later childhood.

Psoriasis

Incidence

Uncommon in childhood; when it occurs there is usually a strong family history. Aetiology unknown.

Clinical features

Erythematous, scaly lesions which form plaques (Fig. 144), typically on the elbows, knees, around the hairline and scalp (Fig. 145).

Management and course

The tendency to psoriasis is usually life-long. Treatment depends on severity of the lesions. Corticosteroids, coal-tar and salicylic acid ointments are the mainstay of treatment.

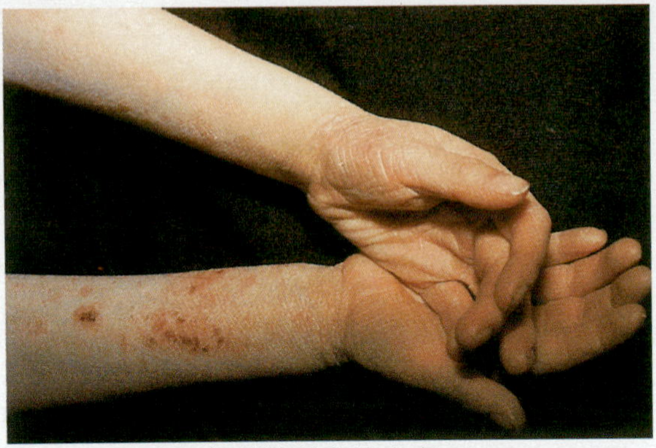

图 143 手臂上典型的湿疹性皮疹
Typical eczematous rash on arms

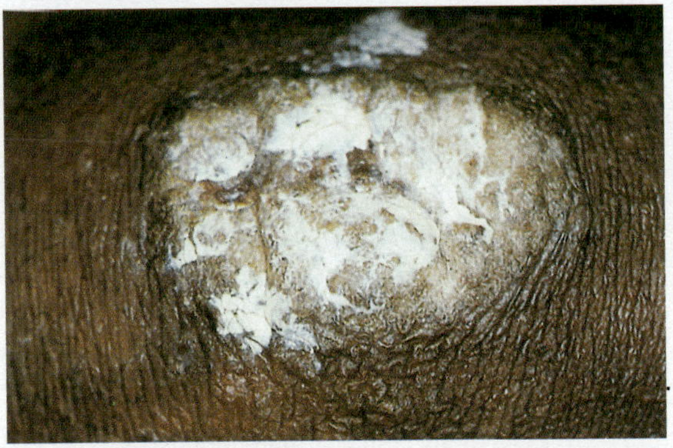

图 144 严重的银屑病
Severe psoriasis

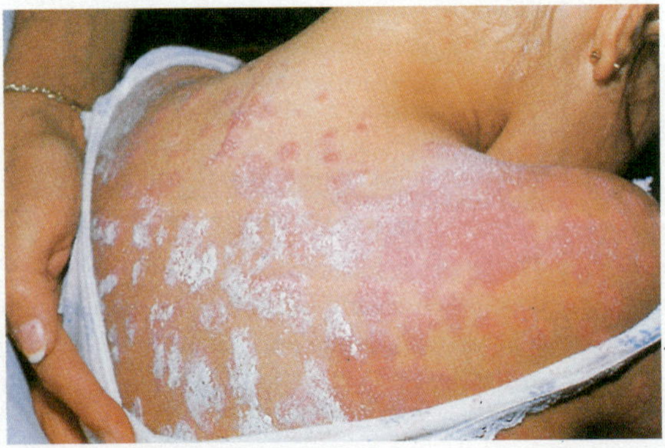

图 145 银屑病多发的斑块
Multiple plaques of psoriasis

荨麻疹

病因学

常常是过敏的表现，但是过敏原一般无法确定。有一些反复发作的病例是由于对食物中的着色剂过敏而引起。

临床特征

有强烈的瘙痒和风团样红斑疹。皮疹的形式会经常变化，并且当风团消退后会留下瘀青。通常有明显的水肿，尤其在眼睛和口唇周围，被称作“血管神经性水肿”(图 146)。

治疗

口唇和舌严重的水肿会导致威胁生命的急性呼吸道阻塞，此时应该皮下注射肾上腺素。全身性抗组织胺类药对于荨麻疹也有效。避免食用会引起过敏的食物对于反复发作的荨麻疹有所帮助。一些慢性或反复发作的病例是由于家族性乙酰胆碱酯酶缺乏。

多形性红斑和斯-约综合征

病因学

通常是对药物（如青霉素或磺胺类药物）的特异质反应。

临床特征

多形性红斑显示为分布广泛的靶形皮损（图 147）。斯-约综合征是一种更严重的疾病，它最初是一种大疱疹，然后迅速进展为广泛的皮肤脱落（图 148）。它常常会累及口唇、肛门、阴道黏膜或结膜。

治疗

停止刺激性药物。隔离护理、严格补液、保持电解质平衡和预防感染很重要。斯-约综合征的死亡率很高，尤其是当出现败血症时。

Urticaria

Aetiology

Common allergic manifestation, but the offending allergen is often not identified. Some recurrent cases are caused by sensitivity to food colouring agents.

Clinical features

Intensely itchy, erythematous rash with wheals. The pattern of the rash is constantly changing and may leave areas of bruising when the wheals subside. There is often marked oedema, particularly around the eyes and mouth, where it is called 'angioneurotic oedema' (Fig. 146).

Management

Acute respiratory obstruction caused by severe swelling of the mouth and tongue may be life-threatening; it responds to subcutaneous adrenaline. Systemic antihistamines may be helpful in urticaria. Food exclusion diets may help some children with recurrent urticaria. Some cases of chronic or recurrent urticaria are due to familial acetylcholinesterase deficiency.

Erythema multiforme and Stevens-Johnson syndrome

Aetiology

Idiosyncratic reactions, often to drugs (e.g. penicillin or sulphonamides).

Clinical features

Erythema multiforme shows widespread target lesions (Fig. 147). Stevens-Johnson is a more severe illness; it begins as a bullous eruption which rapidly progresses to widespread skin loss (Fig. 148). There is always involvement of the mucous membranes of the mouth, rectum, vagina or conjunctiva.

Management

Discontinue the offending drug. Barrier nursing, strict fluid and electrolyte balance and prevention of infection are important. In severe Stevens-Johnson syndrome mortality is high, particularly if septicaemia occurs.

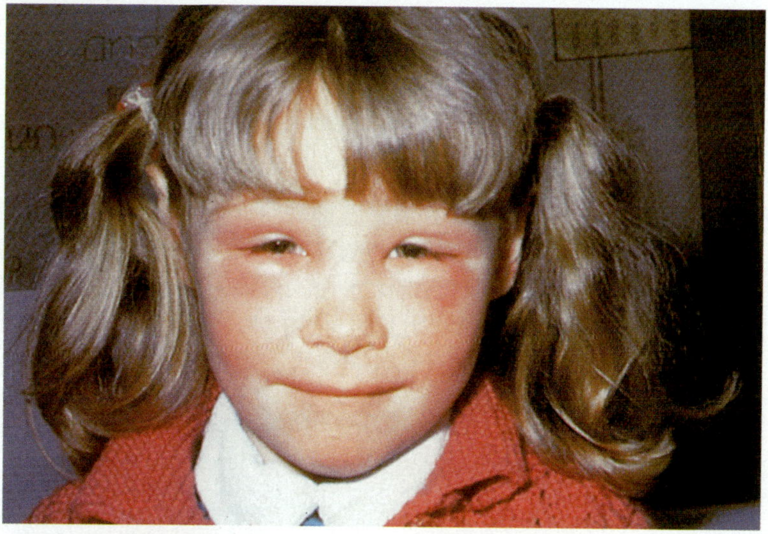

图 146 血管神经性水肿
Angioneurotic oedema

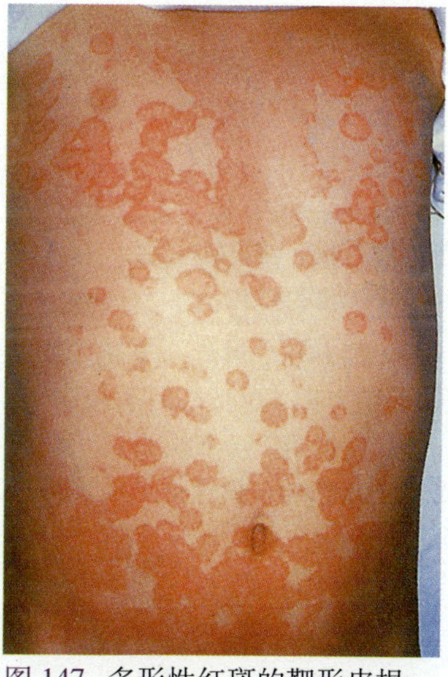

图 147 多形性红斑的靶形皮损
Target lesions of erythema multiforme

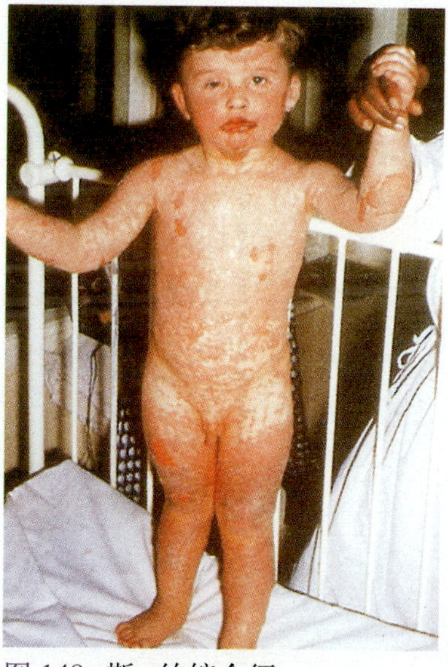

图 148 斯-约综合征
Stevens-Johnson syndrome

亨-舍紫癜综合征（过敏性紫癜）

发病率 常见，通常有一定的流行性。

病因学 不明原因的弥漫性血管炎，此前通常有上呼吸道的病毒感染史。

临床特征 特殊表征是臀部、腿部伸肌表面（图 149、150 和 151）、手臂、有时是脸部的紫癜样皮疹。皮损通常是丘疹，有时会有大水疱。典型的皮疹通常会伴有脸部、手、脚和阴囊的局部水肿，并且一般会有累及外周大关节的迁移性关节炎。腹部绞痛是很麻烦的症状。在少数病例中会发生咯血、黑粪或肠套叠。将近 70% 的病例会有血尿，但是进行性肾病的发生率 <1%。

治疗 应该排除紫癜的其他原因。治疗是针对症状的。如果有严重的胃肠道症状或进行性肾脏疾病，可以应用皮质类固醇。

病程和预后 大多数病例都恢复迅速，虽然今后几周常会偶有发作或复发。如果有急性肾炎或肾病综合征，那么预后较差。

结节性红斑

发病率 常见，尤其是在黑人孩子中。

病因学 通常与链球菌感染、结核病、结节病、支原体感染、药物过敏（尤其对磺胺类药物）或肠炎有关。在大多数病例中，并没有潜在的疾病。

临床特征 大多数在胫骨前区域会出现剧烈的触痛、隆起、红斑性结节（图152），但也可以出现在肘部周围和前臂。皮疹经常会在数周，偶尔在数月内分批出现；可能会伴随有发热和关节痛，尤其当结节累及关节时。皮损愈合后会留下瘀青痕迹。

Henoch-Schönlein purpura (anaphylactoid purpura)

Incidence
Common; often occurs in small epidemics.

Aetiology
Diffuse vasculitis of unknown aetiology; there is often a history of a recent viral upper respiratory tract infection.

Clinical features
Pathognomonic feature is a purpuric rash on buttocks, extensor surfaces of legs (Figs 149, 150 and 151), arms, and sometimes face. Lesions are often papular and bullae sometimes occur. Localized oedema of face, hands, feet and scrotum often accompany the typical rash, and flitting arthritis affecting peripheral joints is common. Colicky abdominal pain is a troublesome symptom. Haematemesis, melaena or intussusception occur in a minority of cases. Haematuria occurs in approximately 70% but progressive renal disease occurs <1%.

Management
Other causes of purpura should always be excluded. Treatment is symptomatic. Corticosteroids may be indicated if there are severe gastrointestinal symptoms or progressive renal involvement.

Course and prognosis
Majority resolve rapidly, although further episodes or recurrences are common in the first few weeks. Prognosis is more serious if acute nephritis or nephrotic syndrome occurs.

Erythema nodosum

Incidence
Common, particularly in black children.

Aetiology
May be associated with streptococcal infection, tuberculosis, sarcoidosis, mycoplasma infection, drug sensitivity (particularly to sulphonamides), or inflammatory bowel disease. In the majority of cases, no underlying condition will be found.

Clinical features
Exquisitely tender, raised, erythematous nodules most frequently occurring over the pretibial region (Fig. 152), but may also occur around the elbows and on the forearms. Often occur in crops over several weeks or occasionally months; may be associated with fever and arthralgia, particularly when nodules occur over joints. Skin lesions resolve with the same colour changes as a bruise.

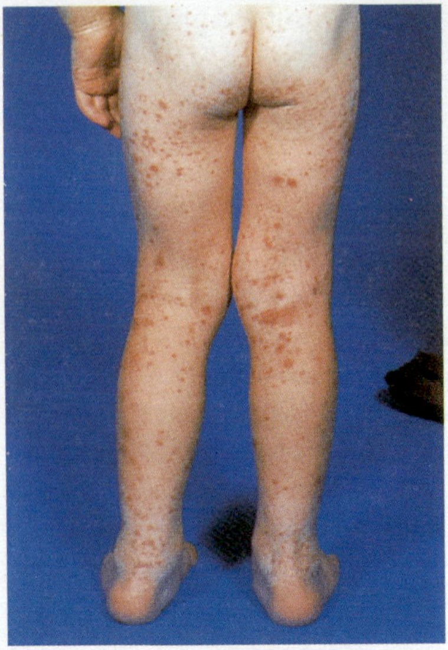

图 149 亨-舍紫癜综合征的典型分布
Classic distribution of Henoch-Schönlein purpura

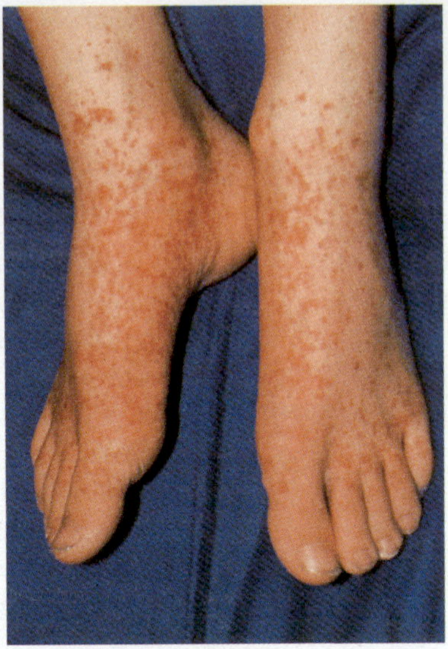

图 150 脚上的紫癜
Purpura on feet

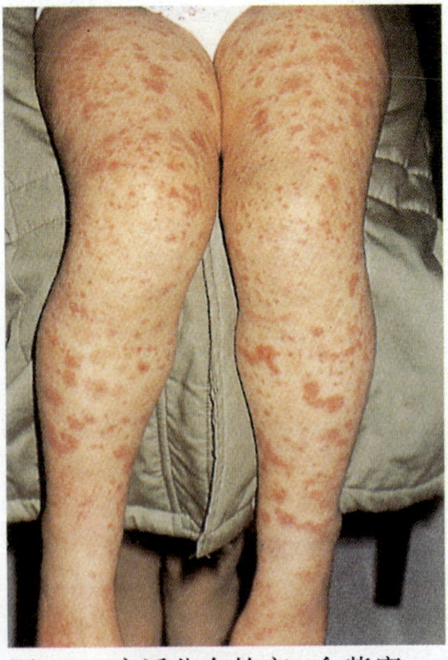

图 151 广泛分布的亨-舍紫癜
Widespread Henoch-Schönlein purpura

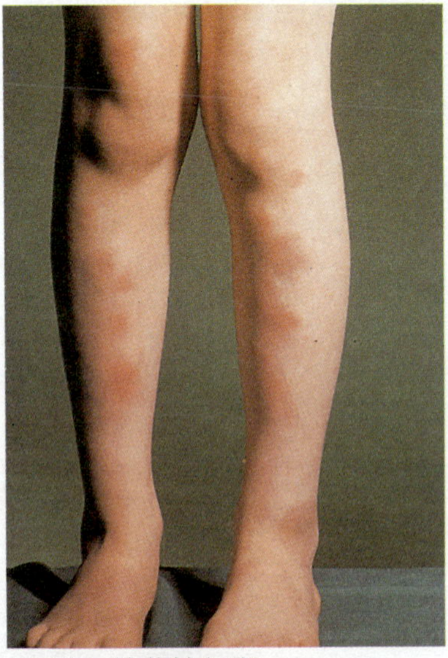

图 152 结节性红斑
Erythema nodosum

川崎病

发病率 在日本最常见，但是在世界范围内都有报道。

临床特征 持续很长时间的发热，伴有短暂的红斑疹、舌痛、唇皲裂和淋巴结病。在热退后的第二周会有典型的手和脚的脱皮（图 153）。

治疗 在少数婴儿中会出现伴有血小板增多的冠状动脉瘤。水杨酸盐和静脉应用丙种球蛋白可以预防这个严重的并发症。

真菌感染

疥螨病（疥疮）

剧烈的瘙痒，脱皮，红色斑丘疹（图 154），有时有肉眼可见的小洞。疥疮可发生于身体的任何部位，但常见于手指之间和手腕周围。它会在密切接触的人群中传播，所以全家都应进行局部林旦治疗。衣服和床单都应该彻底的清洗，这样可以避免复发。

癣

可引起圆形红斑，中央有鳞屑。当癣累及头皮时，可能会有脱发，留下圆形的脱发斑。体癣通常主要应用局部抗真菌药物进行治疗，如咪康唑。当广泛累及毛发和指甲时，全身应用灰黄霉素是有必要的。

念珠菌感染（鹅口疮）

口腔的真菌性感染（图 155），通常出现于小婴儿。念珠菌感染也会引起特征性的尿布疹，形成卫星样溃疡性红斑皮损。在儿童晚期，当应用皮质类固醇激素或患有免疫缺陷综合征时可能会发生鹅口疮。

Kawasaki disease

Incidence

Most common in Japan, but reported worldwide.

Clinical features

Prolonged febrile illness with fleeting erythematous rash, sore tongue, cracked lips and lymphadenopathy. During the second week after the fever has subsided, there is typical peeling of the hands and feet (Fig. 153).

Management

Coronary artery aneurysms associated with thrombocytosis occur in a minority of infants. Salicylates and intravenous gamma globulin prevent this serious complication.

Fungal infections and infestations

Scabies

Intensely itchy, excoriated, erythematous papular rash (Fig. 154), sometimes with burrows visible to the naked eye. Scabies may occur anywhere on the body, but is most common between the fingers and around the wrists. It is spread by close human contact, so the whole family should be treated with topical lindane. Clothes and bed-linen should be thoroughly washed if recurrence is to be avoided.

Tinea (ringworm)

Causes circular erythematous patches with a scaly centre. When tinea affects the scalp, there may be hair loss with circular patches of baldness. Tinea corporis usually responds to topical antifungals such as miconazole. Systemic griseofulvin may be necessary when there is extensive hair or nail involvement.

Monilia

Oral thrush (Fig. 155) is common in young infants. Candida also gives rise to a characteristic napkin rash with erythematous ulcerated satellite lesions. In later childhood, oral thrush may occur when the child is taking corticosteroids or when there is an immunodeficiency syndrome.

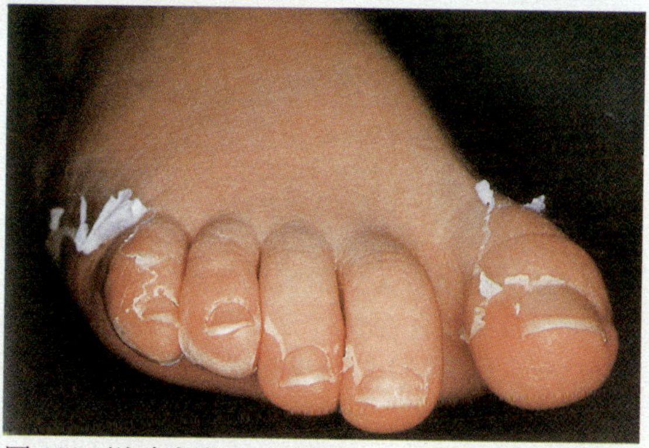

图 153 川崎病脚趾的脱皮
Peeling toes in Kawasaki disease (courtesy of Dr R. Briggs)

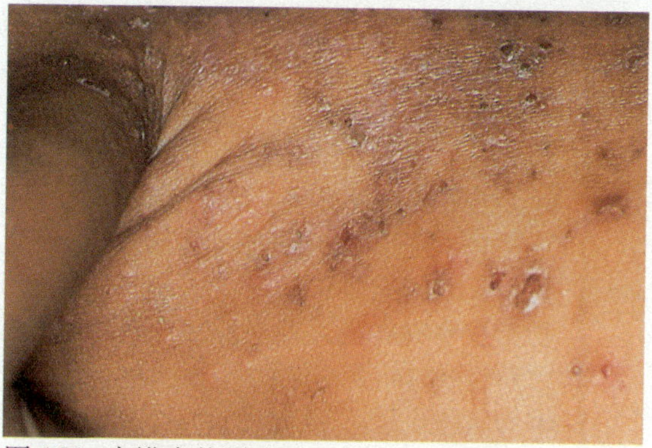

图 154 疥螨病伴脱皮
Scabies infestation with excoriation

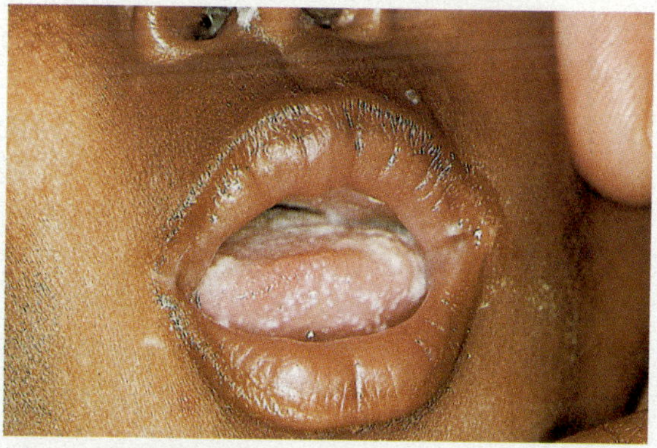

图 155 轻度鹅口疮
Mild oral thrush

医源性皮肤损害

发病率

医源性皮肤损害与新生儿重症监护有关，随着低出生体重儿的存活率不断提高，医源性皮肤损害变得越来越常见。

临床特征

皮肤擦伤与使用胶带（图 156）、新生儿姓名带或浆硬的床单有关。辐射加热器会增加低出生体重儿通过皮肤的不显性水分丢失，而使柔嫩的皮肤变得干燥。O_2和CO_2的经皮皮肤监测器会留下暂时、浅表、粉色的灼伤，而通常不会引起瘢痕形成，除非电极被长时间地遗留在原位，但是在深肤色婴儿的皮肤表面经常可看到留有脱色圆形区域。外周动脉穿刺和反复的足后跟穿刺采血都可能留下瘢痕。用肋间导管进行气胸引流应该小心定位，为了防止损伤乳房，要避开乳头周围区域（图 157）。在大血管中的导管偶尔会引起阻塞、四肢末端的缺血性坏死、血栓形成或栓塞。在插入脐动脉导管后有时可以看到暂时性的下肢发绀，但是如果它没有很快缓解，或者如果伴随有苍白或动脉搏动消失，应该立即取出导管。长时间的导管插入会增加感染和坏死性小肠结肠炎发生的危险。外周静脉输液部位可能会出现水肿和输液的外渗。输液中若含有刺激性成分，如钙或钠的碳酸氢盐，可能会引起严重的组织坏死，导致溃疡和今后的瘢痕形成。

治疗和预防

尽可能的避免过度使用胶带。保护性的遮盖可以限制生后通过皮肤蒸发所引起的不显性水分丢失。在生后数天内，婴儿的皮肤变得较厚而不易受到外伤，即使是未成熟儿。应该小心选择外周静脉输液位点，避免关节附近的静脉，以防止今后因瘢痕挛缩而影响关节功能（图 158）。如果有持续性的四肢末端发绀，或有导管阻塞征象，或四肢、肾、肠道的循环受损，就应该经常更换中心动、静脉导管。一旦患儿临床情况改善，并且血气分析采血操作需求减少，就应该马上拔除动脉导管。

Iatrogenic skin lesions

Incidence

Iatrogenic skin lesions associated with neonatal intensive care are becoming more common with increasing survival of low birth weight infants.

Clinical features

Abrasions are often associated with the use of adhesive tape (Fig. 156), name bands or starched sheets. Radiant heaters increase insensitive water loss through the skin of low birth weight infants and may cause drying of fragile skin. Transcutaneous skin monitors for monitoring O_2 and CO_2 leave a transient, superficial, pink burn which does not usually cause scarring unless the electrode has been left in situ for a prolonged period, but depigmented circular areas are often seen later in dark-skinned infants. Peripheral artery puncture and repeated heel pricking may leave scars. Intercostal catheters for draining pneumothoraces should be sited carefully, avoiding the area around the nipple in order to prevent damage to the breast (Fig. 157). Catheters in major vessels may occasionally cause obstruction and ischaemic necrosis of distal extremities, thrombosis or embolism. Transient cyanosis of the leg is sometimes seen after insertion of an umbilical arterial catheter, but if it does not resolve rapidly or if there is associated pallor or absence of arterial pulses, the catheter should be removed immediately. With prolonged catheterization, the risk of infection and necrotizing enterocolitis increases. Peripheral intravenous infusion sites may be associated with oedema or extravasation of infusion fluid. Infusions containing irritants such as calcium or sodium bicarbonate may cause serious tissue necrosis and lead to ulceration and later scar formation.

Management and prevention

Avoid excessive use of adhesive plasters whenever possible. Protective covering may limit insensible water loss by evaporation soon after birth. Within a few days of birth, the skin becomes thicker and less prone to traumatic damage, even in very immature infants. Care should be taken in siting peripheral infusions to avoid veins near joints because contractures may occur later if there is scarring (Fig. 158). Central catheters should always be removed if there is persistent cyanosis of extremities, or if there are signs of catheter occlusion or impaired circulation to the limbs, kidneys or gut. Arterial catheters should be removed as soon as the infant's clinical condition improves, and when sampling for blood gas analysis is required less often.

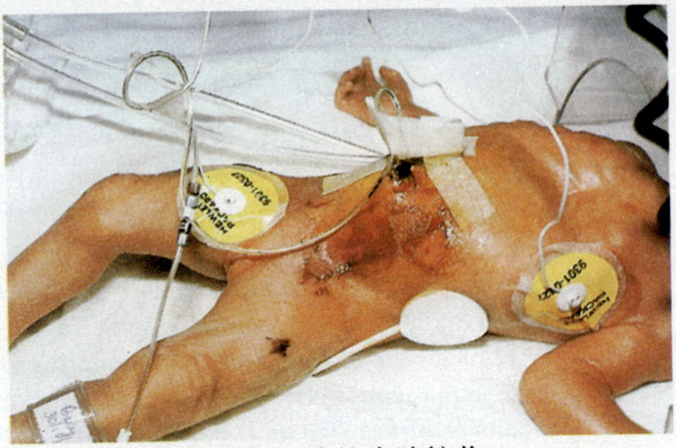

图 156　使用胶带所导致的皮肤擦伤
Skin abrasions from adhesive tape

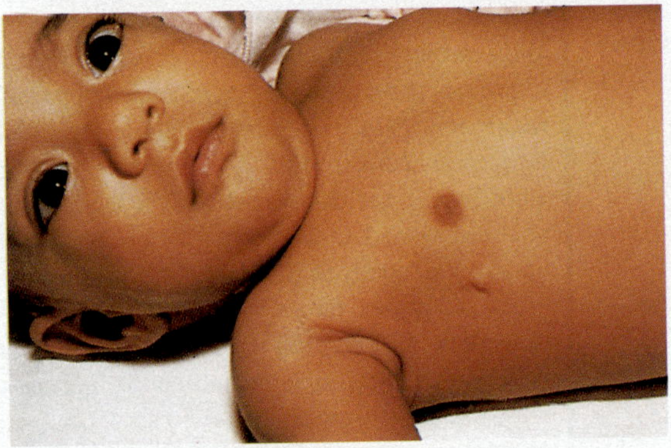

图 157　气胸引流的瘢痕
Scar from a drain for pneumothorax

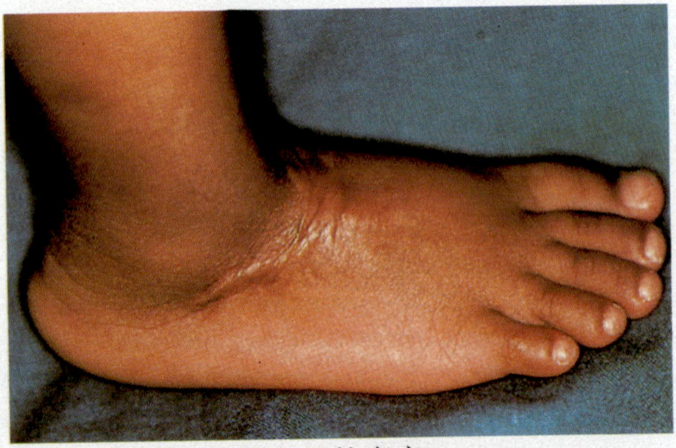

图 158　溃疡愈合后留下的瘢痕
A scar after an ulcer had healed

新生儿眼炎

发病率

小而有黏稠分泌物的眼睛极其常见。

病因学

结膜炎可能与多种微生物有关，多数是在分娩时从母亲产道感染而来的革兰阴性菌（如大肠埃希杆菌）。新生儿结膜炎最严重的原因是性传播微生物，如淋病奈瑟球菌和沙眼衣原体。

临床特征

临床表现轻重不等，从轻度的眼睛发黏（图 159），到严重的有脓性分泌物和眶周组织水肿的结膜炎。淋球菌性眼炎（图 160）会在生后 48 小时内引起严重的症状。一般衣原体感染（图161）一直到生后第二周才会有明显的表现，并且有可能合并有淋球菌感染。

诊断

应该选用合适的拭子采集标本，并进行快速革兰染色。如果怀疑淋球菌感染，应该立即开始用大剂量的青霉素或头孢噻肟进行治疗。

治疗

小而有黏稠分泌物的眼睛通常没有被感染，可以用盐水清洗眼睛。淋球菌性眼炎应该用大剂量的青霉素或头孢噻肟进行局部和全身的用药。沙眼衣原体感染应该局部使用金霉素眼膏，并全身应用红霉素进行治疗。很多其他较轻的感染可以用新霉素或氯霉素眼滴液或软膏。一旦被诊断为淋球菌或衣原体感染，其父母都应该进行生殖器的拭子化验和治疗。

并发症

淋球菌性眼炎的不适当治疗可能会导致角膜瘢痕和失明。在发展中国家，频发的衣原体感染引起的颗粒性结膜炎会导致失明，但是这在发达国家并不常见。这种相同微生物引起不同结果的原因目前尚不清楚。

Neonatal ophthalmia

Incidence

Minor sticky eye is extremely common.

Aetiology

Conjunctivitis may be due to a variety of organisms, most commonly Gram-negative organisms (e.g. Escherichia coli) acquired from the maternal genital tract during birth. The most serious causes of neonatal conjunctivitis are the sexually transmitted organisms, Neisseria gonorrhoeae and Chlamydia trachomatis.

Clinical features

Manifestations vary from a mild sticky eye (Fig. 159), to severe conjunctival inflammation with a purulent discharge and periorbital oedema. Gonococcal ophthalmia (Fig. 160) causes severe signs within 48 h of birth. Chlamydia infection (Fig. 161) often does not become apparent until the second week of life and may coexist with gonorrhoea.

Diagnosis

Appropriate swabs should be taken and an urgent Gram stain should be done. Treatment with high dose penicillin or cefotaxime should be commenced immediately if gonorrhoea is suspected.

Mangement

Minor sticky eyes are usually non-infective and respond to saline eye washes. Gonococcal ophthalmia should be treated with high-dose penicillin or cefotaxime, given both topically and systemically. Chlamydia trachomatis infection will be eradicated with chlortetracycline eye ointment and systemic erythromycin. Most other minor infections will respond to neomycin or chloramphenicol eye drops or ointment. When gonorrhoea or chlamydia are diagnosed, both parents will require genital swabs and treatment.

Complications

Inadequate treatment of gonococcal ophthalmia may lead to corneal scarring and blindness. In developing countries, chlamydia frequently causes blindness from trachoma, but this is uncommon in developed countries. The reason for this different outcome from the same organism is unclear.

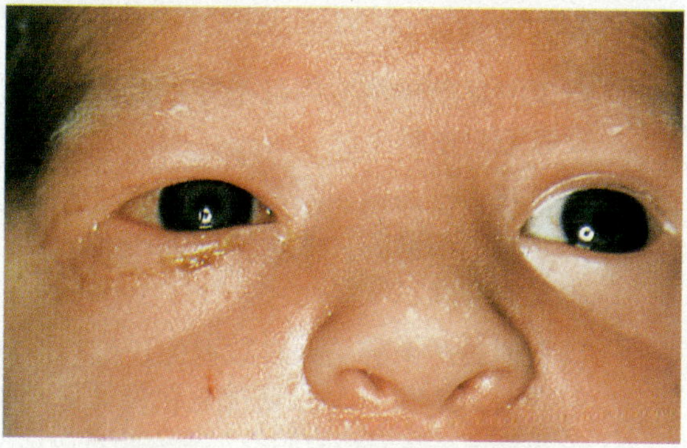

图 159 结膜炎小而有黏稠分泌物的眼睛
Minor sticky eye with conjunctival inflammation

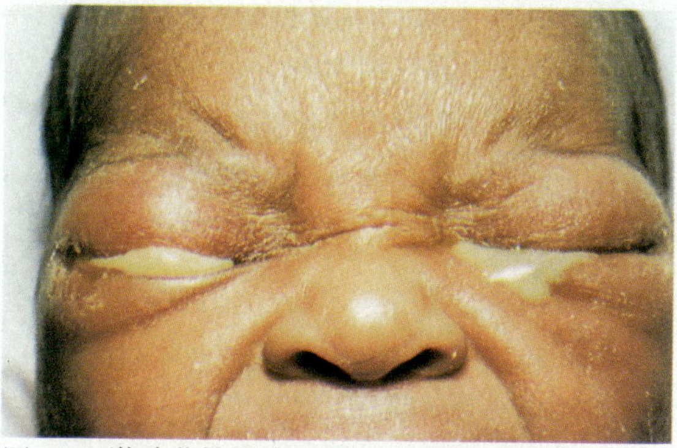

图 160 淋球菌性眼炎明显的脓性分泌物
Frank pus discharge in gonococcal ophthalmia

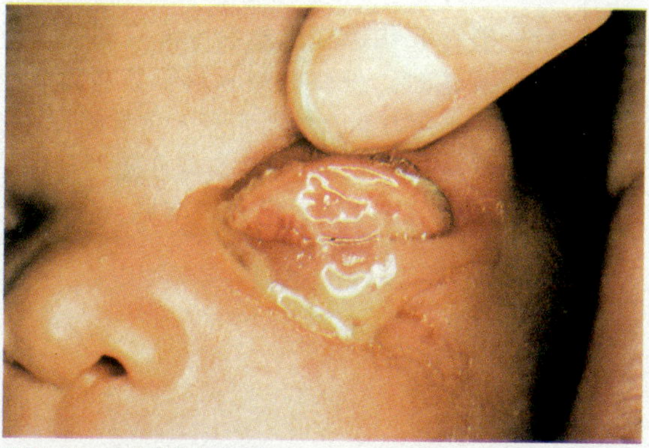

图 161 衣原体性眼炎
Chlamydia ophthalmia

葡萄球菌感染

发病率

严重的葡萄球菌感染目前并不常见，但是较小的浅表感染仍很常见。

病因学

由革兰阳性球菌——金黄色葡萄球菌引起的细菌感染。这型细菌的一些菌株可以产生一种名叫表皮剥脱素的毒素。

临床特征

浅表葡萄球菌感染会导致身体任何部位皮肤的小脓疱（图 162 和 163）。脐部化脓很常见，如果有明显的分泌物或脐周蜂窝织炎，需要全身应用抗生素。指（趾）甲沟炎，即使是很小的感染，如果没有及时治疗也可能引起很严重的脓毒病。偶尔，中毒性表皮坏死溶解（烫伤样皮肤综合征或里特尔病）可发生广泛的表皮分离（图 164）。

并发症

败血病、脑膜炎和骨髓炎。

治疗

小婴儿所有的浅表感染都应在正确的拭子采样和培养后，及时用广谱抗生素进行全身治疗。

骨髓炎

临床特征

大约 90% 的病例是由金黄色葡萄球菌引起。长骨干骺端常会被累及。会有急性炎症反应的局部体征和强烈骨触痛。经常会有发热和毒血症。

诊断和治疗

通常用血培养鉴别致病菌。磁共振和放射性同位素骨扫描成像比 X 线片能更早地发现感染部位，X 线片一般在起病第二周前很少能发现任何异常。当血培养阴性时，外科抽吸术对于鉴别致病菌会有所帮助。在治疗方面，外科引流术常常是有必要的。至少全身性应用6周的抗生素。现在通过合理的治疗，慢性骨髓炎（图 165）已经较罕见。

Staphylococcal infection

Incidence

Serious staphylococcal infection is now uncommon, but not minor superficial infections.

Aetiology

Bacterial infection caused by Gram-positive cocci, Staphylococcus aureus. Some strains of this bacterium produce a toxin called exfoliatin.

Clinical features

Superficial staphylococcal infections result in small pustules anywhere on the skin (Figs 162 and 163). Umbilical sepsis is common, and if there is a frank discharge or periumbilical cellulitis, systemic antibiotics will be required. Paronychiae of the fingers and toes, although apparently minor infections, may cause more serious sepsis if not promptly treated. Occasionally, toxic epidermal necrolysis (scalded skin syndrome or Ritter disease) with extensive epidermal separation may develop (Fig. 164).

Complications

Septicaemia, meningitis and osteomyelitis.

Management

All superficial infections in young infants should be promptly treated with broad-spectrum systemic antibiotics after appropriate swabs and cultures.

Osteomyelitis

Clinical features

About 90% of cases are caused by Staphylococcus aureus. The metaphyses of the long bones are usually affected. There are local signs of acute inflammation and exquisite bony tenderness. Fever and toxaemia often occur.

Diagnosis and management

Blood cultures usually identify the organism. Magnetic resonance imaging and radioisotope bone scans will reveal the site of infection earlier than X-rays which rarely show any abnormality before the second week. Surgical aspiration is helpful for identifying the organism especially when blood cultures are negative. Surgical drainage is sometimes necessary. Systemic antibiotics are given for at least 6 weeks. With adequate treatment, chronic osteomyelitis (Fig. 165) is now rare.

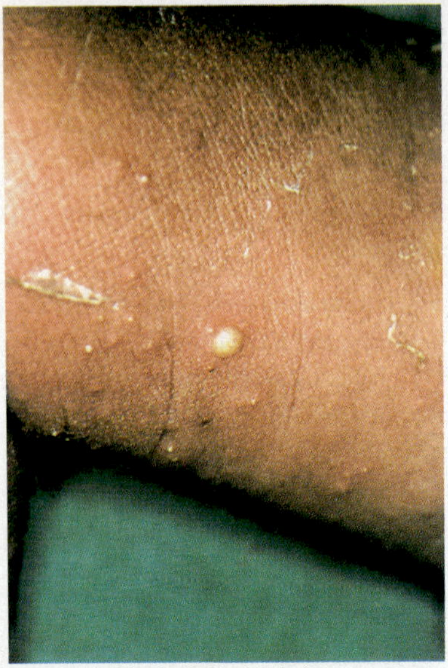

图 162　葡萄球菌小脓疱
Staphylococcal pustule

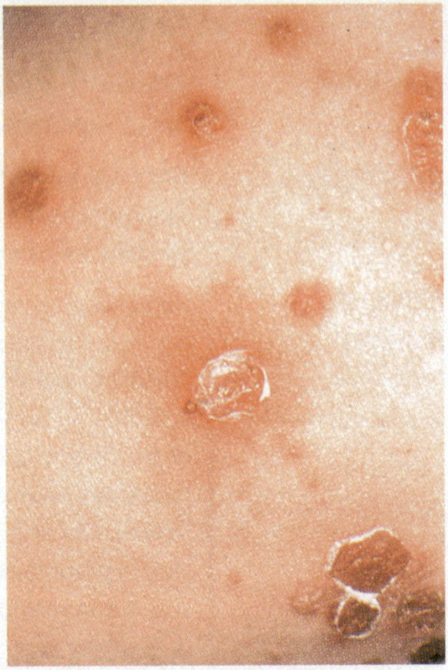

图 163　葡萄球菌脓疱病皮损
Impetiginous staphylococcal lesions

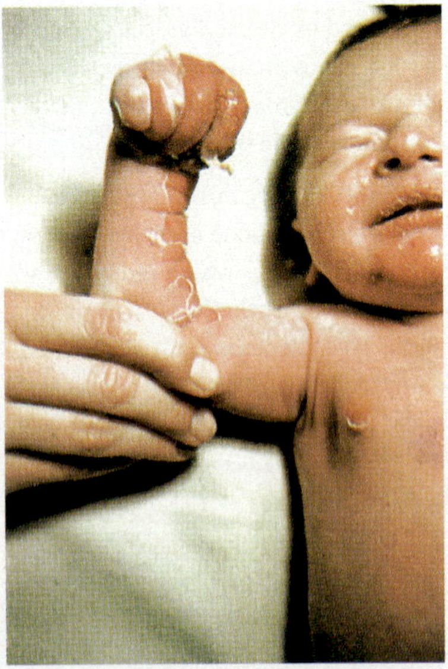

图 164　中毒性表皮坏死溶解
Toxic epidermal necrolysis

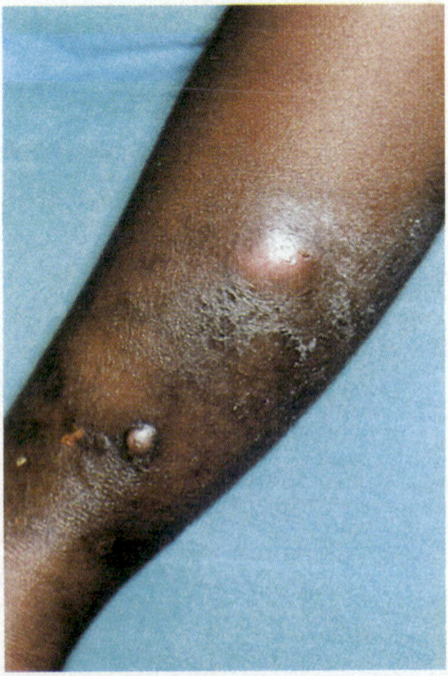

图 165　慢性骨髓炎
Chronic osteomyelitis

丹毒

病因学 链球菌性皮肤感染。

临床特征 边界清楚的广泛蜂窝织炎（图 166）。沿淋巴管分布区域有时可见有红色蔓延。

治疗 大剂量静脉应用青霉素。

脑膜炎球菌血症

临床特征 伴有休克和紫癜的急性暴发性败血症（图 167）。脑膜炎球菌性败血症有较高的致死率。

诊断 应该进行血培养。抗原试验很有用，尤其当抗体已经产生。应该考虑进行腰椎穿刺，但是对于很虚弱的患儿则是禁忌的。

治疗 应该立即对任何有可疑皮疹的儿童大剂量肌注或静脉使用青霉素或头孢噻肟。循环衰竭的早期支持性治疗是存活的关键。

脑（脊）膜炎

病因学 在小于5岁的孩子中，引起细菌性脑（脊）膜炎的常见微生物有流感嗜血杆菌、脑膜炎球菌和肺炎球菌。免疫接种可以降低 B 型流感嗜血杆菌和 C 型脑膜炎球菌感染的发病率。

临床特征 特异性体征，如头痛和颈项强直，可发生于大龄儿童，但在小婴儿中常常没有。婴儿经常表现出易激惹、嗜睡、呕吐、厌食、抽搐或发热等非特异性体征。囟门膨隆、高调哭闹和弓形背（角弓反张；图 168）都是晚期症状。

诊断 对于任何有无法解释的发热或抽搐的患儿都高度怀疑脑（脊）膜炎。脑脊液检查和培养将进一步确诊。

治疗 在致病菌和药敏试验结果出来之前应该先用广谱抗生素进行治疗。

Erysipelas

Aetiology

Streptococcal skin infection.

Clinical features

Spreading cellulitis with a well-defined edge (Fig. 166). A red flare is sometimes seen spreading along the draining lymphatics.

Management

High dose intravenous penicillin.

Meningococcaemia

Clinical features

Acute fulminating septicaemia with shock and a purpuric rash (Fig. 167). Meningococcal septicaemia has a high mortality.

Diagnosis

Blood cultures should always be taken. Antigen testing is very useful, particularly when antibiotics have already been given. Lumbar puncture should be considered, but may be contraindicated in a very ill child.

Management

High dose intramuscular or intravenous penicillin or cefotaxime should be given immediately to any child with a suspicious rash. Early support of circulatory failure is critical to survival.

Meningitis

Aetiology

Common organisms causing bacterial meningitis in children <age of 5 years are Hacmophilus influenzae, meningococci and pneumococci. The incidence of Haemophilus influenzae B and meningococcal C infection can be reduced by immunization.

Clinical features

Specific signs such as headache and neck stiffness occur in older children but are often absent in young infants. Infants often present with non-specific signs of irritability, drowsiness, vomiting, anorexia, convulsions or fever. Bulging fontanelle, high pitched cry and arching of the back (opisthotonos; Fig. 168) are late signs.

Diagnosis

High index of suspicion in any ill child with unexplained fever or convulsions. Cerebrospinal fluid examination and culture will confirm the diagnosis.

Management

Broad-spectrum antibiotics should be given until the organism and sensitivities are known.

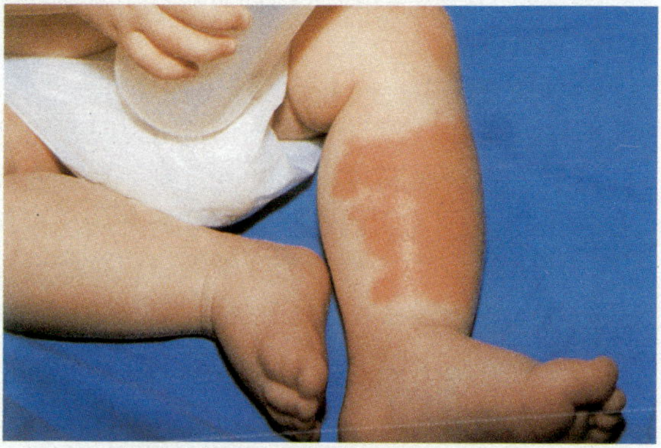

图 166 边界清楚的红斑（丹毒）
Well-defined erythema (erysipelas)

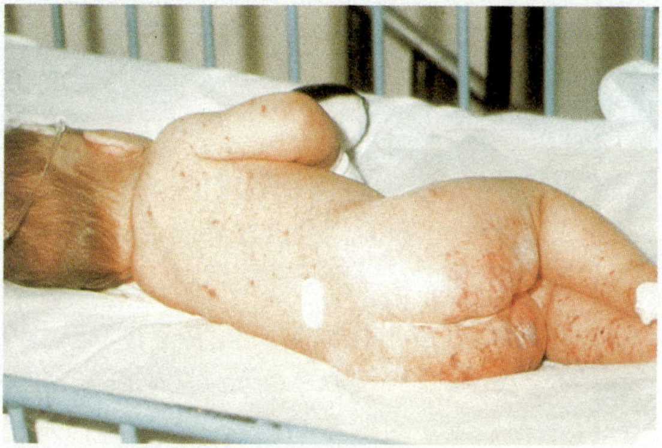

图 167 脑膜炎球菌性败血症
Meningococcal septicaemia

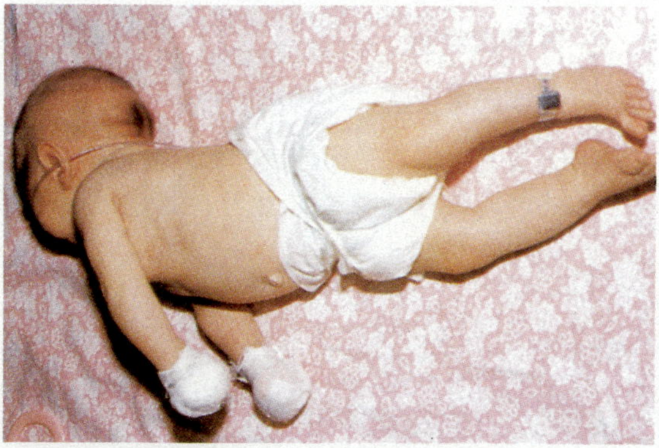

图 168 角弓反张
Opisthotonos

麻疹

临床特征

潜伏期是 10 ~ 14 天。前驱症状有发热、卡他症状、结膜炎和咳嗽。当皮疹开始出现时，患儿会极度痛苦。在颊黏膜可见鲜红色背景上有小白斑（Koplik 斑）。3 ~ 4 天后，脸上和耳后开始出现鲜红的斑丘疹（图 169）。皮疹会逐渐融合成片状，沿躯干向下蔓延。一般会在 7 天后变成褐色并出现脱屑。

并发症

支气管肺炎和中耳炎很常见；1000个患儿中会有1个发生脑炎。在有营养不良或免疫缺陷的患儿中死亡率较高。很少情况下，在急性麻疹后数年会发生慢性进行性神经变性疾病（亚急性硬化性全脑炎）。

免疫接种

麻疹、流行性腮腺炎和风疹三联疫苗（MMR）是很有效的，一般在出生后约 12 ~ 15 个月进行接种。

风疹

临床特征

潜伏期为14 ~ 21天。轻度的、暂时的、非特异性斑疹，持续仅数天。全身性淋巴结病，尤其枕下淋巴结较为常见。

并发症

偶尔会有血小板减少。关节炎在女性青少年中较常见。妊娠期前三个月，先天性风疹综合征会影响胎儿发育，是最有破坏性的并发症。

免疫接种

在英国，MMR 疫苗常规在出生后 12 ~ 15 个月进行接种。所有的女性都应该在妊娠前进行接种。

传染性软疣

临床特征

由痘病毒引起的珍珠样丘疹，中央有凹陷（图170）。

治疗

通常无症状，无须治疗。如果皮损较为广泛，或者对外观有较严重影响，用冷冻疗法或针刺术对于减少病程有帮助。

Measles

Clinical features

Incubation period 10-14 days. Prodromal illness with fever, coryza, conjunctivitis and cough. The child is extremely miserable as the rash begins to appear. Tiny white spots on a bright red background (Koplik's spots) may be seen on the buccal mucosa. After 3-4 days, a florid, maculopapular rash appears initially on the face and behind the ears. (Fig. 169). The rash becomes more confluent as it spreads down the trunk; bronzing and desquamation occur after about 7 days.

Complications

Bronchopneumonia and otitis media are common; encephalitis occurs in 1 in 1000 children. Mortality is high in children with malnutrition or immunodeficiency. Rarely, a slowly progressive neurodegenerative disorder (subacute sclerosing panencephalitis) occurs some years after acute measles.

Immunization

A triple vaccine with mumps and rubella (MMR) is very effective and usually given around 12-15 months of age.

German measles (rubella)

Clinical features

Incubation period 14-21 days. Mild illness with transient, non-specific macular rash lasting only a few days. Generalized lymphadenopathy, particularly of suboccipital nodes, is common.

Complications

Thrombocytopenia occasionally occurs. Arthritis is more common in adolescent females. Congenital rubella syndrome affecting the developing fetus in the first trimester of pregnancy is the most devastating complication.

Immunization

In the UK, MMR vaccine is given routinely at 12-15 months of age. All girls should be vaccinated before pregnancy.

Molluscum contagiosum

Clinical features

Pearly papules with a central punctum (Fig. 170) caused by pox virus.

Treatment

Usually asymptomatic and no treatment required. Cryotherapy or needling reduces the duration and is useful if the lesions are widespread, or cosmetically unacceptable.

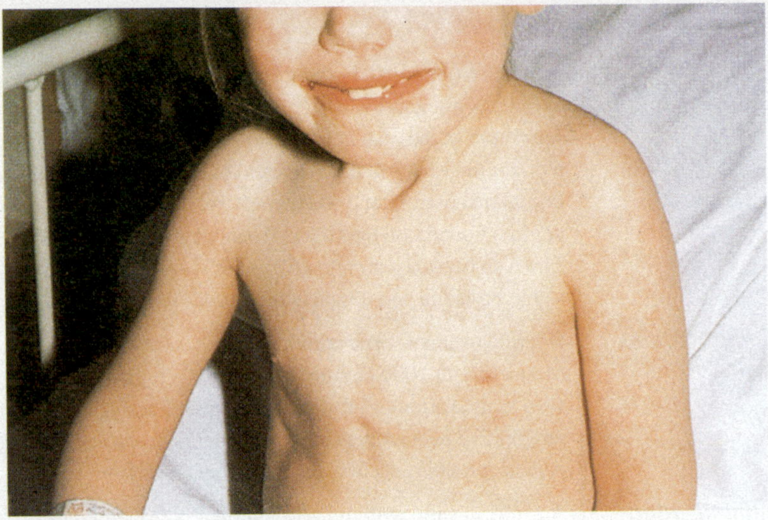

图 169 麻疹
Measles rash

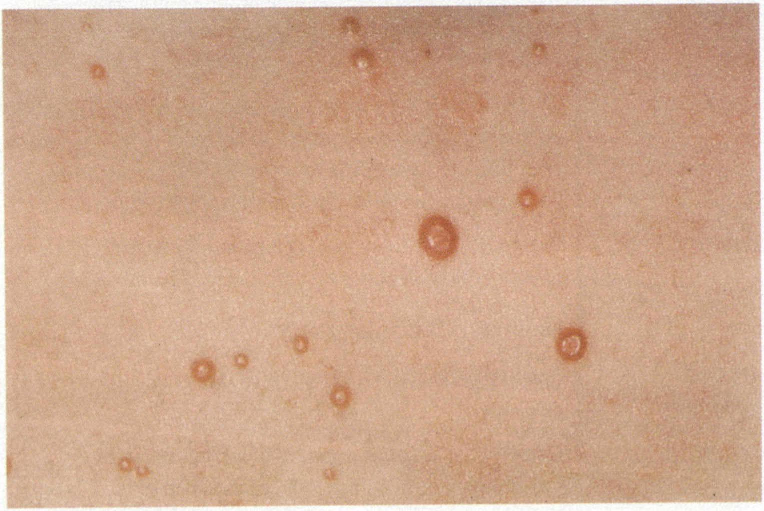

图 170 传染性软疣典型的斑点样皮损
Typical punctate lesions of molloscum contagiosum

腮腺炎

临床特征 在接触传染源后的14～21天会有发烧和单侧或双侧的腮腺肿大（图 171）。隐性感染比较常见。结实、肿胀的腺体有疼痛感、触痛，并且经常伴有耳痛和牙关紧闭。颌下唾液腺也可能受累。

并发症 常有轻度脑（脊）膜炎，可能在腮腺肿胀之前或没有腮腺肿胀症状时发生。胰腺炎和附睾-睾丸炎较多发生于成人。

免疫接种 在出生后 12 ～ 15 个月进行 MMR 疫苗接种。

嗜血杆菌性蜂窝织炎

临床特征 流感嗜血杆菌可能会引起严重的面部蜂窝织炎，尤其是颊部、眶周和颈部（图 172）。目前，由于 B 型嗜血杆菌的免疫接种，该病已不常见。

治疗 合理应用抗生素（如全身应用氨苄西林或头孢菌素）。

传染性单核细胞增多症（腺热）

临床特征 由EB病毒引起的散发感染，潜伏期为4～14天。厌食、身体不适、发热和全身性淋巴结肿大都是主要的症状。经常会有腭部瘀点和严重的渗出性扁桃体炎。在将近20%的病例中会出现斑疹；如果给予氨苄西林治疗，90%的病例会出现斑疹（图173）。

诊断 在血涂片上会有非典型单核细胞，并且在病程前几周，凝集试验［如保-邦试验（嗜异性抗体反应)］可能为阳性。

并发症 肝炎较常见。非特异性的发烧和身体不适可能会持续数周，甚至数月。

Mumps

Clinical features

Fever and enlargement of one or both parotid glands (Fig. 171) occur 14-21 days after contact by a susceptible individual. Subclinical infection is common. The brawny, swollen glands are painful, tender and often accompanied by earache or trismus. Submandibular salivary glands may also be affected.

Complications

Mild meningitis is common and may precede or occur in the absence of parotid swelling. Pancreatitis and epididymo-orchitis occur more often in adults.

Immunization

Part of routine MMR at 12-15 months of age.

Haemophilus cellulitis

Clinical features

Haemophilus influenzae may cause severe cellulitis affecting the face, particularly the check, periorbital region and neck (Fig. 172). Now uncommon as a result of haemophilus B immunization.

Management

Responds to an appropriate antibiotic (e.g. systemic ampicillin, or a cephalosporin).

Infectious mononucleosis (glandular fever)

Clinical features

Sporadic infection caused by the Epstein-Barr virus after an incubation period of 4-14 days. Anorexia, malaise, fever and generalized lymphadenopathy are prominent symptoms. Petechiae on the palate, and severe exudative tonsillitis often occur. A macular rash occurs in approximately 20% of cases, and in 90% if ampicillin is given (Fig. 173).

Diagnosis

Atypical mononuclear cells appear in the blood film, and agglutination tests (e.g. Paul-Bunnell test) may be positive in early weeks.

Complications

Hepatitis is common. Non-specific symptoms of fever and malaise may persist for several weeks or occasionally months.

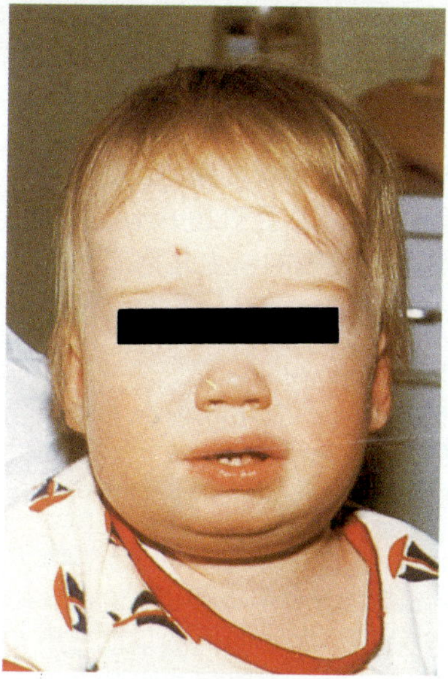

图 171　腮腺炎腮腺肿大
Parotid swelling in mumps

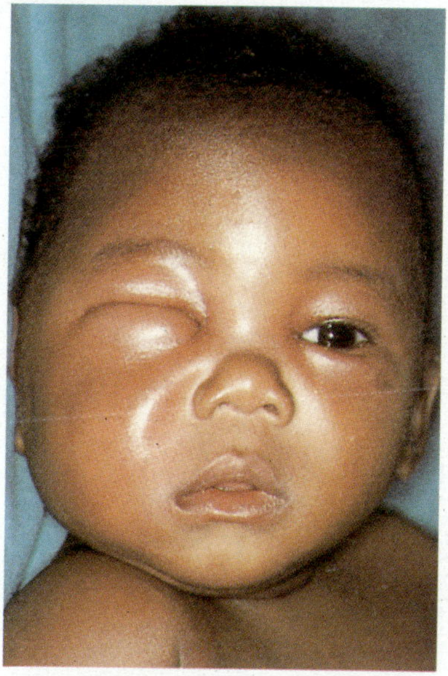

图 172　面部嗜血杆菌性蜂窝织炎
Haemophilus cellulitis of the face

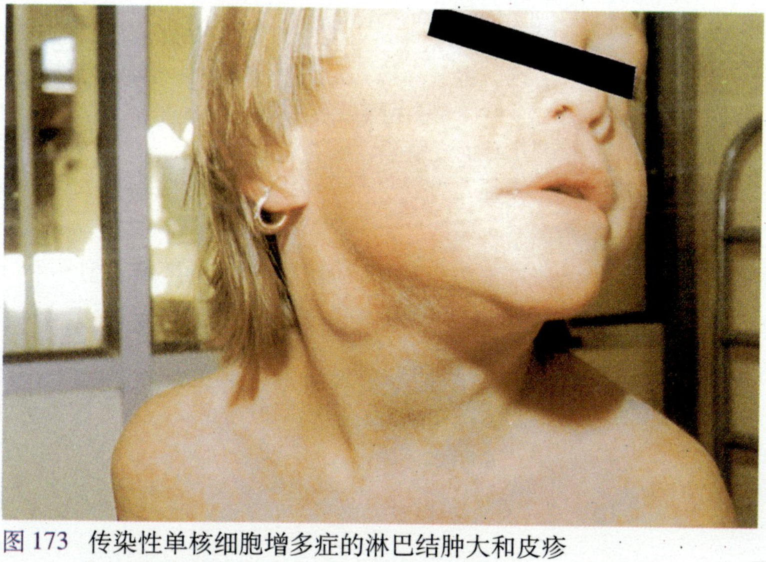

图 173　传染性单核细胞增多症的淋巴结肿大和皮疹
Lymphadenopathy and rash in infectious mononucleosis

单纯性疱疹

临床特征

I型病毒的原发感染可能会引起严重的龈口炎。会在嘴唇（图 174）、颊黏膜出现多发性、疼痛的大水疱或溃疡。患儿通常极度痛苦，伴有多涎、发烧、易激惹和吞咽困难。复发性单纯疱疹会引起单纯、普通的唇疱疹。出有全身性水泡性疹的新生儿疱疹感染一般是Ⅱ型病毒，是新生儿通过产道分娩时获得的急性疱疹感染。

并发症

由于口唇疼痛和吞咽困难，若有水分摄入不充足会发生脱水。单纯性疱疹脑炎是严重的并发症，但较少见，致死率高，即便存活，也有较高的神经系统发育障碍的危险。

治疗

富有同情心的护理，止痛和充分的液体摄入。原发感染一般在 2 周内有自限性。48 小时内的早期感染，需要局部应用阿昔洛维。静脉应用阿昔洛维也用于治疗全身并发症。如果母亲在妊娠晚期有活动性外阴疱疹感染应该考虑选择性剖宫产。

带状疱疹：水痘

临床特征

潜伏期为14～21天。皮疹会成群出现，迅速从斑疹进展到丘疹，再到小囊泡（图 175 和 176）。小囊泡会结痂，患儿具有传染性，直到10～14天后痂皮脱落，而且通常会留下凹陷性瘢痕。一般病情较轻，除非患儿有免疫缺陷。脑炎较罕见，但是一旦发生，主要的体征是共济失调，会在水痘急性发病数周后发生。

并发症

出血性水痘较罕见，但却是该病的严重类型。

带状疱疹

在儿童不常见，小囊泡具有典型的皮区分布（图 177)。瘙痒是常见的症状，但是带状疱疹后神经痛在儿童并不常见。

Herpes simplex

Clinical features

Primary infection with type 1 virus may cause severe gingivostomatitis. Multiple painful blisters or ulcers occur around the mouth, on the lips (Fig. 174) and buccal mucous membranes. The child is usually extremely miserable with excessive dribbling and salivation, fever, irritability and difficulty in swallowing. Recurrent herpes simplex causes the simple common cold sore. Neonatal herpes infection with a generalized vesicular eruption, usually type II virus, is acquired by the infant during delivery through a genital tract with active herpes infection.

Complications

Dehydration may occur when there is inadequate fluid intake because of the painful mouth and difficulty in swallowing. Herpes encephalitis is a rare but serious complication with high mortality and high risk of neurodevelopmental disability in survivors.

Management

Sympathetic nursing, analgesia and adequate fluid intake. Primary infection is usually self-limiting within 2 weeks. Early infection within 48 h of onset may respond to topical acyclovir. Intravenous acyclovir is also used for systemic complications. Elective Caesarean section should be considered if active maternal genital herpes has been present in late pregnancy.

Herpes zoster: chicken pox (varicella)

Clinical features

Incubation period 14-21 days. The spots occur in crops which rapidly progress from macules to papules to vesicles (Figs 175 and 176). The vesicle becomes crusted and the child remains infectious until the scales separate 10-14 days later, often leaving pitted scars. Usually a mild illness, except when the child is immunodeficient. Encephalitis is rare, but when it occurs, the predominant sign is ataxia with onset several weeks after the acute illness.

Complications

Haemorrhagic chicken pox is a rare, but severe form of the illness.

Shingles (herpes zoster)

Uncommon in children. Vesicles have the typical dermatome distribution (Fig. 177). Itching is a common symptom, but post-herpetic neuralgia is uncommon in children.

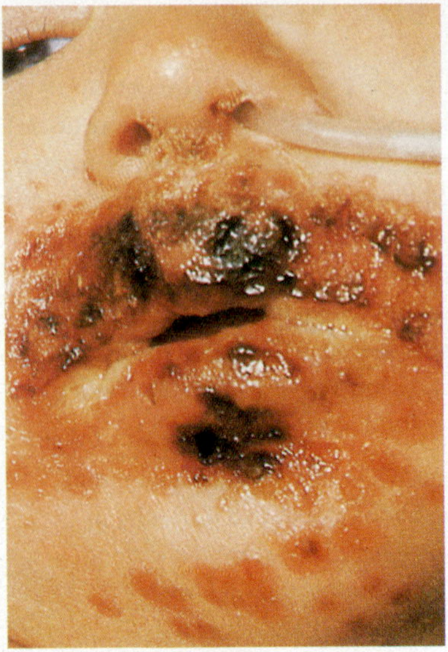

图 174 疱疹性口炎
Herpes stomatitis

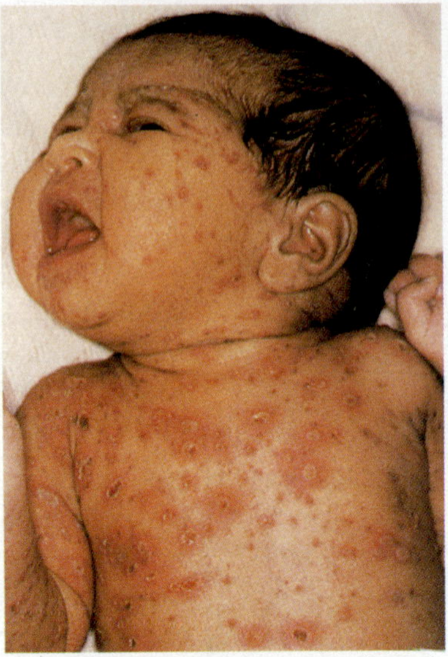

图 175 未免疫母亲生的患有水痘的小婴儿
Chicken pox in a young infant born to a non-immune mother

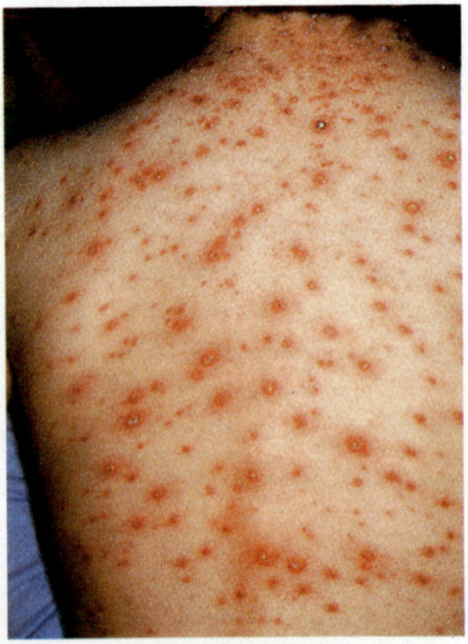

图 176 大龄儿童典型的水痘
Typical chicken pox in an older child

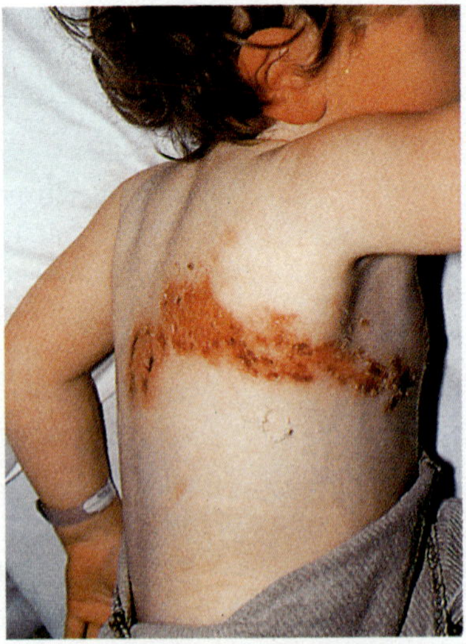

图 177 带状疱疹的皮区分布
Shingles involving dermatome

人类免疫缺陷病毒（HIV）感染

发病率

由于在世界范围内的传播，该病变得越来越常见。大多数患儿是通过阴道分娩垂直传播而患病的。母乳喂养会增加感染的危险。

临床特征

大多数感染 HIV 病毒的婴儿在出生时都很健康。疾病通常在孩子出生数月后开始发展。复发性念珠菌感染、复发性腮腺炎、发育停滞、卡氏肺囊虫性肺炎、全身性淋巴结肿大（图178）和慢性腹泻都很常见。

预防

如果妊娠时通过抗逆转录病毒治疗，母亲的病毒载量减少，那么围产期传播的危险性可以减少到＜2%。避免产后母乳喂养和选择剖腹产也可以减少感染的危险，但是在发展中国家也许并不适用。

结核病

病因学

结核分支杆菌（图 179）。原发感染可能在肺部或肿大的淋巴结。它通常是无症状患病人群通过飞沫传播。

临床特征

原发性结核病通常都是无症状的。血性播散和脑（脊）膜炎常见于较小年龄儿童以及患有营养不良或间发性感染的儿童。肺结核在病程晚期有慢性咳嗽。

诊断

在感染后的 4 ～ 8 周结核菌素试验呈阳性反应（图180）。胸部 X 光片会有肺门淋巴结肿大和肺叶损伤的表现。

治疗

用异烟肼和利福平进行 6 ～ 12 个月的联合化疗，有时也可能用其他药物，尤其当有粟粒性播散或结核性脑（脊）膜炎时。

预防

接种卡介苗可以提供 80% 的保护性。

Human immunodeficiency virus (HIV) infection

Incidence

Becoming more common as a result of the epidemic throughout the world. Most children are infected by vertical transmission during vaginal delivery. Breast-feeding increases the risk of infection.

Clinical features

Most babies with HIV infection are healthy at birth. AIDS-defining illness does not usually develop until the baby is several months old. Recurrent candida infection, recurrent parotitis, failure to thrive, pneumocystis pneumonia, generalized lymphadenopathy (Fig. 178), and chronic diarrhoea are common.

Prevention

If maternal viral load is reduced by anti-retroviral therapy during pregnancy, the risk of perinatal transmission can be reduced to < 2%. Avoidance of breast-feeding and elective Caesarean section, also reduce the risk of infection, but may not be appropriate in developing countries.

Tuberculosis

Aetiology

Mycobacterium tuberculosis (Fig. 179). Primary infection may present in the lung or as enlarged lymph nodes. It is contracted by droplet spread, usually from asymptomatic adults.

Clinical features

Primary tuberculosis is usually asymptomatic. Haematogenous spread and meningitis are most common in the very young, and in children with malnutrition or intercurrent infection. Pulmonary tuberculosis with chronic cough occurs in later life.

Diagnosis

Sensitivity to tuberculin as shown by a positive Mantoux reaction (Fig. 180) develops within 4-8 weeks after infection. Chest X-ray may show hilar lymphadenopathy or a segmental lesion.

Management

Combination chemotherapy with isoniazid and rifampicin for 6-12 months, and occasionally other drugs, particularly if there is miliary spread or tuberculous meningitis.

Prevention

Bacille Calmette-Guérin vaccination provides up to 80% protection.

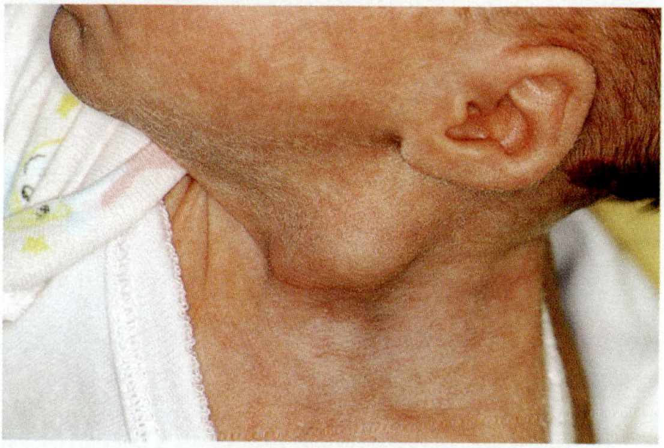

图 178 明显的颈部淋巴结肿大
Marked cervical lymphadenopathy

图 179 结核分支杆菌的抗酸杆菌
Acid fast bacilli of *Mycobacterium tuberculosis*

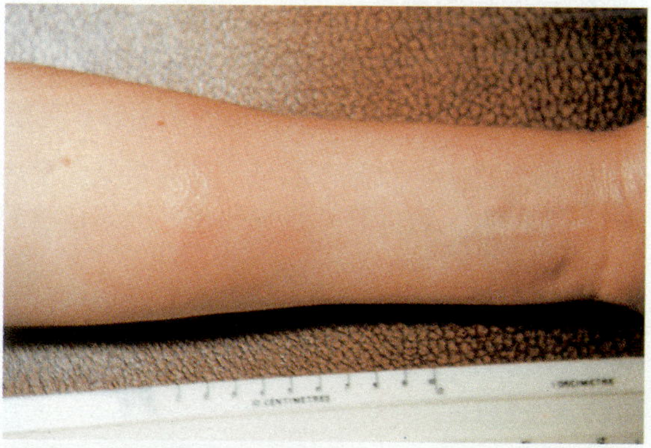

图 180 结核菌素试验阳性
Positive Mantoux reaction

巨细胞病毒（CMV）

临床特征 表现为小头、贫血、肝脾大、紫癜（图181）、黄疸、淋巴结肿大、颅内钙化和肺炎。耳聋、精神残障、脑性麻痹，和癫痫可以在病程后期发生。

预后 大约1%的无症状新生儿通过尿液排泄CMV病毒，大多数没有后遗症。大约5%的患儿会有耳聋，1%的患儿则有更为严重的神经系统表现。

弓形虫病

发病率 相对于欧洲的其他国家，该病在英国并不常见。通过猫的粪便或食用被感染的生肉可感染此病。

临床特征 肝脾大，紫癜，黄疸，生长发育迟缓，颅内损伤（图182）和钙化，脉络膜视网膜炎和脑积水。神经系统的损害更为严重，但是较罕见。

诊断 弓形虫特异性的IgM可以证实有感染，但是IgM阴性的孩子可能仍有感染，需要随访数月。

治疗 对经被证实有感染的母亲在妊娠期应用螺旋霉素，并且出生后对孩子继续应用。在新生儿期以后对婴儿应用乙胺嘧啶和磺胺嘧啶。针对脉络膜视网膜炎的治疗尤为重要。

预后 多变。许多儿童仅有眼部损害，很少情况下，神经系统的损害可能较为严重。

李斯特菌病

发病率 在法国比在英国更常见。该病菌存在于多种食物中，如软的未经高温消毒的奶酪或者色拉中。

临床特征 宫内感染导致流产或早产较为常见。常表现为新生儿肺炎、脑（脊）膜炎和皮肤上不连续的溃疡（图183）。

治疗和预后 通过氨苄西林进行早期治疗可以使所有患儿生存。

Cytomegalovirus (CMV)

Clinical features

Microcephaly, anaemia, hepatosplenomegaly, purpura (Fig. 181), jaundice, lymphadenopathy, intra-cranial calcification, and pneumonia. Deafness, mental handicap, cerebral palsy and epilepsy may occur later.

Prognosis

Some 1% of asymptomatic neonates excrete CMV in urine, majority have no sequelae. Approximately 5% develop deafness, and 1% more serious neurological manifestations.

Toxoplasmosis

Incidence

Less common in the UK than in continental Europe. Infection is acquired from eating raw infected meat or from cat faeces.

Clinical features

Hepatosplenomegaly, purpura, jaundice, growth retardation, intra-cranial lesions (Fig. 182) and calcification, chorioretinitis and hydrocephalus. Rarely, neurological damage may be severe.

Diagnosis

Toxoplasma-specific IgM confirms infection, but IgM-negative babies may still be infected and need follow-up for many months.

Management

Spiramycin is used in pregnancy after proven infection and continued after birth. Pyrimethamine and sulphadiazine are used for infants after the neonatal period. Treatment is particularly important in chorioretinitis.

Prognosis

Variable. Many children only have eye lesions, and rarely, neurological damage may be severe.

Listeriosis

Incidence

More common in France than in the UK. The bacterium is present in many foods, such as soft unpasteurized cheeses or in salads.

Clinical features

Intra-uterine infection resulting in abortion or premature delivery is common. Neonatal pneumonia and meningitis and discrete ulceration of the skin (Fig. 183).

Management and prognosis

Early treatment with ampicillin may provide intact survival.

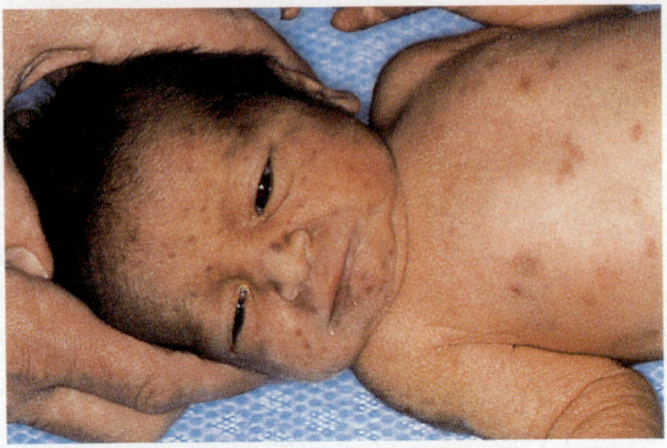

图 181　宫内病毒感染婴儿身上的紫癜
Infant with purpura and an intra-uterine viral infection

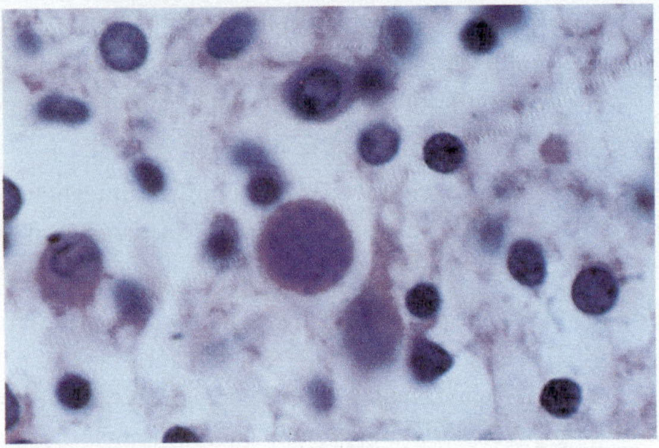

图 182　显微镜下一个新生儿脑内的弓形虫包囊
Microscopic view of toxoplasma cysts in a new born brain

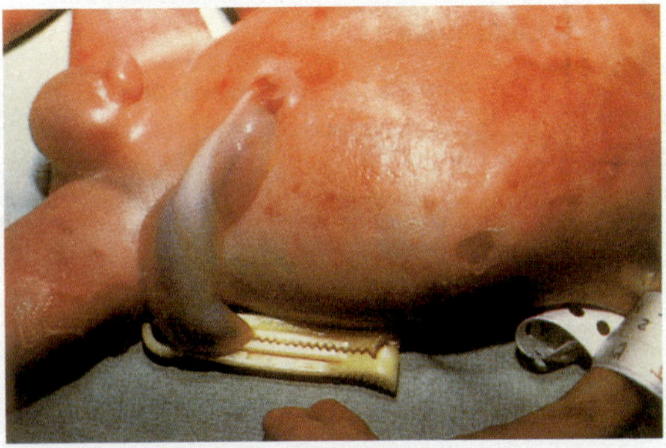

图 183　李斯特菌病的皮肤溃疡
Skin ulcers in listeriosis

白血病

发病率 是最常见的儿童恶性肿瘤，约有 85% 为急性淋巴母细胞性白血病（ALL）。

临床特征 苍白、嗜睡、反复感染、发烧和自发性瘀青很常见。有时会有肝脾大、淋巴结肿大和骨触痛。新生儿白血病虽然很罕见，但是可有特征性的皮下沉积物（图184）。贫血，血小板减少，并且在外周血中出现原始细胞。在骨髓中发现过多的原始细胞（图185）可以进一步确诊。

治疗 与家属就治疗和预后进行充分的讨论很重要。经常有必要输全血、血小板或粒细胞。用几种细胞毒性药物进行化疗要持续数年。骨髓移植正变成重要的治疗方法。

预后 目前 ALL 至少有 70% 的 5 年生存率。

朗格汉细胞组织细胞增生症

病理学 组织细胞的异常增生；多变的疾病谱有时会有恶性病程。

临床特征 界限清晰的溶解性骨损伤，常累及颅骨，但一般是良性的（嗜酸细胞肉芽肿）。伴有发烧、肝脾大、淋巴结肿大、脂溢性皮疹（图186）或皮肤沉积物的全身性疾病较为严重。

治疗 用类似急性白血病的细胞毒性药物进行化疗来治疗全身性疾病。

Leukaemia

Incidence

The most common childhood malignancy; 85% have acute lymphoblastic leukaemia (ALL).

Clinical features

Pallor, lethargy, recurrent infections, fever and spontaneous bruising are common. Hepatosplenomegaly, lymphadenopathy and bone tenderness sometimes occur. Neonatal leukaemia, though rare, may present with characteristic subcutaneous deposits (Fig. 184). Anaemia, thrombocytopenia and blast cells in peripheral blood. Excessive blast cells (Fig. 185) in bone marrow confirm the diagnosis.

Management

Full discussion of treatment and prognosis with the family is very important. Transfusions of blood, platelets or granulocytes are often necessary. Maintenance chemotherapy with several cytotoxic drugs will continue for several years. Bone marrow transplantation is becoming an important method of treatment.

Prognosis

At least 70% 5-year survival now occurs in ALL.

Langerhan cell histiocytosis

Pathology

Abnormal proliferation of histiocytes; variable disease spectrum which sometimes runs a malignant course.

Clinical features

Clearly defined lytic bone lesions, often involving the skull, are usually benign (eosinophilic granuloma). Systemic disease with fever, hepatosplenomegaly, lymphadenopathy, seborrhoeic rash (Fig. 186) or skin deposits is more serious.

Management

Systemic disease may respond to cytotoxic chemotherapy similar to treatment for acute leukaemia.

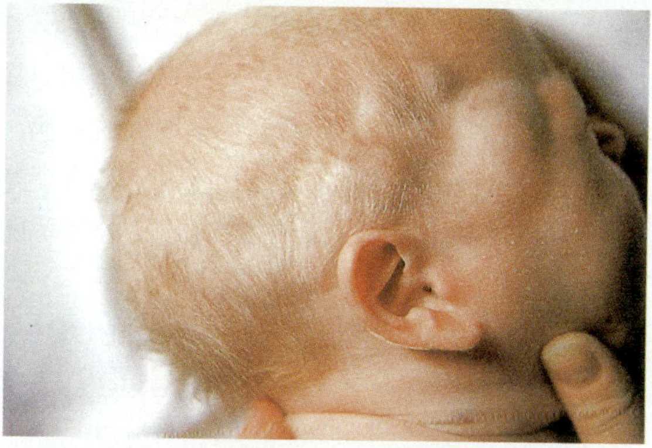

图 184 新生儿白血病的皮下沉积物
Subcutaneous lesions of neonatal leukaemia

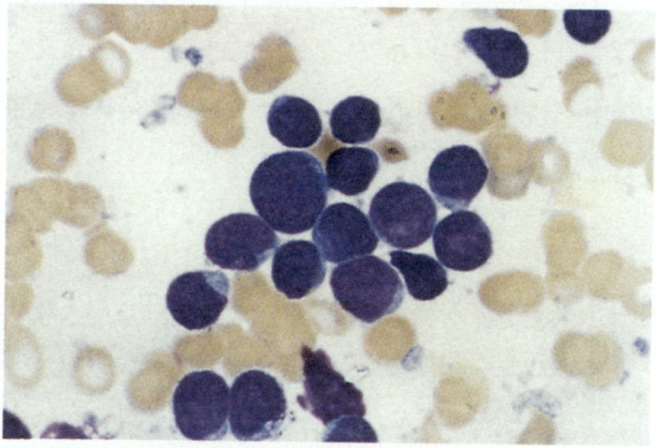

图 185 骨髓中可见许多原始细胞
Bone marrow showing many blast cells

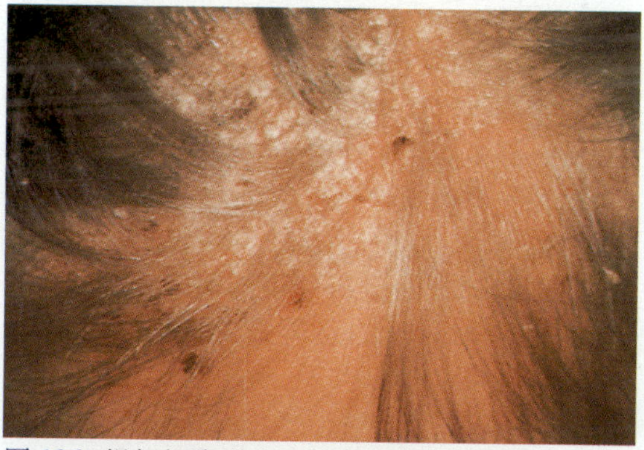

图 186 组织细胞增生症的脂溢性头皮损伤
Seborrhoeic scalp lesions of histiocytosis

镰形细胞（贫血）病

病因学 常见。血红蛋白病，具有镰刀样细胞特征，可见于15%的黑人中。是常染色体隐性遗传病。

临床特征 慢性贫血，反复的骨痛伴触痛和肿胀，发烧和黄疸(图187)。慢性腿部溃疡、血尿、胸部和腹部疼痛都很常见。

治疗 疼痛危象的对症治疗。及时应用抗生素控制感染。预防性应用青霉素和肺炎球菌疫苗都可以预防严重的肺炎球菌感染。

特发性血小板减少性紫癜（ITP）

病因学 通常发生于病毒感染后，尤其是风疹病毒。一般可发现有血小板抗体。

临床特征 自发性瘀点和表面瘀青（图 188)。必须排除其他更为严重的引起血小板减少的原因。

预后 大多数会在数月内自行恢复；偶尔有慢性病情，需要进行脾切除。

治疗 如果血小板计数下降到＜30 000，就需输注血小板。应用类固醇和静脉输注丙种球蛋白也会对病情有所帮助。

再生障碍性贫血

临床特征 苍白，贫血，多毛症和腭部瘀点（图 189)。

诊断 血常规显示有贫血、血小板减少和中性粒细胞减少。骨髓检查可进一步证实血细胞前体的缺乏。

治疗 骨髓或脐血干细胞的配对移植可以治愈该疾病，目前已经作为优先治疗方法。输血和血小板进行支持治疗，用皮质类固醇、环孢素、抗胸腺细胞或抗淋巴细胞球蛋白进行免疫抑制治疗，或采用雄激素治疗。用广谱抗生素对败血症进行早期积极的治疗。

Sickle cell disease

Aetiology

Common. Haemoglobinopathy with sickle cell trait is found in 15% of black people. Inheritance is autosomal recessive.

Clinical features

Chronic anaemia, recurrent bone pains with tenderness and swelling, fever and jaundice (Fig. 187). Chronic leg ulcers, haematuria, chest and abdominal pain are common.

Management

Symptomatic treatment of painful crises. Prompt antibiotic treatment of infection. Prophylactic penicillin and pneumococcal vaccines to prevent serious pneumococcal infections.

Idiopathic thrombocytopenic purpura (ITP)

Aetiology

Often occurs after viral infections, especially rubella. Platelet antibodies are usually detectable.

Clinical features

Spontaneous petechiae and superficial bruising (Fig. 188). Other more serious causes of thrombocytopenia must be excluded.

Prognosis

Majority recover spontaneously within a few months; occasionally chronic, requiring splenectomy.

Management

Platelet transfusions if count falls <30 000. Steroids and intravenous gammaglobulin may also be helpful.

Aplastic anaemia

Clinical features

Pallor, anaemia, hirsutism, and palatal petechiae (Fig. 189).

Diagnosis

Blood tests show anaemia, thrombocytopenia, and neutropenia. Bone marrow confirms absence of precursors.

Management

Matched bone marrow transplant or stem cells from umbilical blood may be curative and are now the preferred treatment. Supportive treatment includes blood and platelet transfusions, immunosuppression with corticosteroids, ciclosporin, and antithymocyte or antilymphocyte globulin, or androgens. Early aggressive management of sepsis with broad spectrum antibiotics.

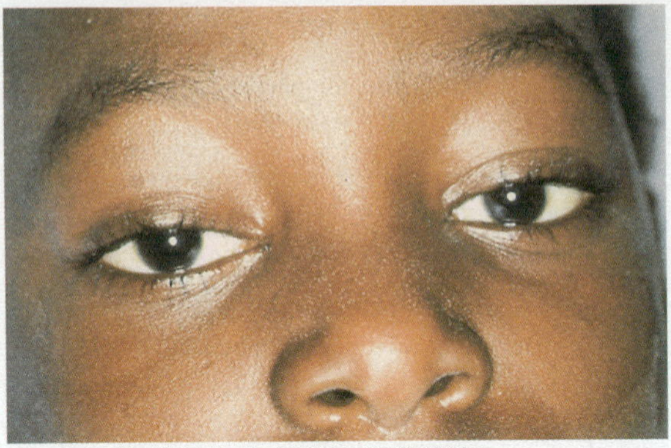

图 187 镰形细胞贫血病的巩膜黄染
Jaundiced sclera in sickle cell anaemia

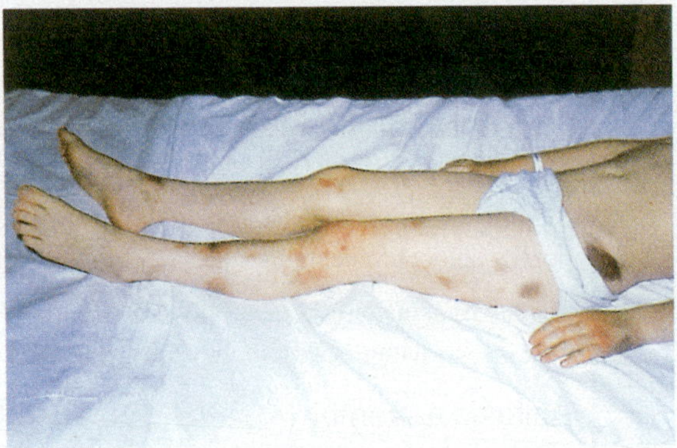

图 188 ITP 的瘀青
Bruising in ITP

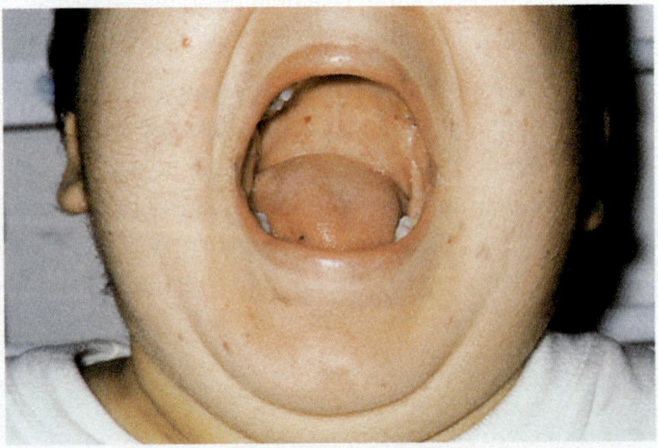

图 189 苍白、多毛症以及脸部和腭的瘀点
Pallor, hisutism and petechiae on face and palate

地中海贫血

病因学和遗传特性

不能合成珠蛋白的α链和β链。是常染色体隐性遗传疾病，如果父母有地中海贫血遗传特性，那么他们的孩子有1/4有纯合子型重型地中海贫血的危险。

临床特征

α地中海贫血在亚洲较为常见。纯合子型α地中海贫血会导致胎儿水肿（图190），并且在宫内或新生儿早期死亡。β地中海贫血主要出现于地中海人群中。当出生后前几个月胎儿血红蛋白水平下降，就会出现严重的贫血，以及由于髓外造血引起的肝脾大，并且有时会发生心力衰竭。代偿性的骨髓增生在大龄儿童会产生特征性的颅骨和面骨增大（图191）。颅骨X光片显示有特征性的垂直短发样骨刺表现。

治疗

终生需规律输血。骨髓配型移植可以治愈疾病，但是可能很难找到合适的供体。

并发症

频繁的输血会引起慢性铁沉积。皮下输注铁螯合剂（去铁敏）可以改善生存情况。如果没有及时治疗慢性铁沉积会在成年早期出现心肌病、生长和青春期发育不良、糖尿病、皮肤色素沉着和肝损害等表现。

产前诊断

可以通过分析胎儿血液珠蛋白链的合成情况或者对绒膜绒毛样本进行DNA检测从而发现患病的胎儿。

出血障碍

病因学

A型血友病（Ⅷ因子缺乏）是最常见的类型。

临床特征

自发性瘀青或在轻微损伤后过度出血而引起关节积血（图192）、深部血肿或黏膜出血。

治疗

外伤的早期治疗和手术操作时静脉输注Ⅷ因子浓缩物可以减少慢性关节损伤。

Thalassaemia

Aetiology and inheritance

Failure of synthesis of alpha or beta globin chains. Autosomal recessive; 1 in 4 risk of homozygous major disease in infants of parents with thalassaemia trait.

Clinical features

Alpha-thalassaemia is more common in Asians. Homozygous α -thalassaemia results in hydrops fetalis (Fig. 190) with intrauterine or early neonatal death. Beta-thalassaemia occurs mainly in Mediterranean populations. When fetal haemoglobin levels decline after the first few months, severe anaemia, hepatosplenomegaly due to extramedullary haemopoiesis, and sometimes cardiac failure occur. Compensatory bone marrow hyperplasia produces characteristic expansion of the skull and facial bones in older children (Fig. 191). Skull X-rays show characteristic hair-on-end appearance.

Management

Lifelong regular blood transfusions. Matched bone marrow transplant is curative, but a suitable donor may be difficult to find.

Complications

Frequent transfusions cause chronic iron overload. Subcutaneous infusions of an iron chelating agent (desferrioxamine) improve survival. Cardiomyopathy occurs in early adult life; growth and puberty failure, diabetes mellitus, skin pigmentation and liver damage are other manifestations of untreated chronic iron overload.

Antenatal diagnosis

Affected fetuses may be detected by analysis of globin chain synthesis of fetal blood or DNA analysis of chorionic villus samples.

Bleeding disorders

Aetiology

Haemophilia A (factor VIII deficiency) is the most common.

Clinical features

Spontaneous bruising or excessive bleeding after minimal trauma cause haemarthrosis (Fig. 192), deep haematomas or mucosal haemorrhage.

Management

Early treatment of trauma and surgical procedures with intravenous factor concentrates may reduce chronic joint damage.

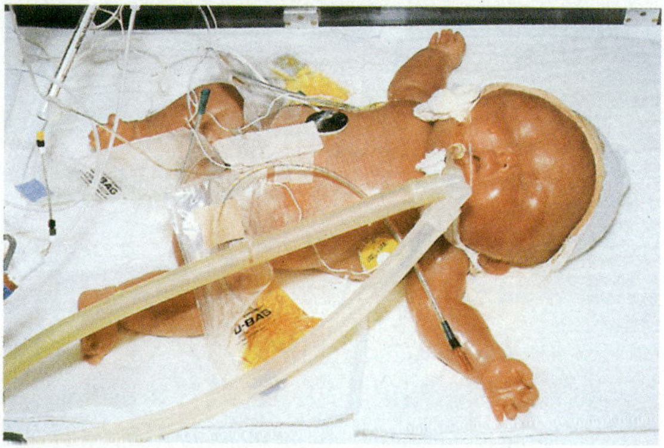

图 190 几乎全身水肿的胎儿水肿
Gross generalized oedema of hydrops fetalis

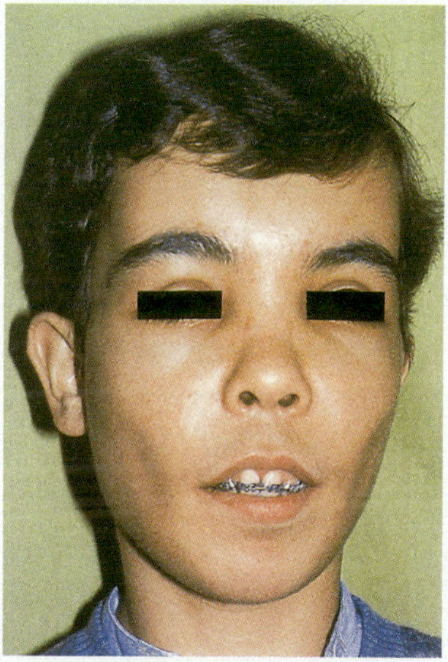

图 191 β 地中海贫血的骨增生
Bone hyperplasia in β-thalassaemia intermedia

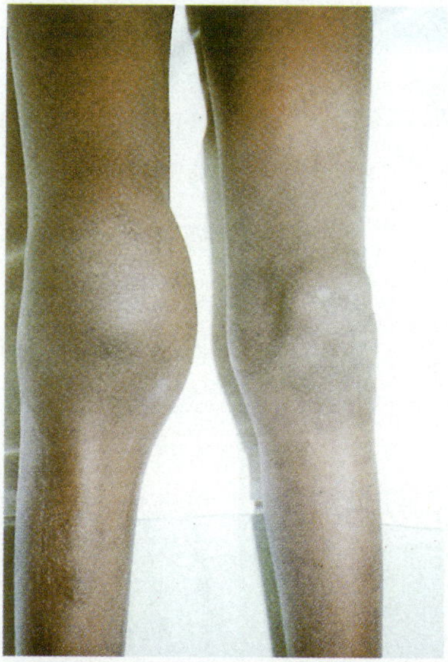

图 192 血友病的关节积血（经由 Dr A. Kilby 许可）
Haemarthrosis in haemophilia (courtesy of Dr A. Kilby)

Wilms瘤（肾母细胞瘤）和神经母细胞瘤

临床特征

无症状的腹部肿块（图193）。在Wilms瘤中通常会有血尿和腹痛。

诊断

在Wilms瘤中，超声显示肾盂肾盏系统变形。在神经母细胞瘤中，腹部X线片显示肿瘤钙化。肾上腺肿瘤使肾移位，但是通常并不会使肾盂肾盏系统变形。尿液儿茶酚胺［香草扁桃酸（VMA）和高香草酸（HVA）］水平升高可对90%的病例确诊神经母细胞瘤的诊断，并且它们也是复发的敏感指标。神经母细胞瘤有时会发生骨转移（图195）。

治疗和预后

Wilms瘤：在手术前进行化疗可以缩小肿块。有时可在术后进行放疗。5年生存率至少是80%。转移较为常见，但是经常对治疗有效。神经母细胞瘤：在放疗后进行外科切除。5年生存率是60%；偶尔有自行恢复的报道。

脑肿瘤

发病率

是儿童恶性肿瘤的第二大肿瘤。

临床特征

头痛、呕吐、共济失调或视物障碍都是较常见的症状。有时会有行为障碍、性格改变、惊厥发生。在脑干肿瘤中会经常发生颅神经麻痹（图194）。

治疗和预后

可进行外科切除，但是通常较困难。髓母细胞瘤对放疗较为敏感，并且目前的5年生存率至少是60%。肿瘤或治疗的长期并发症，尤其是生长和内分泌紊乱，在每一个生存者都会出现。

其他恶性肿瘤

儿童的实体瘤不常见，但可能会有视网膜母细胞瘤、横纹肌肉瘤、骨肉瘤、霍奇金病和淋巴瘤。双侧视网膜母细胞瘤有较高的家族发病率，并且早期治疗的远期生存预后较理想。

Wilms tumour (nephroblastoma) and neuroblastoma

Clinical features

Asymptomatic abdominal mass (Fig. 193). Haematuria and abdominal pain common in Wilms tumour.

Diagnosis

Ultrasound shows distortion of renal pelvicalyceal system in Wilms tumour. Abdominal X-ray may show tumour calcification in neuroblastoma. Adrenal tumours displace the kidney but do not usually distort the pelvicalyceal system. Elevated urinary catecholamine levels (VMA and HVA) confirm diagnosis of neuroblastoma in 90% cases and are a sensitive indicator of recurrence. Bony metastases (Fig. 195) sometimes occur in neuroblastoma.

Management and prognosis

Wilms tumour: chemotherapy reduces tumour mass before surgery. Sometimes postoperative radiotherapy. The 5-year survival is at least 80%. Metastases are common, but frequently respond to therapy. Neuroblastoma: surgical excision followed by radiotherapy. The 5-year survival is 60%; occasional spontaneous recovery reported.

Cerebral tumour

Incidence

Second most common childhood malignancy.

Clinical features

Headache, vomiting, ataxia or visual disturbance are common presenting symptoms. Behavioural disturbance, mood change, convulsions sometimes occur. Cranial nerve palsies (Fig. 194) are often found in brain stem tumours.

Management and prognosis

Surgical resection, but often difficult. Medulloblastomas are often radiosensitive and 5-year survival is now at least 60%. Long-term complications of tumour or treatment, particularly growth and endocrine disturbance, are almost invariable in survivors.

Other malignancies

Solid tumours are uncommon in childhood, but retinoblastoma, rhabdomyosarcoma, osteosarcoma, Hodgkin`s disease, and lymphoma may occur. Bilateral retinoblastoma has a strong familial incidence and a good prognosis for survival with early treatment.

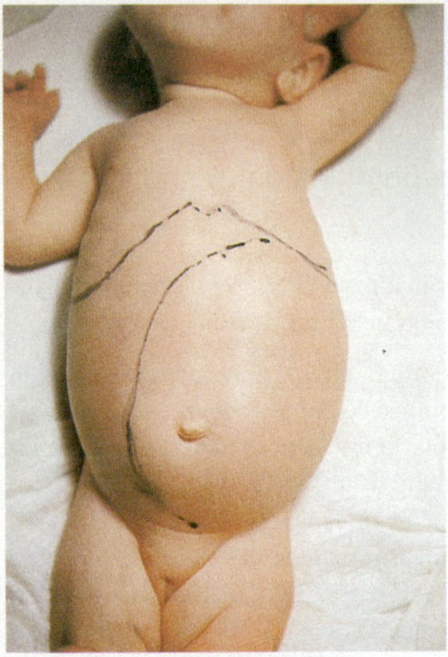

图 193　Wilms 瘤的腹部膨隆
Wilms tumour presenting as abdominal distension

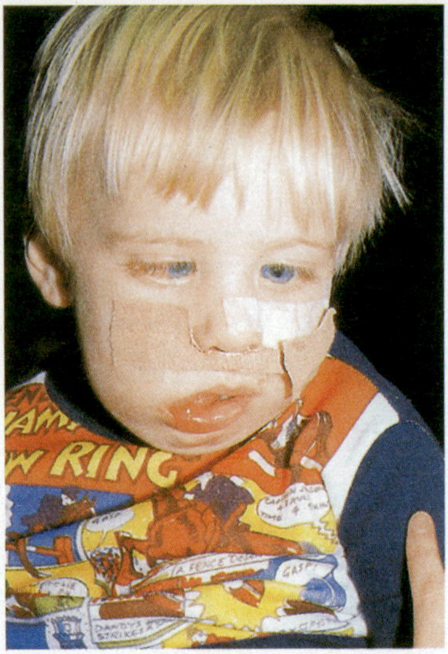

图 194　由于脑干神经胶质瘤导致VI和VII对颅神经麻痹
VI and VII nerve palsies due to brain stem glioma

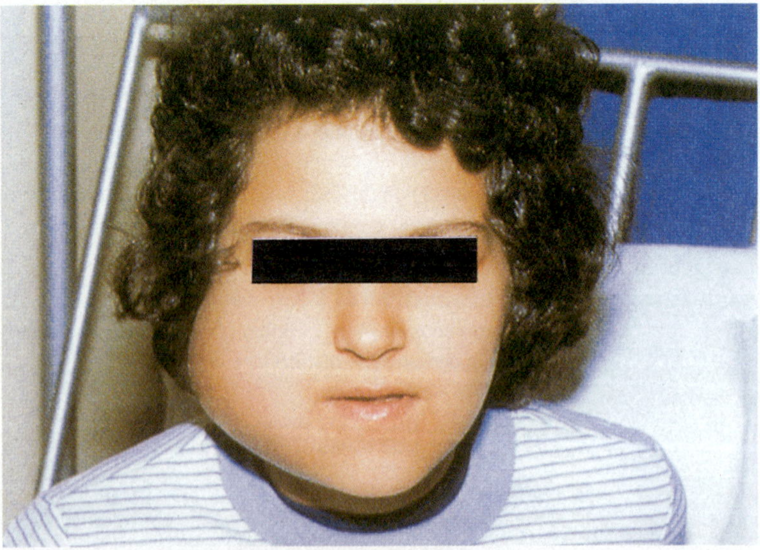

图 195　继发于神经母细胞瘤的下颌骨转移
Secondary neuroblastoma of mandible

常见临床类型

化脓性关节炎

通常突然发作，累及单个关节。受累关节发热、肿胀、疼痛，且因疼痛而使活动受限。金黄色葡萄球菌是最常见的致病菌。外科引流是诊断和治疗较为常用的方法。

风湿热

在发达国家，该病的发生率明显减少。典型的表现为急性游走性多关节炎，伴有发热、皮疹和皮下结节。心脏炎是最严重的长期并发症，会导致永久性的瓣膜损伤。

亨-舍紫癜（过敏性紫癜）

常见的过敏性血管炎，其临床表现较易识别。有特征性的紫癜性皮疹（图 149、150、151 和 198）、迁移性关节炎和关节痛、腹痛和血尿。大多数能够迅速消退，只需要休息和止痛治疗。偶尔经过数月后会有复发。

青少年慢性关节炎(JCA)

该系统性疾病(Still 病)的发病高峰是 1 ～ 5 岁，可同时伴有发热、体重减轻和轻度贫血。在大龄儿童常有大关节（图 197 和 198）和小关节（图 196）反复发作的疼痛性肿胀和僵直。少部分有关节炎的儿童会伴发银屑病，在疾病早期皮肤和指甲的表现可能比较轻微。通过选择合适的抗炎药物进行治疗可以减轻关节炎症。锻炼、理疗、水疗和夜间用夹板固定可以帮助限制关节畸形。急性关节炎症通常会自行缓解，但是有时仅在多年之后才会缓解。

Common clinical forms

Pyogenic arthritis

Usually sudden onset of a single, hot, swollen, tender joint with painful restriction of movement. Staphylococcus aureus is the most common infective organism. Surgical drainage is often necessary for diagnosis and treatment.

Rheumatic fever

There has been a dramatic reduction in the incidence of this disease in developed countries. Classically there is an acute migratory polyarthritis associated with fever, rash and sometimes subcutaneous nodules. Carditis is the most serious long-term complication, resulting in permanent valvular damage.

Henoch-Schönlein purpura

A common allergic vasculitis which causes an easily recognizable clinical picture. There is a characteristic purpuric rash (Figs 149, 150, 151, 198), flitting arthritis or arthralgia, abdominal pain and haematuria. The majority resolve rapidly and require only rest and analgesia. Occasionally recurrent over a period of several months.

Juvenile chronic arthritis (JCA)

The peak incidence of systemic disease (Still's disease) is between 1-5 years of age. Fever, weight loss and mild anaemia are associated findings. Recurrent painful swelling and stiffness of both small (Fig. 196) and large joints (Figs 197 and 198) is common in older children. Psoriasis is associated with a small number of children presenting with arthritis, and skin and nail manifestations may be subtle in the early years of the disease. Joint inflammation can be reduced by appropriate choice of anti-inflammatory drugs. Exercise, physiotherapy, hydrotherapy and night splints help to limit deformity. Acute inflammatory episodes often remit spontaneously, but sometimes only after many years.

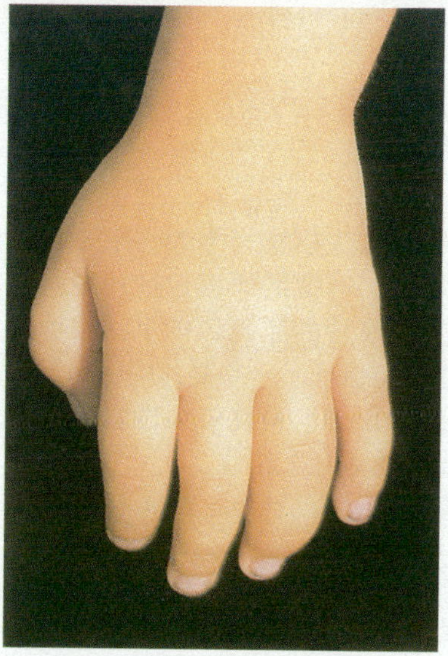

图 196 JCA的手部小关节肿胀(经由 Dr B.Ansell 许可)
Swelling of small joints of the hand in JCA (courtesy of Dr B. Ansell)

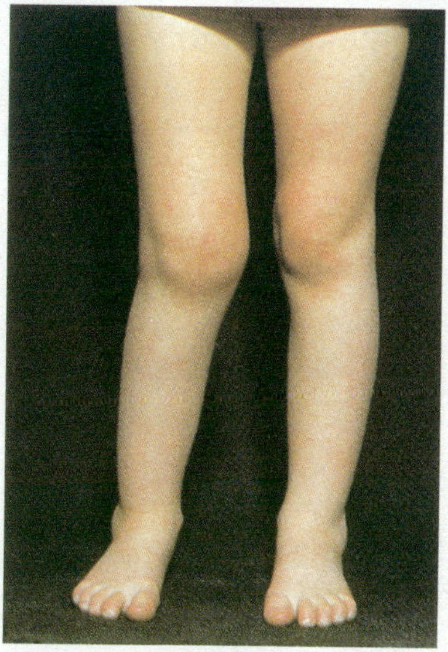

图 197 膝部的单关节炎（经由 Dr B. Ansell 许可)
Monoarthritis of knee (courtesy of Dr B. Ansell)

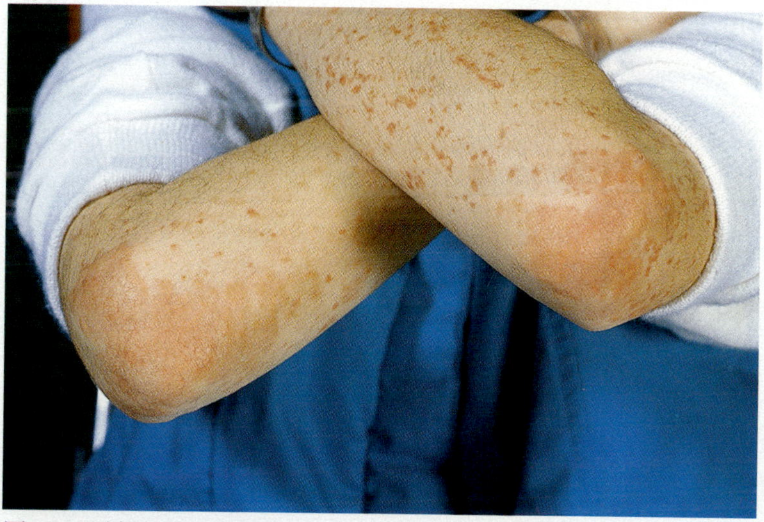

图 198 肘部的亨-舍紫癜
Henoch-Schönlein purpura on the elbows

婴儿松软症

病因学

描述肌张力减退的婴儿在生后第一年的临床表现。有许多可能的潜在原因。麻痹的原因包括神经肌肉障碍和大脑性麻痹。非麻痹的原因包括甲状腺功能减退、营养不良和唐氏综合征。一些婴儿的运动发育虽然延迟，但最终仍然正常（良性先天性肌张力减退）。良性肌张力减退通常有家族性。

临床特征

评估的有效方法是将新生儿从仰卧位拉起到坐位（图 199）。

脊髓性肌萎缩症（韦-霍病）

遗传特性和发病率

常染色体隐性遗传；每 20 000 名出生存活儿中就有 1 名患有该病。

临床特征

通常婴儿自出生后就有软弱无力和全身肌肉松弛（图 200）。一般在生后 12 ~ 18 个月会因为进行性呼吸衰竭而迅速死亡。

产前诊断

目前在一些患病家族中开展。

先天性多关节弯曲

临床特征

屈曲性挛缩、有时会有关节脱臼（图201）以及大肌肉萎缩的临床综合征。

病因学

精确的诊断可能较困难。有时是原发性肌肉发育不全或继发于羊水过少。

预后和治疗

取决于肌肉发育不良的严重程度。长期的理疗可以减轻挛缩。后期的外科治疗可能会有所帮助。

The floppy baby

Aetiology

Describes the clinical condition of the hypotonic infant in the first year of life. There are many possible underlying causes. Paralytic causes include neuromuscular disorders and cerebral palsy. Non-paralytic causes are hypothyroidism, malnutrition and Down syndrome. A few may have delayed, but eventually normal motor development (benign congenital hypotonia). Benign hypotonia is often familial.

Clinical features

A useful method of assessment is to hold the young infant in ventral suspension and pull the infant from supine to sitting posture (Fig. 199).

Spinal muscular atrophy (Werdnig-Hoffmann disease)

Inheritance and incidence

Autosomal recessive inheritance; occurs in 1 in 20 000 live births.

Clinical features

Infants are often weak and floppy from birth (Fig. 200)
Rapidly progressive with death from respiratory failure within 12-18 months.

Antenatal diagnosis

Now available for some affected families.

Arthrogryposis multiplex congenita

Clinical features

Clinical syndrome of flexion contractures and sometimes dislocation of joints (Fig. 201), and gross muscle wasting.

Aetiology

Precise diagnosis may be difficult. Sometimes primary muscle hypoplasia or secondary to oligohydramnios.

Prognosis and management

Depends on severity of muscle hypoplasia. Long-term physiotherapy reduces contractures. Surgery may be helpful later.

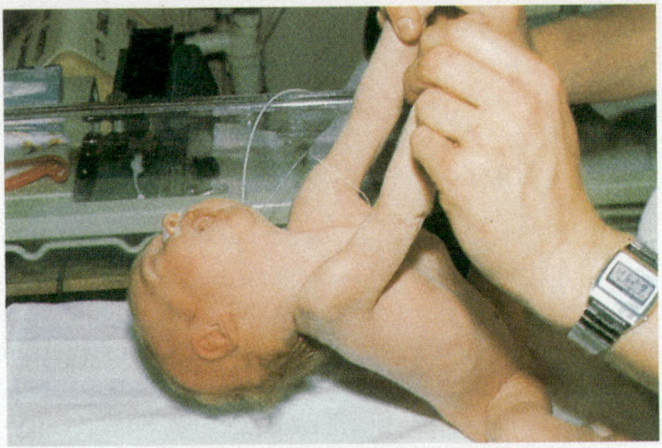

图 199 婴儿松软症明显的头部抬起迟滞
Marked head lag of floppy newborn infant

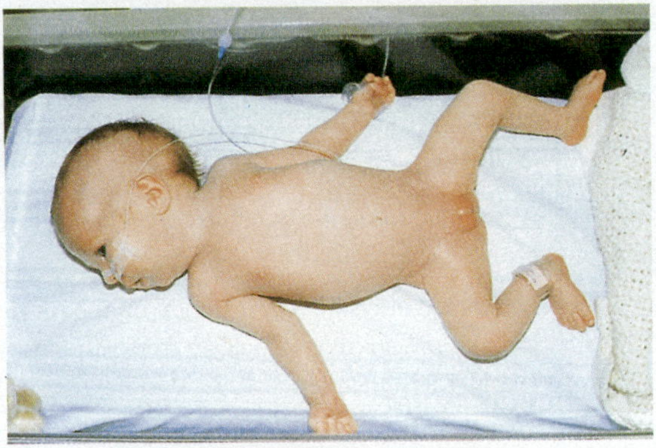

图 200 脊髓性肌萎缩症婴儿的蛙样体位
Frog-like posture of infant with Werdnig-Hoffmann disease

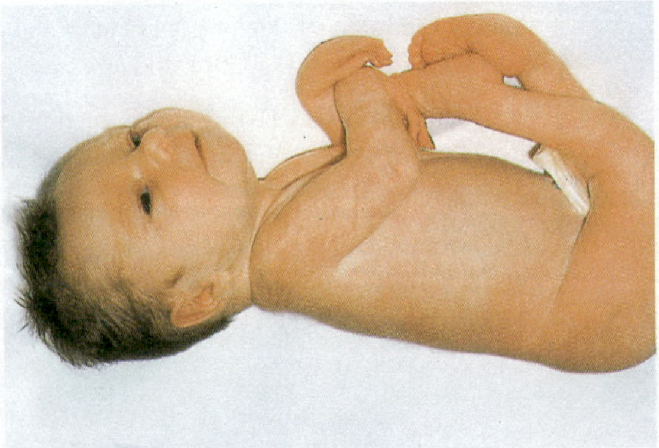

图 201 先天性多关节弯曲
Arthrogryposis multiplex congenita

大脑性瘫痪

发病率和病因学

在出生的存活儿中大约有2‰的发病率。原因一般不明。一些是由于胎儿期或新生儿早期大脑的缺氧性损伤。新生儿卒中发作导致的轻度偏瘫患儿中越来越确定有血栓形成的趋势（如蛋白C、蛋白S、抗凝血酶Ⅲ和Ⅴ因子Leiden）。痉挛性双侧偏瘫在早产儿中较为常见。

临床特征

永久性的、但非进行性的运动和体位障碍。由于患儿在不断地生长发育，所以临床特征经常变化。婴儿通常表现出吮吸无力、喂养困难、肌张力减退、肌张力过高或易激惹。大约 70% 的大脑性瘫痪患儿有痉挛表现：剪刀腿、角弓反张、肌张力过高（图 202）、阵挛和腱反射活跃。可能会累及一个或多个肢体，引起偏瘫、双瘫或四肢瘫痪。约有 10% 的患儿会发生共济失调性大脑性瘫痪伴肌张力减退和肌肉无力。另有 10% 的患儿为舞蹈手足徐动症，表现为特征性的不规则、非自主性运动，并且有时伴有高胆红素血症（核黄疸）。

诊断

大脑性瘫痪一般在出生后前几个月表现并不明显，直到出现运动发育延迟或异常，才变得越来越明显。高危婴儿（早产儿和有无法解释的新生儿癫痫发作史的婴儿）应该在新生儿期进行常规的超声检查和长期的神经发育随访。脑部磁共振检查或CT检查对于寻找病因也有所帮助，但是并不作为常规检查。

并发症

60% 的大脑性瘫痪患儿会有精神发育迟缓、癫痫和感觉障碍。

治疗

进行多学科的评估和长期治疗是有必要的。理疗可以促进正常的运动发育和预防肌肉挛缩。应该避免因长期制动而产生的“风蚀样”畸形（图 203）。

Cerebral palsy

Incidence and aetiology

Approximately 2 per 1000 live births. Cause is often obscure. A few are due to hypoxic brain damage in fetal or early neonatal life. Increasingly, thrombotic tendencies (e.g. protein C, protein S, anti-thrombin 3 and factor V Leiden), are being identified in children with hemipareses secondary to neonatal stroke. Spastic diplegia is more common in preterm infants.

Clinical features

Permanent, but non-progressive disorder of movement and posture. Clinical features often change because the child is continuing to grow and develop. Infants often show poor sucking, feeding difficulties, hypotonia, hypertonia, or irritability. About 70% of children with cerebral palsy have spastic manifestations with scissoring of legs, opisthotonos, hypertonia (Fig. 202), clonus and brisk tendon reflexes. One or several limbs may be involved, giving rise to hemiplegia, diplegia or quadriplegia. Ataxic cerebral palsy with hypotonia and weakness occurs in approximately 10%. Choreoathetosis characterized by irregular involuntary movements accounts for another 10% and is sometimes associated with hyperbilirubinaemia (kernicterus).

Diagnosis

Cerebral palsy is often not apparent for several months, until delayed or abnormal motor development become more obvious. Infants at high risk (e.g. preterm and infants with unexplained neonatal seizures) should have routine ultrasonography in the neonatal period and long-term neurodevelopmental follow-up. Magnetic resonance imaging or computed tomography brain scans are also helpful in establishing a cause, but may not be routinely available.

Complications

Mental retardation, epilepsy and sensory handicap are present in at least 60% of children with cerebral palsy.

Management

A multidisciplinary approach to assessment and long-term management is essential. Physiotherapy may encourage normal motor development and prevent contractures. The 'wind-swept' deformity (Fig. 203) seen after prolonged immobilization should be avoidable.

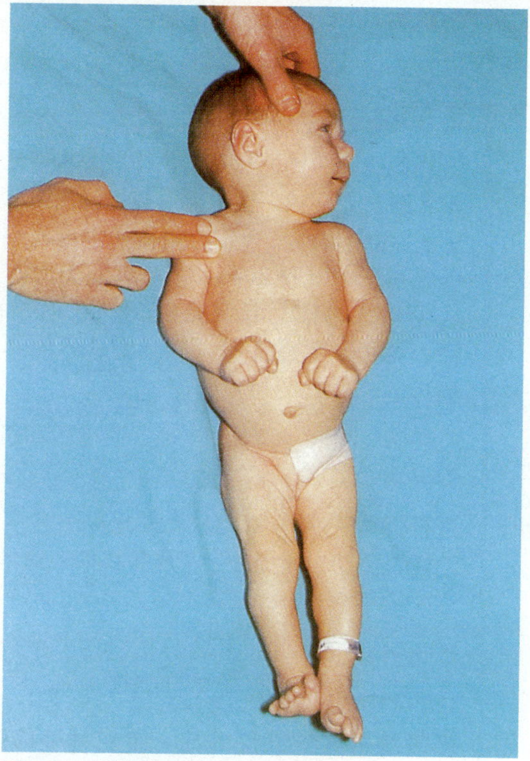

图 202 大脑性瘫痪患儿的夹钳拳
Clenched fists in cerebral palsy

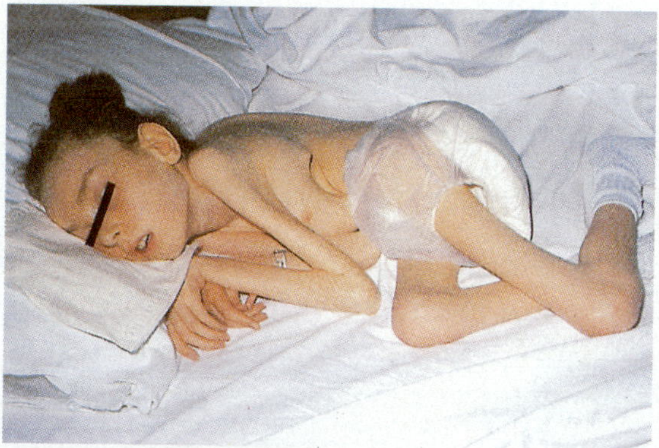

图 203 “风蚀样”畸形
‘Wind-swept’ deformity

进行性假肥大性肌营养不良

发病率 是最常见的肌肉萎缩症，在4000名男婴中就有1名患有此病。

遗传特性 性连锁隐性遗传，但是染色体突变也很常见。女性携带者通常无症状，但是可以被检测出来。通常在出生后前5年内发病，表现为爬楼梯困难和经常摔倒。腓肠肌很肥大（图204），但是软弱无力。当患儿尝试从坐位或躺位立起到站位时，他须先转为俯卧屈膝，再用双手撑住胫、膝及大腿才能站起（Gower征）。

诊断 肌酸磷酸激酶（CPK）生高，肌电图和肌肉活组织检查异常。

病程和预后 进行性肌无力导致大多数患儿在十几岁时只能坐在轮椅里活动。死亡发生于成年早期，通常是由于呼吸道感染引起。

产前诊断 患病男胎可以通过DNA分析检测出来。一些携带异常染色体的女婴有轻度的CPK升高。

多发性神经纤维瘤（冯·雷克林豪森病）

发病率 每3000名出生存活儿中有1名患此病。

遗传特性 常染色体显性遗传，但是至少有50%是由于新的突变而患病。

临床特征 大多数都有皮肤色素沉着不足或色素沉着过度（咖啡牛奶色斑）（图205）。腋窝的色素沉着斑很有特征性。皮下纤维瘤、脊柱侧凸（图206）、外周神经和内脏的神经纤维瘤较为常见。大多数都有骨骼异常和假关节。偶尔可见肢体的偏侧肥大（图207）。

并发症 嗜铬细胞瘤和神经胶质瘤常见。至少50%的患者会发生不同程度的神经系统损害。

Duchenne muscular dystrophy

Incidence

Most common muscular dystrophy; occurs in 1 in 4000 male infants.

Inheritance

Sex-linked recessive, but mutations are frequent. Female carriers are usually asymptomatic but can often be identified. The disorder usually presents within the first 5 years because of difficulty in climbing stairs and frequent falls. The calf muscles are prominent (Fig. 204) though weak. When attempting to rise to standing from sitting or lying position, the boy 'climbs up' his legs using his hands for support (Gower's sign).

Diagnosis

Elevated creatine phosphokinase (CPK); abnormal electromyogram and muscle biopsy.

Course and prognosis

Progressive weakness resulting in most boys being confined to a wheelchair by teenage years. Death, usually from respiratory infections, occurs in early adult life.

Antenatal diagnosis

An affected male fetus can be identified using DNA analysis. Some carrier females have a mildly elevated CPK .

Neurofibromatosis (Von Recklinghausen's disease)

Incidence

1 in 3000 live births.

Inheritance

Autosomal dominant; but at least 50% due to new mutation.

Clinical features

Most have areas of skin hypo- or hyperpigmentation (café-au-lait spots) (Fig. 205). Pigmented spots in the axillae are characteristic. Subcutaneous fibromata, scoliosis (Fig. 206), neurofibromata of peripheral nerves and viscera are common. Many have skeletal abnormalities and pseudoarthroses. Limb hemi-hypertrophy (Fig. 207) occasionally occurs.

Complications

Phaeochromocytoma and glioma are common. At least 50% develop some neurological impairment.

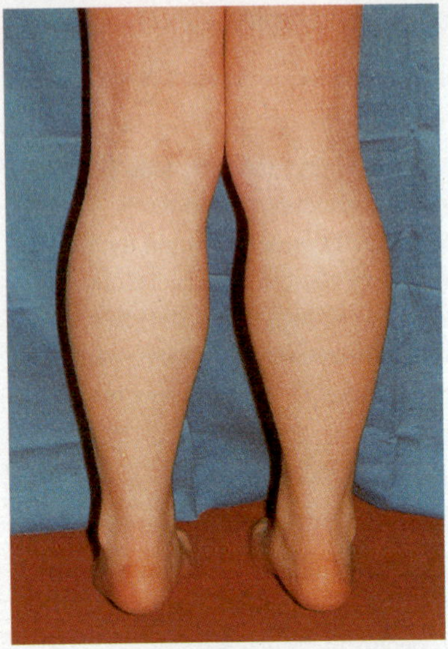

图 204 Duchenne肌营养不良的腓肠肌肥大
Hypertrophied calf muscles in Duchenne muscular dystrophy

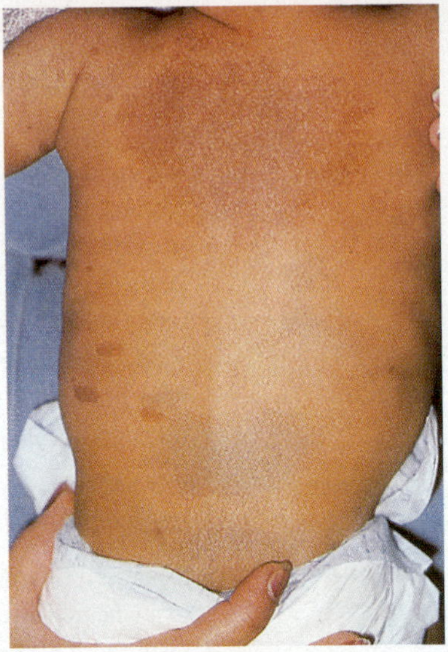

图 205 多发性神经纤维瘤的咖啡牛奶色斑和鲨革斑
Café-au-lait spots and shagreen patch in neurofibromatosis

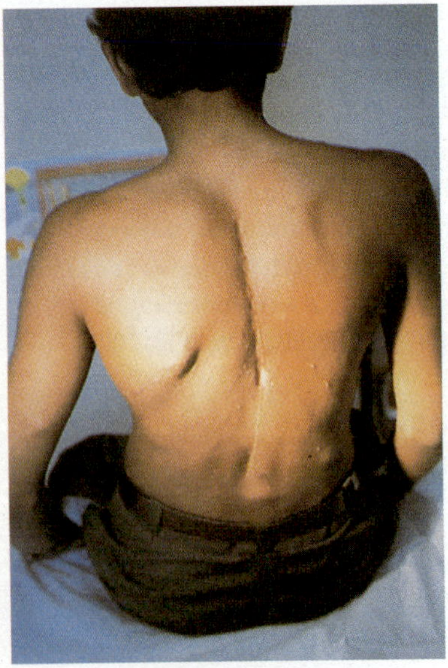

图 206 脊柱侧凸术后
Scoliosis after surgery

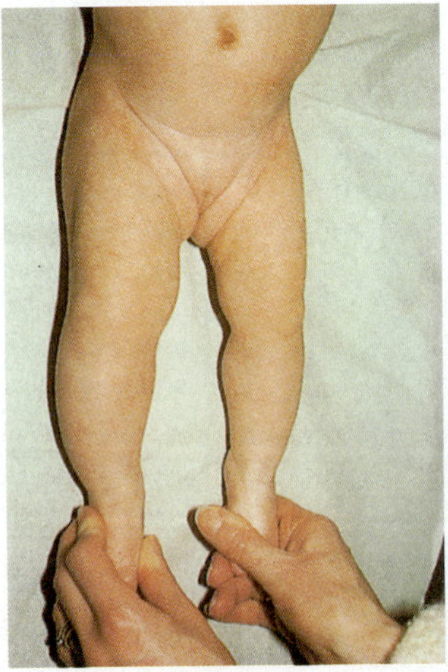

图 207 右腿的偏侧肥大
Hemi-hypertrophy of right leg

脊髓灰质炎

发病率 在免疫接种政策实施较好的国家中并不常见。

临床特征 最初只是轻度病毒感染性疾病，表现为发烧、嗓子痛、头痛和呕吐，持续数天。大约1周后，大约30%的病例会出现更为严重的头痛、颈部僵硬、腿和背部疼痛，以及由于前角细胞损伤导致肌肉麻痹而引起的进行性不对称肌肉软弱无力。

病程和预后 在一些严重的病例中，可能会由于呼吸衰竭和急性延髓性麻痹而死亡。大多数病例在12～18个月后，会逐渐改善。许多孩子会残留肌肉萎缩和麻痹（图208）。

重症肌无力

发病率 在儿童早期不常见。发病高峰期为青春期的女孩儿。

病因学 是自身免疫性疾病，在大多数病例中可以检测到抗胆碱酯酶抗体。

临床特征 逐步进展的肌肉无力，早期表现为疲劳。面部表情丧失、手臂无力、咀嚼困难和上睑下垂（图209）都很常见。如果母亲有此病，那么抗体会通过胎盘进入胎儿体内，从而使新生儿有暂时性的重症肌无力。

诊断 临床上通过静脉注射乙基二甲胺（滕西隆，Tensilon）能使症状迅速改善，从而进一步确诊该病。

治疗 运用长效抗胆碱酯酶药，如吡斯的明。进行胸腺切除术也有所帮助。

Poliomyelitis

Incidence

Uncommon in countries with a successful immunization policy.

Clinical features

Initially a mild viral illness with fever, sore throat, headache and vomiting, lasting several days. About 1 week later, in approximately 30% of cases, there are more severe symptoms of headache, neck stiffness, leg and back pains, and progressive asymmetrical weakness with muscular paralysis due to anterior horn cell damage.

Course and prognosis

In severe cases, death may occur from respiratory failure and bulbar paralysis in the acute illness. In the majority there is gradual improvement over 12-18 months. Many children have residual muscle wasting and paralysis (Fig. 208).

Myasthenia gravis

Incidence

Uncommon in early childhood. Peak incidence in adolescent girls.

Aetiology

Autoimmune disorder; anticholinesterase antibodies can be demonstrated in the majority.

Clinical features

Gradual onset of muscle weakness, with early fatigue. Loss of facial expression, arm weakness, chewing difficulty and ptosis (Fig. 209) are common. A transient form of myasthenia gravis occurs in newborn infants of mothers with the disease due to transplacental passage of antibodies.

Diagnosis

Clinically confirmed by showing prompt improvement with intravenous edrophonium (Tensilon).

Management

Long-acting anticholinesterase drugs such as pyridostigmine. Thymectomy often helpful.

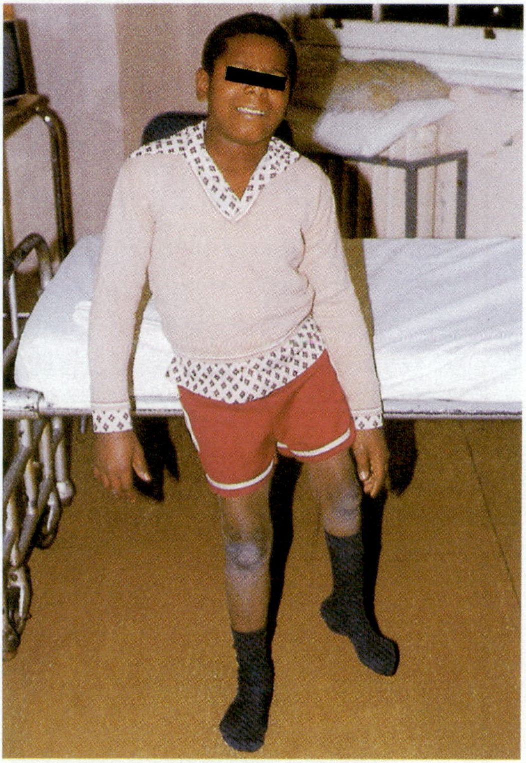

图 208 陈旧性脊髓灰质炎患腿变短
Old poliomyelitis with shortening of leg

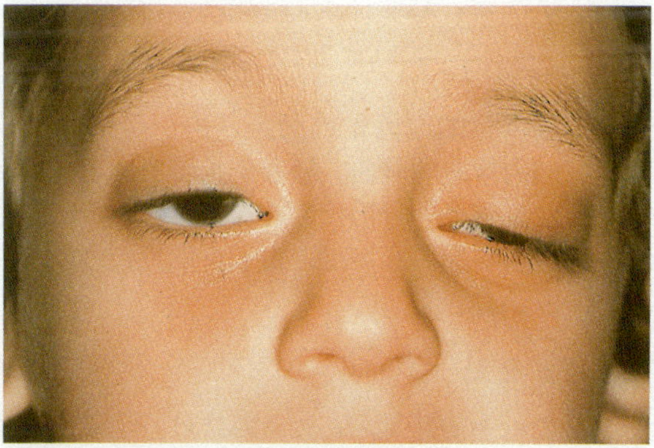

图 209 重症肌无力的上睑下垂
Ptosis in myasthenia gravis

脊柱侧凸

病因学 通常为特发性，主要发生在青春期的女孩儿。

临床特征 让孩子向前弯腰就能很明显的察觉脊柱弯曲。通常是无症状的，但是有外观上的畸形。严重的脊柱侧凸可以引起呼吸困难或脊髓并发症。中线损伤，如血管瘤（图 210）、多毛痣或脂肪瘤，可能暗示有潜在的脊椎异常，尤其当这些症状出现于腰骶位时。

治疗 给予支架治疗，或当畸形进行性加重时给予外科矫正。

腿和脚的姿态性畸形

常见临床类型

弓形腿

在出生后前2年，正常孩子的胫骨有向外弯曲和内旋的趋势。当开始学习走路时，这种弓形腿外观（图 211）常常更为明显。一般会自行改善。

膝外翻

2岁以后，可能会由于股骨髁的生长不相同而引起膝外翻体位（图 212）。女孩的发病率较高。一般会逐渐改善，到 6~7 岁时腿通常会变直。

趾朝内

最常见的原因是内翻跖，由于足前段内收使得脚有向内弯曲的倾向。随着生长会有改善的趋势，但是偶尔也需要外科治疗。在女孩股骨过度内旋很常见，它也会引起内八字足，由于可以自行缓解，所以没有必要治疗。

重叠趾

小趾重叠于第4趾上（图213） 很常见，而且大多是双侧的。如果有穿鞋不适时，可以进行外科纠治，一般在儿童后期会有胼胝形成。

Orthopaedic problems

Scoliosis

Aetiology

Usually idiopathic; occurs mainly in adolescent girls.

Clinical features

Spinal curvature is best detected by asking the child to bend forwards. Usually asymptomatic, but is a cosmetic deformity. Severe scoliosis may cause respiratory embarrassment or spinal cord complications. Midline lesions, such as haemangiomas (Fig. 210), hairy naevi, or lipomas, may indicate an underlying vertebral anomaly, particularly when they occur in the lumbosacral region.

Management

Bracing or surgical correction when deformity progresses.

Postural deformities of the leg and foot

Common clinical types

Bow legs

In the first 2 years of life, the tibia of the normal child has an outward curve and internal rotation. This bow-legged appearance (Fig. 211) is often more apparent when walking begins. Spontaneous improvement occurs.

Knock-knees

After 2 years of age, there may be unequal growth of the femoral condyles which gives rise to the knock-knee posture (genu valgum) (Fig. 212). Girls are more commonly affected. Gradual improvement occurs and by 6-7 years of age, the legs are usually straight.

In-toeing

The most common cause is metatarsus varus. The feet tend to curve medially because of adduction of the forefoot. The natural tendency is for improvement with growth, although surgery is occasionally necessary. Excessive internal rotation of the femora is common in girls and this also causes in-toeing. Treatment is unnecessary because spontaneous resolution occurs.

Overlapping toes

Overlapping of the little toe over the fourth toe (Fig. 213) is common and often bilateral. Surgical correction may be required as shoes may be uncomfortable and callous formation is common in later childhood.

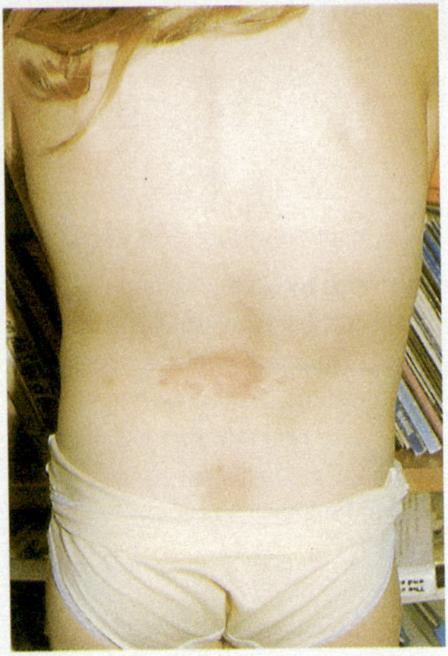

图 210 脊柱侧凸和中线血管瘤
Scoliosis and midline haemangioma

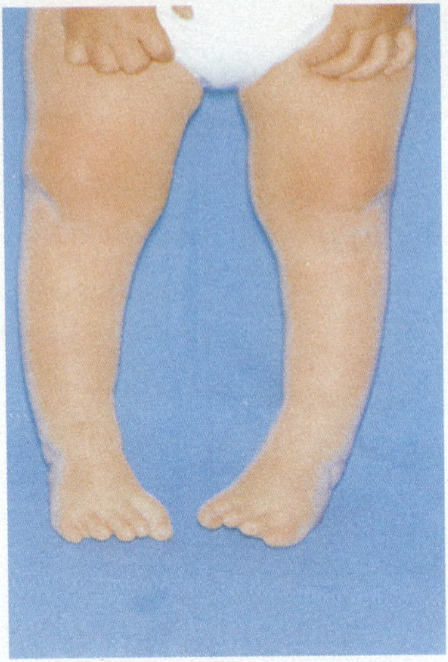

图 211 婴儿正常的弓形腿
Normal bow legs in infancy

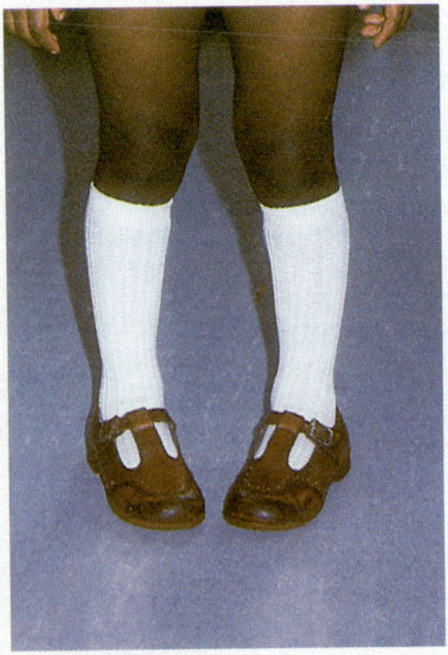

图 212 膝外翻
Knock-knee

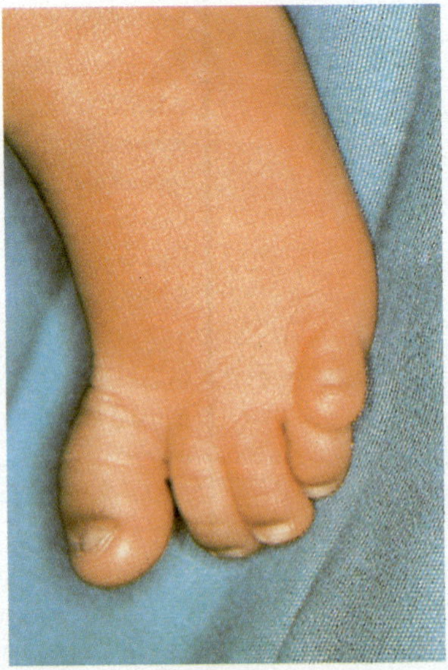

图 213 小趾重叠
Overriding little toe

肢体的发育异常

发病率	常见，尤其是手臂和手的异常。
病因学	一般不明。桡骨缺失或肢体缺如方面的缺陷可能是由于胎儿时期大血管的破坏损伤而引起。母亲在孕早期服用药物如反应停，会造成短肢畸形。
临床特征	**多指（趾）畸形**：额外的手指（图214）和脚趾非常常见，并且一般是常染色体显性遗传。
治疗	手上额外的手指一般需要在生后早期进行外科切除。脚的多趾畸形当儿童长大穿鞋不适时，就需要进行外科切除。
临床特征	**并指（趾）畸形**：并指，尤其在第2和第3脚趾间极为常见，并且没有功能上的影响。
治疗	手的并指畸形不常见，但是如果影响到功能和外观时，就需要外科治疗。
临床特征	**缺肢畸形**：有时可见桡骨和拇指缺失，并伴随有血小板减少或贫血。有时会发生手指缺失（图 215)。手部的完全缺失是最常见的肢体缺如畸形。有时几乎整个肢体都缺失——短肢畸形（图 74)。
治疗	当有上肢的缺失异常时，应该在学习需要手部协调性技能的年龄之前安装替代的假肢。
临床特征	**爪样畸形**：爪样手（图216）和脚都是不常见的畸形，严重影响功能。
治疗	一般考虑进行外科手术，但并非都有必要。

Developmental limb anomalies

Incidence

Common, particularly anomalies of the hand and arms.

Aetiology

Usually unknown. Absent radius or limb reduction defects may occur after a major vascular catastrophe in fetal life. Phocomelia is known to occur with maternal ingestion of drugs such as thalidomide in early pregnancy.

Clinical features

Polydactyly: extra digits of the hands (Fig. 214) and feet are extremely common and are often of autosomal dominant inheritance.

Management

Extra digits on the hand usually require surgical excision in early life. Polydactyly of the toes may require excision as the provision of comfortable footwear is difficult when the child is older.

Clinical features

Syndactyly: webbing, particularly of the 2nd and 3rd toes is extremely common and is never of any functional significance.

Management

Syndactyly of the fingers is uncommon, but surgery will be necessary as it is of functional as well as cosmetic significance.

Clinical features

Amputation deformities: absent radius and thumb is sometimes found in association with thrombocytopenia or anaemia. Missing digits (Fig. 215) sometimes occur. Complete absence of the hand is the most common limb reduction deformity. Sometimes almost the whole limb is missing — phocomelia (see Fig. 74).

Management

When there are upper limb reduction anomalies, prosthetic substitutes should be provided before the age of acquisition of skills requiring hand coordination.

Clinical features

Claw deformities: claw hand (Fig. 216) and foot are uncommon anomalies of major functional significance.

Management

Surgery is usually considered, but is not always necessary.

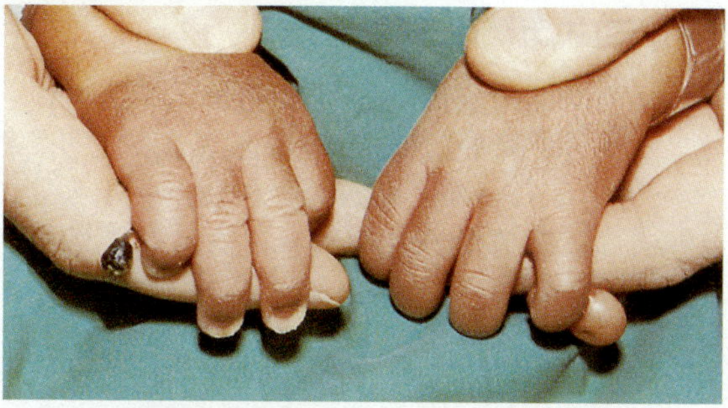

图 214 双侧的多指畸形
Bilateral polydactyly

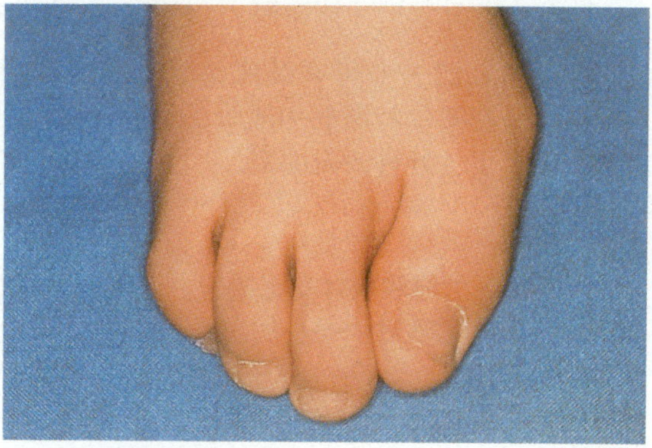

图 215 脚趾缺失
Missing digit

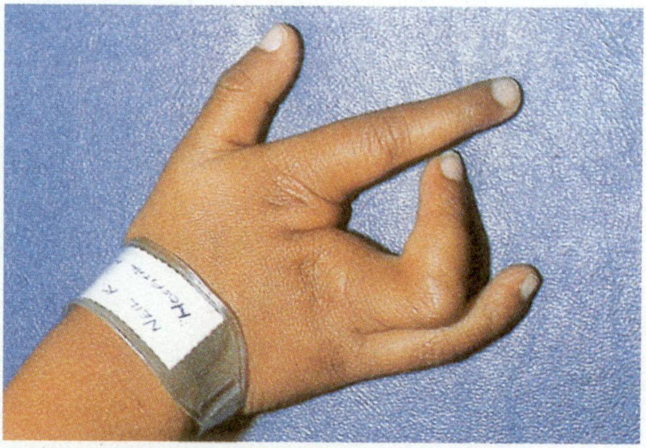

图 216 爪样手
Claw hand

髋关节障碍

发病率和病因学

暂时的滑膜炎（髋关节刺激）或外伤都是跛行和髋关节疼痛最常见的原因。股骨头缺血性坏死（佩尔特斯病，Perthes' disease）一般发生于5～10岁的男孩儿。肥胖的十几岁男孩儿有股骨上端骨骺滑脱的危险。

临床特征

通常是突然发生的跛行和髋关节疼痛。下肢外展、伸展和内旋受限。

诊断

X线片可以诊断佩尔特斯病（图217）和股骨头骨骺滑脱。刺激性髋关节需要在排除了感染和特殊的关节和骨异常后才能诊断。

治疗

刺激性髋关节可在卧床休息数天或数周后得到恢复。在佩尔特斯病和股骨头骨骺滑脱中可能需要肢体牵引、外科或内固定。

骨折

临床特征

疼痛、肿胀和肢体功能缺失。并不一定总能得到其外伤史，尤其对于很小的患儿。对于＜1000g的极低出生体重儿(extremely low birth weight， ELBW)和＜26孕周的婴儿，尤其是那些需要长期胃肠外营养的婴儿，早产骨质减少（新生儿佝偻病）和病理性骨折的危险性比较高。

治疗

在儿童，由于在生长过程中最终都会有较好的重新塑形结果，所以最佳的解剖复位一般没有太大的必要。小婴儿的肱骨骨折（一般是由于产伤）仅需要衣领－袖口样悬带吊挂（图218）即可。小儿骨痂的形成和愈合较为迅速。甚至是股骨骨折也能在支架牵引制动（图219）数周后快速治愈。ELBW婴儿应该每天至少给予400U的维生素D，以及长期充分的磷酸盐摄入。

并发症

动脉缺血或神经损伤都是任何骨折的主要并发症。

Hip disorders

Incidence and aetiology

Transient synovitis (irritable hip), or trauma is most common cause of limp or hip pain. Avascular necrosis of femoral head (Perthes' disease) occurs in boys 5-10 years of age. Obese teenage boys are at risk of slipped upper femoral epiphyses.

Clinical features

Usually sudden onset of limp and hip pain. There is restriction of abduction, extension and internal rotation.

Diagnosis

X-rays are diagnostic in Perthes' disease (Fig. 217) and slipped femoral epiphyses. Irritable hip is diagnosed after exclusion of infection and specific joint and bone disorders.

Management

Irritable hip recovers with a few days or weeks of bed-rest. Limb traction, surgery or internal fixation may be necessary in Perthes' disease and slipped femoral epiphyses.

Fractures

Clinical features

Pain, swelling and loss of function of a limb. A history of trauma is not always obtained, particularly in the very young. Extremely low birth weight infants (ELBW) <1000 g birth weight and <26 weeks' gestation, particularly those requiring prolonged parenteral nutrition, are at high risk of osteopenia of prematurity (neonatal rickets) and pathological fractures.

Management

Exact anatomical repositioning is not always necessary in children, as efficient remodelling ensures a good end result. Fracture of the humerus in young infants (usually due to birth trauma) requires only a collar-and-cuff sling (Fig. 218). Callus formation and healing is more rapid in young children. Even a major fracture of the femur will heal rapidly after a few weeks of immobilization in gallows traction (Fig. 219). ELBW infants should receive at least 400 U vitamin D daily and adequate long term phosphate intake.

Complications

Arterial ischaemia or nerve injury are the major complications of any fracture.

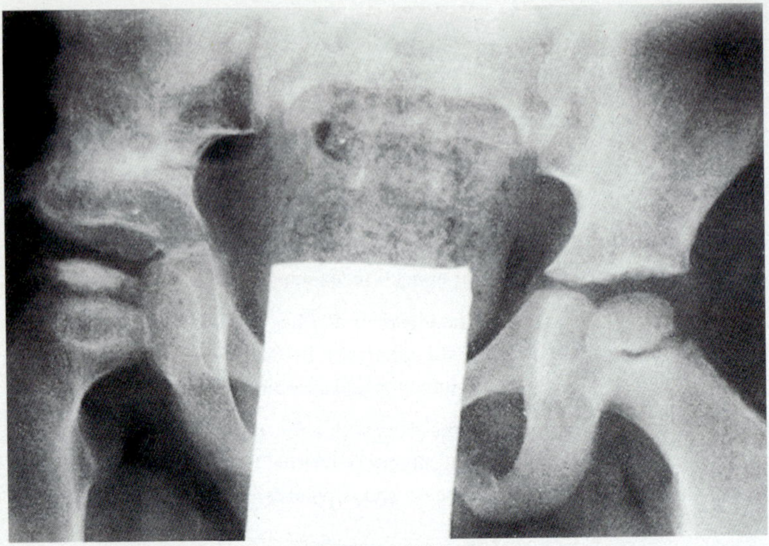

图 217　佩尔特斯病右侧髋关节的 X 线片
X-ray of Perthes' disease of right hip

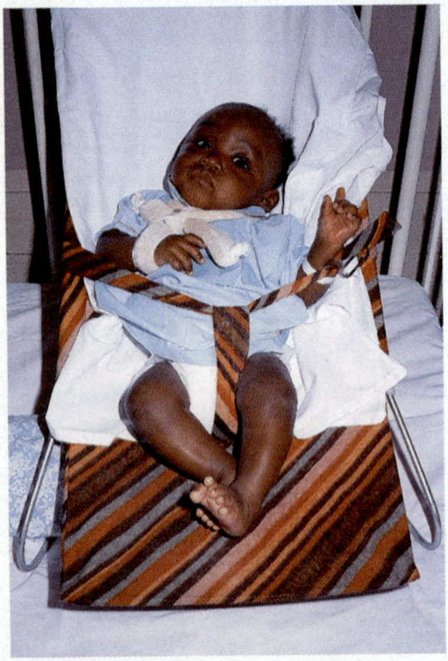

图 218　衣领－袖口样悬带
Collar-and-cuff sling

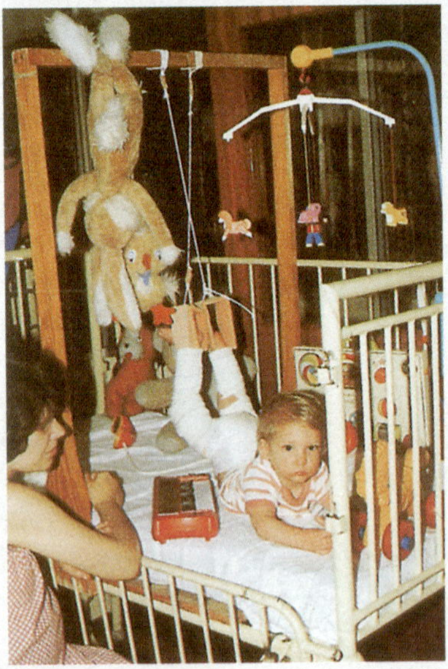

图 219　支架牵引。下肢牵引，但是仍有部分可以活动
Gallows traction. Legs in traction, but still partly mobile

腹股沟疝

发病率

非常常见的疾病，需要在婴儿期进行外科治疗。每50个出生存活男婴中就有1个，最高发病率出现于出生后的前3个月内。

病因学

鞘状突持续性的开放，伴随有小肠的疝出。

临床特征

在婴儿哭闹或用力时，可看到腹股沟区或阴囊部位出现间歇性肿胀（图 220）。疝一般可以较容易地回纳复位，但是如果无法复位，就有较高的绞窄危险性。

治疗

如果一旦诊断为单纯性疝，应立即施行外科修复（疝修补术）。对于有紧张、疼痛、不能复位性肿胀的绞窄疝，有时伴有肠梗阻体征（如呕吐、腹胀），需要外科急症手术。

脐疝

发病率

大约有 20% 的婴儿和 60% 的黑人婴儿会发生脐疝。早产儿有较高的发病率。

临床特征

脐部腹壁中央的缺损，伴有肠疝入冗余皮肤中（图 221）。当哭闹、用力或咳嗽时，覆盖在疝囊表面的皮肤会变得紧绷、发亮和带有蓝色，但是没有疼痛。当孩子安静地平躺或睡觉时，脐疝一般会很容易地复位。

意义

仅仅是外观上的畸形。在中央脐疝绞窄一般很少见，但绞窄可能发生于脐旁疝中临近脐部的（腹白线缺损）。

治疗

大多数在生后前几年内会自行关闭，偶尔需要在3岁左右进行外科修补术。绑扎法不能促进自行关闭。

脐肉芽肿

柔软、有弹性、粉红色的脐部肿块（图 222），常伴有血清血液性分泌物。局部应用硝酸银可能会促进消退，但是大多数不需要治疗。

Inguinal hernia

Incidence
Most common condition requiring surgery during infancy; 1 in 50 live male births, highest incidence in first 3 months of life.

Aetiology
Persistent patency of the processus vaginalis, accompanied by herniation of small bowel.

Clinical features
Intermittent swelling in inguinal region (Fig. 220) or scrotum, often noticed after crying or straining. Herniae are usually easily reducible, but high risk of strangulation if irreducible.

Management
Surgical repair (herniorraphy) as soon as possible after diagnosis of an uncomplicated hernia. Strangulation, with a tense, tender, irreducible swelling sometimes accompanied by signs of gut obstruction (e.g. vomiting, abdominal distension) is a surgical emergency.

Umbilical hernia

Incidence
Approximately 20% of infants and 60% of black infants. High incidence in preterm.

Clinical features
Central defect in abdominal wall at umbilicus, with herniation of bowel into redundant skin (Fig. 221). On crying, straining or coughing, the skin covering the bowel-filled hernia often becomes tense, shiny and bluish but is not painful. Umbilical herniae always reduce easily when the infant is lying quietly or when asleep.

Significance
Cosmetic deformity only. Strangulation is extremely rare in central umbilical herniae, but may occur in para-umbilical herniae (defect in linea alba adjacent to umbilicus).

Management
Most close spontaneously within the first few years of life; occasionally surgical repair around 3 years of age. Strapping does not hasten spontaneous resolution.

Umbilical granuloma

Soft, spongy, pink umbilical mass (Fig. 222) which is often accompanied by sero-sanguinous discharge. Topical application of silver nitrate may hasten resolution but most do not require treatment.

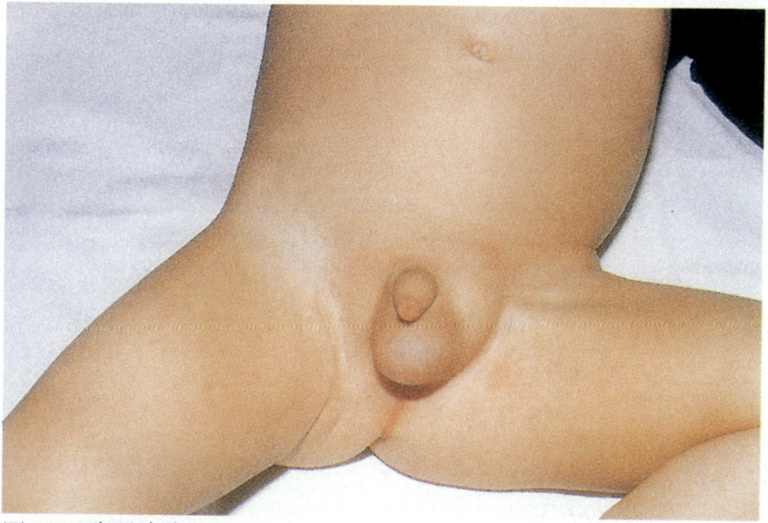

图 220 腹股沟疝
Inguinal hernia

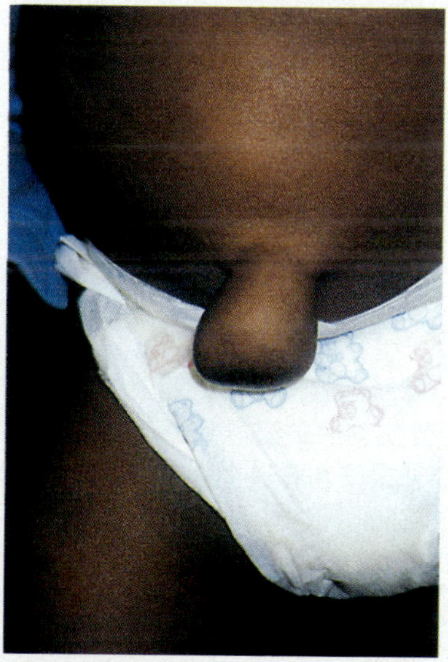

图 221 脐疝
Umbilical hernia

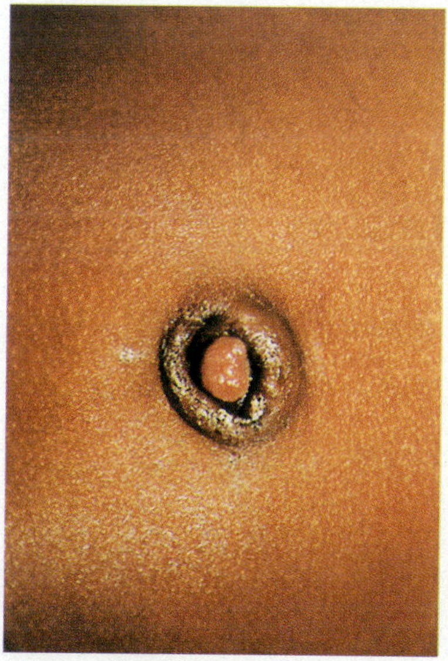

图 222 脐肉芽肿
Umbilical granuloma

睾丸鞘膜积液

发病率和病因学 常见，鞘状突开放未闭。

临床特征 在睾丸前方有无痛、充满液体的囊肿，睾丸通常可在阴囊里很容易触及。半透明，可透光（图223）；其内容物不能被压力排空，虽然在大小上会有所变化。由于它不能进入腹股沟环而能与疝相鉴别。

治疗 大多数可以在出生后第1年自行恢复，但是那些持续时间较长的患儿则需要外科手术治疗。

尿道下裂

发病率 阴茎头尿道下裂较为常见；每350个男性婴儿中就有1个。

临床特征 尿道口位于阴茎腹侧，接近正常的开口位置（图224）。下裂严重程度不同，从阴茎头口到阴囊或会阴部位。通常伴有冗长的背侧包皮覆盖，有时还会伴有阴茎向腹侧弯曲，称为痛性阴茎勃起（图 225）。

治疗 轻度的阴茎头尿道下裂不伴痛性阴茎勃起通常无关紧要，但是一般需要进行小的矫形外科手术。如果尿道口的位置接近阴茎头，或者如果有痛性阴茎勃起，则提示需进行外科修复手术。包皮环切术应该在外科矫正手术完成后再进行，因为包皮有可能用于尿道成形术中。

膀胱外翻

发病率 很罕见，男性较为常见。

临床特征 耻骨联合广泛分离，膀胱向腹侧疝出，膀胱黏膜暴露（图226），并且由于骨盆盆底缺陷导致直肠脱垂。通常伴有尿道上裂、睾丸未降和腹股沟疝。在女性，阴蒂常被隔膜分开或具有两个阴蒂。

治疗 外科重建比较困难。排尿节制罕见。

Hydrocele

Incidence and aetiology

Common; patent processus vaginalis.

Clinical features

Painless, fluid-filled cyst anterior to testes which is usually easily palpable within the scrotum. Brightly translucent (Fig. 223) and not emptied by pressure, although it may vary in size. Can be differentiated from a hernia because it does not extend up to the inguinal ring.

Management

Majority resolve spontaneously in the first year of life, but those presenting later often require surgery.

Hypospadias

Incidence

Glandular hypospadias is common; 1 in 350 male infants.

Clinical features

The urethral orifice is situated on the ventral aspect of the penis at a site proximal to the normal opening (Fig. 224), with severity varying from a glandular orifice to a scrotal or perineal site. Usually accompanied by a redundant dorsal hooded prepuce and sometimes associated with ventral curvature called chordee (Fig. 225).

Management

Mild glandular hypospadias without chordee is usually insignificant but minor cosmetic surgery is usually required. Surgical repair is indicated if the urethral orifice is situated proximal to the glans, or if chordee is present. Circumcision should be delayed until corrective surgery is performed, as the prepuce may be required for urethroplasty.

Ectopia vesicae

Incidence

Very rare; more common in males.

Clinical features

Wide separation of pubic symphysis with ventral herniation of bladder, exposure of bladder mucosa (Fig. 226) and a deficiency of pelvic floor leading to rectal prolapse. The condition is often accompanied by epispadias, undescended testis and an inguinal hernia. In the female, the clitoris is frequently septate or duplicated. Abnormalities of the kidneys are common.

Management

Surgical reconstruction is difficult. Continence is rare.

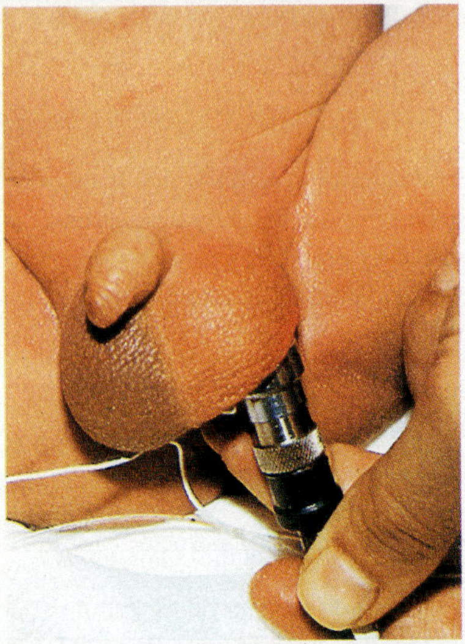

图 223 睾丸鞘膜积液的透照法检查
Transillumination of hydrocele

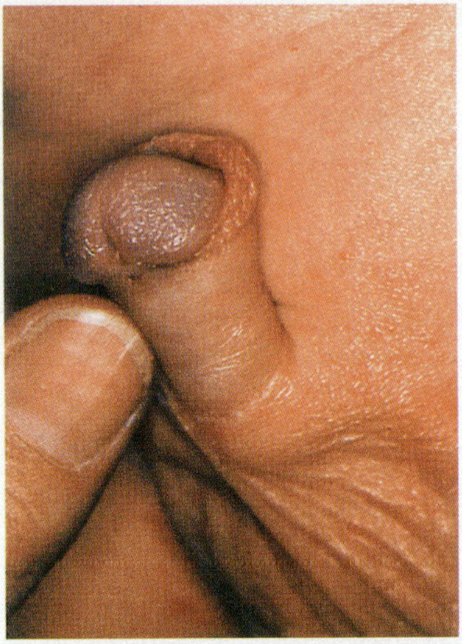

图 224 尿道下裂，背侧有包皮覆盖
Hypospadias with dorsal hooded prepuce

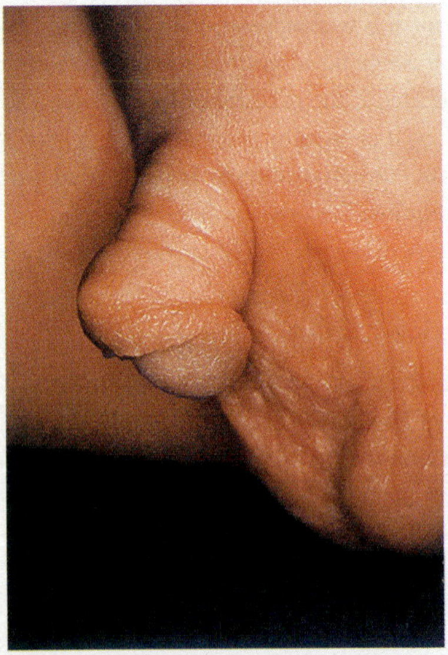

图 225 阴茎向腹侧弯曲（痛性阴茎勃起）
Ventral curvature of penis (chordee)

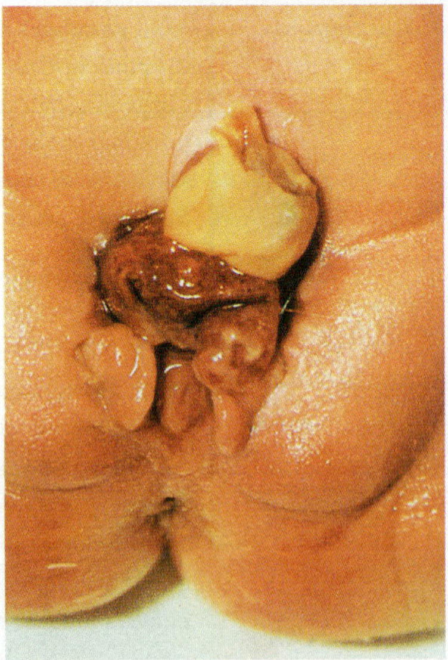

图 226 膀胱外翻
Ectopia vesicae

睾丸未降（隐睾）

发病率 睾丸未降在小婴儿很常见，尤其是早产儿（图227）。

临床特征 活跃的提睾反射引起睾丸回缩极其常见，并且也完全正常。双侧的睾丸未降（隐睾症）常伴有阴囊发育不良（图 228）。

检查 腹股沟区域的超声检查将会提示睾丸在腹股沟管内。有隐睾症的婴儿需要进行染色体分析，排除男性化综合征（如先天性肾上腺增生）。

治疗 98%的病例睾丸会自行下降。如果睾丸到1岁时还未下降就需进行手术探查和睾丸固定术。

包皮环切术

在儿童早期包皮是紧贴在阴茎头上，回缩是没有必要的。几年之后会自行分离。包皮环切术的指征是包茎、嵌顿包茎、反复发作的阴茎头炎和反复发作的尿道感染伴膀胱 - 输尿管反流。

阴道缺损

发病率 不常见。

临床特征 处女膜闭锁是罕见的情况，可能出现在新生儿期，会在闭锁的膜下聚积较多的黏液（阴道黏液蓄积），并在小阴唇间向外膨出。阴道旁囊肿（图229）可能会与处女膜闭锁相混淆，但是前者可以用探针沿着囊肿旁边进入阴道。

治疗 处女膜闭锁需要外科引流和切除膜性组织。阴道旁囊肿通常会自行破裂。

Undescended testes

Incidence

Undescended testes are common in young infants, particularly preterm (Fig. 227).

Clinical features

Retractile testes due to an active cremasteric reflex are extremely common and entirely normal. Bilateral undescended testes (cryptorchidism) are associated with hypoplastic scrotum (Fig. 228).

Investigations

Ultrasound examination of the inguinal region will identify testes in the inguinal canal. Infants with cryptorchidism will require chromosome analysis and exclusion of virilizing syndromes (e.g. congenital adrenal hyperplasia).

Management

Some 98% of testes descend spontaneously. Exploration and orchidopexy is indicated if the testes fail to descend by 1 year of age.

Circumcision

The prepuce is closely adherent to the glans during early childhood and retraction is unnecessary and undesirable. Spontaneous separation occurs after some years. The only medical indications for circumcision are phimosis, paraphimosis, recurrent balanitis and recurrent urinary tract infections associated with vesicoureteric reflux.

Vaginal defects

Incidence

Uncommon.

Clinical features

Imperforate hymen is a rare condition which may present in the neonatal period with an accumulation of mucus beneath the imperforate membrane (mucocolpos) which bulges out between the labia minora. Paravaginal cysts (Fig. 229) may be confused with an imperforate hymen, but it is possible to pass a probe into the vagina alongside the cyst.

Management

Imperforate hymen requires surgical drainage and excision of the membrane. Paravaginal cysts usually rupture spontaneously.

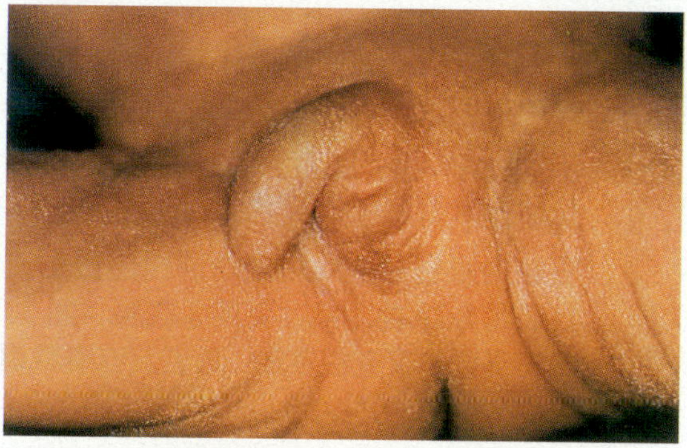

图 227 不成熟的男性外生殖器，阴囊未充分发育和睾丸未降
Immature male genitalia with underdeveloped scrotum and undescended testes

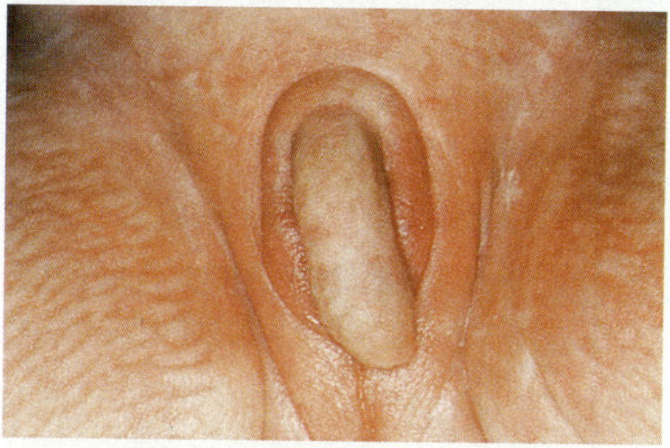

图 228 隐睾症——睾丸未降
Cryptorchidism – undescended testes

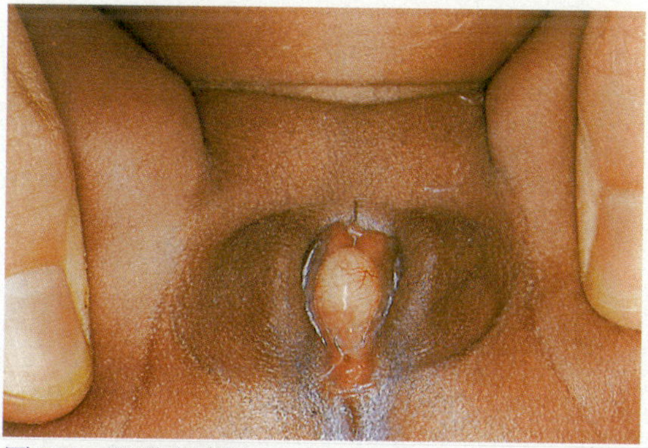

图 229 阴道旁囊肿
Paravaginal cyst

脐膨出

发病率和病因学 不常见的畸形，病因不明。

病理学 在胎儿发育期肠的旋转不良和未能重新回入腹腔。

临床特征 腹腔内脏通过中线腹壁的缺损部位先天性疝出，而且脐带在顶端，有时会覆盖腹膜（图 230 和 231）。脐膨出可与腹裂相鉴别，后者没有囊状组织，并且脐带嵌入在缺损的边缘。

合并症 常见其他的一些先天性异常，尤其是心脏和肠的缺陷。

治疗 外科手术关闭。应该仔细检查肠段，以排除狭窄或闭锁。如果缺损较大，那么最后的修补手术通常要延迟到腹腔能够容纳这些内容物后才能施行。囊和囊内容物通常要封入一个人造膜中，经过几周逐渐缩小后，将内容物慢慢回纳于腹腔中。

肛门闭锁（隐肛，直肠闭锁）

临床特征 一般是在出生后即做的常规检查中被发现并诊断的(图232)，但是偶尔在出现肠梗阻或胎粪延迟排出时才发现。

合并症 在接近 60% 的病例中会有其他的一些先天性异常。肠－生殖器－尿瘘较为常见，尤其是高位直肠闭锁。尿道感染也很常见，尤其当有尿瘘时。

治疗 简单的隐肛可被切开。在新生儿期更多的是进行结肠造口术。应该彻底搜寻是否存在瘘管，尤其是女孩儿。直肠成形术和拖出术可在6~12个月大小时再施行。大约 70% 的病例在最后的手术施行之后，肛门可以有自制性。

Exomphalos (omphalocele)

Incidence and aetiology
Uncommon anomaly of unknown aetiology.

Pathology
Failure of rotation and re-entry of gut into abdominal cavity during fetal development.

Clinical features
Congenital herniation of abdominal viscera through midline abdominal wall defect with umbilical cord at apex, and sometimes with a covering of peritoneum (Figs 230 and 231). Exomphalos can be differentiated from gastroschisis where there is no sac, and the umbilical cord is inserted at edge of the defect.

Associations
Other congenital anomalies are common, particularly cardiac or bowel defects.

Management
Surgical closure. The bowel should be carefully inspected to exclude stenosis or atresia. With large defects, definitive repair is often delayed until the peritoneal cavity is able to accommodate the contents. The sac and contents are usually enclosed in an artificial membrane, and gradually reduced in size over some weeks as the contents are slowly replaced into the abdominal cavity.

Imperforate anus (anal atresia, covered anus, rectal atresia)

Clinical features
Usually diagnosed during routine examination immediately after birth (Fig. 232), but occasionally presents later as intestinal obstruction or delayed passage of meconium.

Associations
Other congenital abnormalities are found in approximately 60% of cases. Recto-genito-urinary fistulae are common, particularly in high rectal atresia. Urinary tract infections are common, particularly when there is a fistula.

Management
A simple covered anus can be incised. More often, colostomy is performed in the neonatal period. A thorough search should be made for fistulae, particularly in females. Rectoplasty and a pull-through procedure are done later, at 6-12 months of age. Continence is achieved in approximately 70% of cases after final surgery.

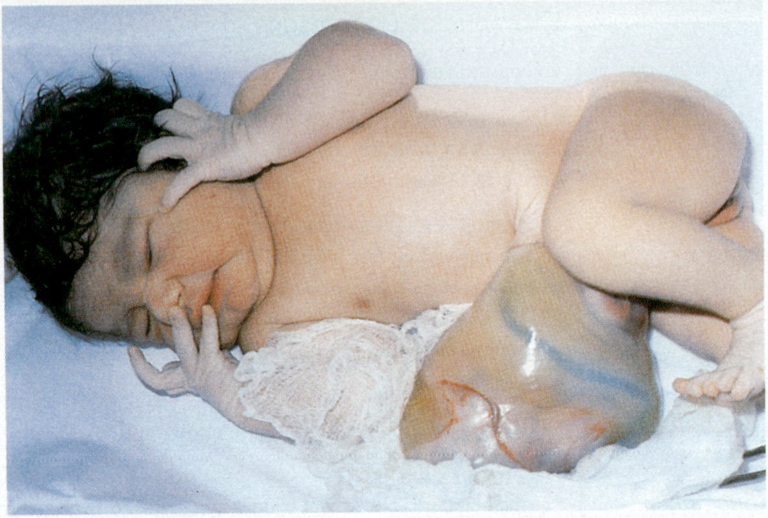

图 230 覆盖有腹膜的脐膨出
Exomphalos with peritoneal covering

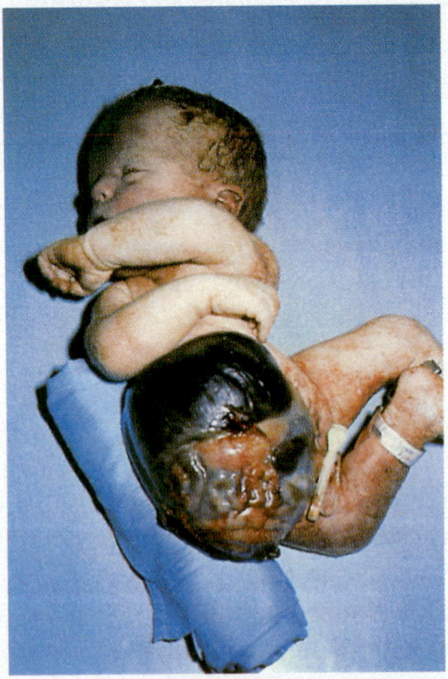

图 231 伴有整个腹腔内容物疝出的巨大脐膨出
Massive exomphalos with herniation of entire abdominal contents

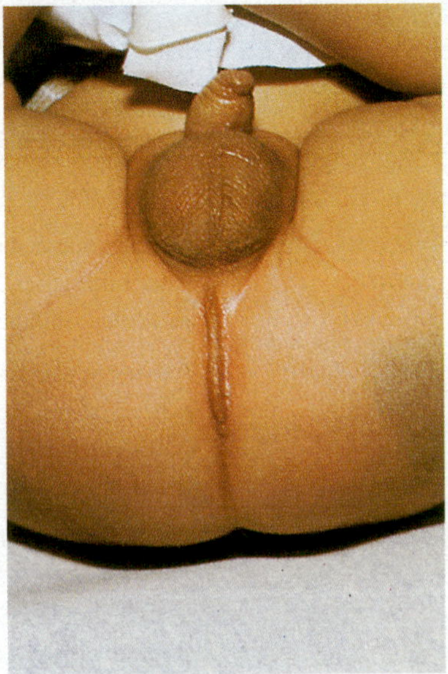

图 232 肛门闭锁
Imperforate anus

坏死性小肠结肠炎（NEC）

发病率 病情多变，更多见于早产儿。伴有严重的宫内生长迟缓，出生窒息，脐插管，需早期喂养和人工喂养。可以有很多病例发生 NEC。

病因学 未知。可能与肠缺血和继发性肠道菌群侵袭感染有关。

病理学 有肠灌注受损、肠缺血和坏死的组织学证据，通常会影响到回肠末端、盲肠和近端横结肠。

临床体征 腹胀、呕吐和排血便。有时会伴有腹膜炎，前腹壁呈现有光泽的浅蓝色和水肿（图 233），腹部静脉曲张或可触及团块。产气菌侵入或管腔内气体进入肠壁会在腹部 X 线片上显示出肠壁囊样积气症的特异病征（壁内囊泡积气）（图 234）。

治疗 应该终止肠道喂养，而给予胃肠外营养。应该使用抗生素，包括抗厌氧菌的抗生素，但是很少能分离到特殊的病原体。可使用机械通气、止痛剂和鼻胃管持续抽吸。给予静脉输液和应用正性肌力药物以保持良好的循环很有必要。持续的代谢性酸中毒、血小板减少或凝血障碍都是预后差的征象。如果保守治疗 48 个小时后没有改善，就需进行剖腹术探查，并切除无活性肠段。肠穿孔（图 235）是急性 NEC 施行剖腹术探查的惟一指征，并且手术死亡率很高。

病程和预后 通过保守治疗，死亡率有所改善，但是在大约25%的幸存者中会发生继发粘连或狭窄的肠梗阻，需要在后期进行外科手术。

Necrotizing enterocolitis (NEC)

Incidence

Variable; more common in preterm infants. Associated with severe intrauterine growth restriction, birth asphyxia, umbilical catheterization, early feeding and artificial milk formulae. Clusters of cases may occur.

Aetiology

Unknown. Probably related to gut ischaemia and secondary infection with invasion by gut flora.

Pathology

Histological evidence of impaired gut perfusion, bowel ischaemia and necrosis, usually affecting terminal ileum, caecum and proximal transverse colon.

Clinical signs

Abdominal distension, vomiting and passage of bloody stools. NEC is sometimes accompanied by peritonitis, shiny bluish discoloration and oedema of anterior abdominal wall (Fig. 233), dilated abdominal veins or a palpable mass. Invasion by gas-forming organisms or diffusion of intraluminal gas into the bowel wall gives rise to the pathognomonic sign of pneumatosis intestinalis (intramural bubbles of gas) on plain abdominal X-ray (Fig. 234).

Management

Enteral feeds should be discontinued and parenteral nutrition will be required. Antibiotics, including those for anaerobes, are usually given, but specific pathogens are rarely isolated. Mechanical ventilation, analgesia and continuous nasogastric suction may be indicated. Maintenance of circulation with intravenous fluid and inotropes is essential. Persistent metabolic acidosis, thrombocytopenia or coagulopathy are signs of poor prognosis. If there is no improvement after 48 h conservative treatment, laparotomy may be indicated to assess and excise non-viable gut. Perforation (Fig. 235) is the only indication for laparotomy in the acute stages of NEC when mortality with surgery is high.

Course and prognosis

With conservative management, mortality has improved, but gut obstruction secondary to adhesions or stricture may require surgical intervention at a later stage in approximately 25% of survivors.

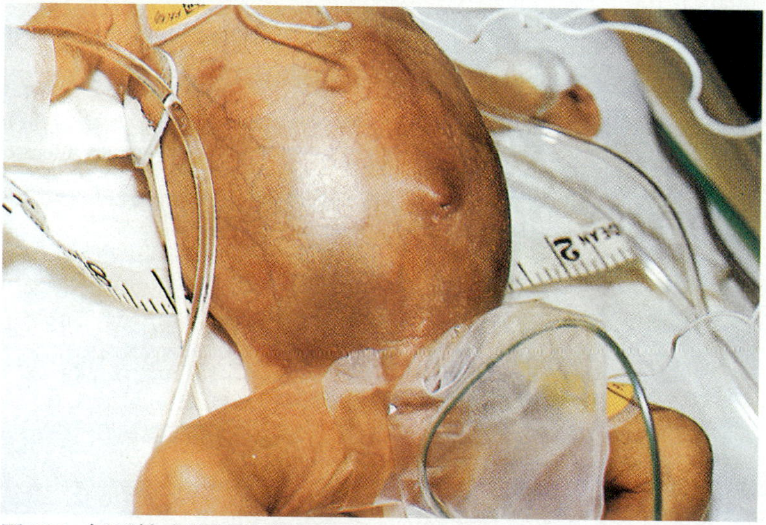

图 233 坏死性小肠结肠炎的腹胀
Necrotizing enterocolitis with distended abdomen

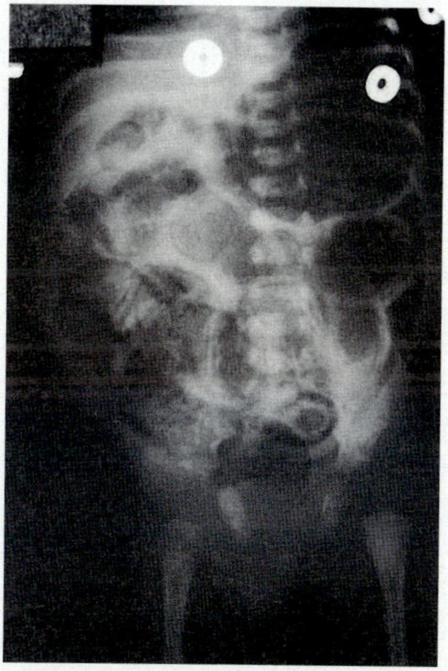

图 234 X 线片显示壁内积气
X-ray showing intramural gas

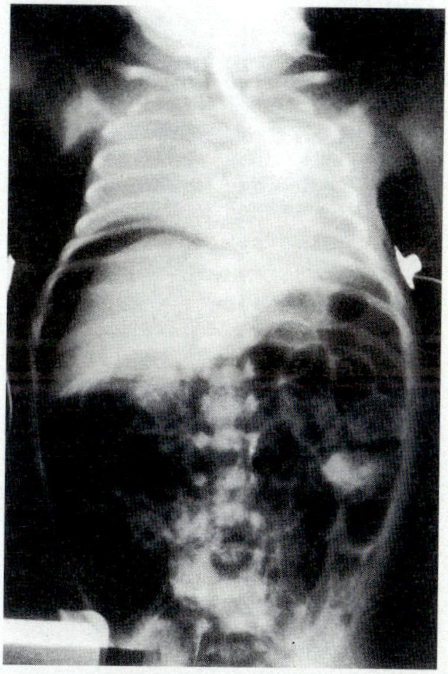

图 235 X 线片显示肠穿孔后腹腔中的气体
X-ray showing gas in the peritoneal cavity from perforation

膈疝

发病率 每 1500 名出生存活儿中就有 1 名发病。

病因学 横膈的前、后叶组织不能融合或肌化。最常见的原因是由于胸腹膜管的持续开放，一般多见于左侧，会引起腹腔内容物通过博赫达勒克孔（foramen of Bochdalek）从膈肌后外侧疝入胸腔。

产前诊断 如果在妊娠早期发生膈疝，那么腹腔内胃泡缺如可通过常规的产前异常超声检查被诊断出来。由于异常出现得较早，肺发育不良的情况可能很严重，所以这些早期发现异常的病例预后较差。如果在妊娠晚期形成疝，那么可能到出生后才发现异常。

临床特征 大部分的膈疝都比较大，而且在出生后都会有心肺症状。症状和体征的严重程度取决于疝的大小，包括是否有呼吸窘迫、发绀、右位心、伴有腹部内容物减少或缺如的舟状腹（图 236）。

合并症 肺发育不良，肠异常。

治疗 母亲应该在有小儿外科部门的围产中心分娩。患儿生后可通过胸部 X 线片（图 237）予以进一步确诊。术前需用较大的鼻胃管进行肠腔减压，并需要进行机械通气。肺高压较常见，如果情况严重，在施行手术修复前应使用肺血管扩张剂，包括吸入一氧化氮。外科手术在技术上并不复杂，但是如果等患儿情况较为稳定再对横隔缺陷实施修复手术，那么会提高生存率。

预后 即使在手术成功的情况下，也有较高的死亡率。生存与否取决于肺发育不良的严重程度。近年来，即使较好的治疗肺高压和延迟手术并不能改善生存率。

Diaphragmatic hernia

Incidence
Occurs in 1 in 1500 live births.

Aetiology
Failure of fusion or muscularization of the anterior and posterior leaves of the diaphragm. The condition is most commonly due to persistence of the pleuroperitoneal canal, usually on the left side and resulting in a posterolateral hernia through the foramen of Bochdalek.

Antenatal diagnosis
When herniation occurs early in gestation, absence of the abdominal stomach bubble may be diagnosed on routine antenatal anomaly ultrasonography. Those detected early have a poor prognosis because pulmonary hypoplasia is likely to be severe. Herniation in later gestation may not be diagnosable until after birth.

Clinical features
Most diaphragmatic herniae are large and produce cardio-respiratory symptoms soon after birth. The signs and symptoms depend on the size of the hernia and include respiratory distress, cyanosis, dextrocardia and scaphoid abdomen with reduced or absent abdominal contents (Fig. 236).

Associations
Pulmonary hypoplasia; gut anomalies.

Management
The mother should be delivered in a perinatal centre with a paediatric surgical service. Confirm the diagnosis with a chest X-ray after birth (Fig. 237). Preoperative decompression of the gut with a large nasogastric tube and mechanical ventilation are usually required. Pulmonary hypertension is common and when significant should be treated with pulmonary vasodilators, including nitric oxide, before surgical repair is undertaken. Surgery is usually not technically difficult, but delay in surgical repair of the diaphragmatic defect until the baby`s condition is stable, improves the chances of survival.

Prognosis
Mortality is high even after successful surgery. Survival depends on the severity of pulmonary hypoplasia. Better treatment of pulmonary hypertension and delayed surgery has not improved survival in recent years.

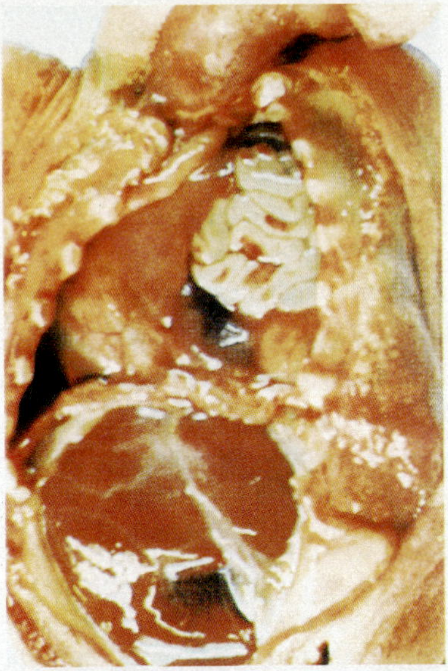

图 236 膈疝患儿的尸体解剖（经由 Dr S. Gould 的许可）
Post-mortem appearance of diaphragmatic hernia (courtesy of Dr S. Gould)

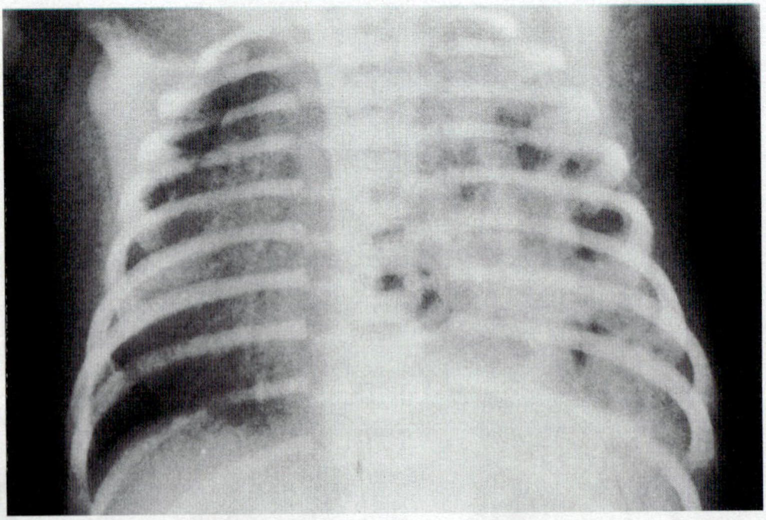

图 237 典型的左侧膈疝 X 线片表现
X-ray appearance of typical left-sided diaphragmatic hernia

幽门狭窄

病因学 幽门平滑肌肥大的原因不明。第一胎男婴经常会受累。

临床特征 在生后几周内出现呕吐。典型症状有喷射性呕吐，伴有生长发育停滞和便秘。在喂养过程中，一般可在上腹部触及幽门团块并看见蠕动（图 238）。超声检查有助于进一步确诊。

治疗 在补充液体和纠正电解质紊乱后进行 Ramstedt 幽门肌切开术。

肠套叠

发病率 是婴儿肠梗阻的常见原因。

临床特征 突然发生的腹部胶痛，粪便松软并且带血（红色果酱样粪便）。在腹部可触及腊肠样肠段。

治疗 轻柔的钡餐或空气灌肠（图 239）可以进一步确诊，也可以对一些病程较短的病例起到治疗效果。对于诊断延迟而病程较长的病例，可能需要外科手术治疗。

希施斯普龙病（先天性巨结肠）

病因学 先天性结肠神经节细胞缺如。

临床特征 可能引起新生儿急性肠梗阻（图 240），在大龄儿童中可引起慢性便秘。

诊断 钡餐灌肠和直肠肛门测压法有助于诊断，须通过直肠活组织检查来确诊。

治疗 结肠造口术可以减轻急性梗阻；可在以后切除无神经节的肠段，并实行肠拖出吻合术。

Pyloric stenosis

Aetiology
Hypertrophy of the smooth muscle of pylorus of obscure aetiology. First born male infants often affected.

Clinical features
Onset of vomiting within a few weeks of birth. Classically, there is projectile vomiting with failure to thrive and constipation. During feeding, a pyloric mass (Fig. 238) can usually be palpated and visible peristalsis may be seen in the upper abdomen. Ultrasound examination is helpful for confirmation of the diagnosis.

Management
Surgery (Ramstedt's pyloromyotomy) after rehydration and correction of electrolyte imbalance.

Intussusception

Incidence
Common cause of gut obstruction in infancy.

Clinical features
Sudden onset of colicky abdominal pain, with loose stools often blood-stained (red-currant jelly stools). A sausage-shaped bowel mass may be palpable.

Management
Gentle barium or air enema (Fig. 239) will confirm the diagnosis and may be curative in cases of recent onset. Surgery may be required for intussusception when the diagnosis is delayed.

Hirschsprung's disease

Aetiology
Congenital absence of ganglionic cells in the colon.

Clinical features
May cause acute neonatal intestinal obstruction (Fig. 240) or chronic constipation in older children.

Diagnosis
Barium enema and anorectal manometry assist in the diagnosis; rectal biopsy is always necessary for confirmation.

Management
Colostomy relieves acute obstruction; resection of the aganglionic segment and a pull-through anastomosis are performed later.

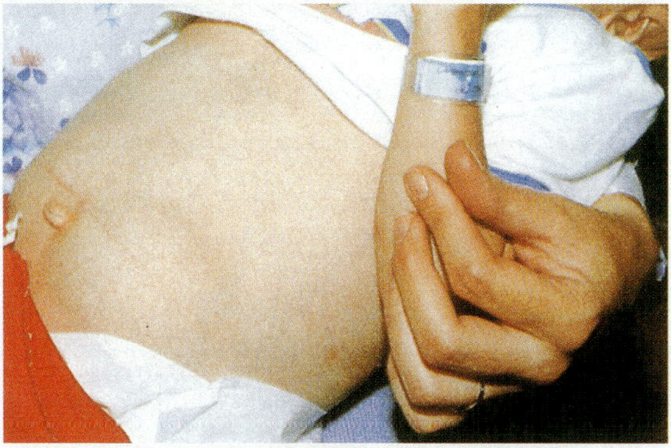

图 238　幽门狭窄可在腹部表面看见蠕动波
Visible peristalsis in pyloric stenosis

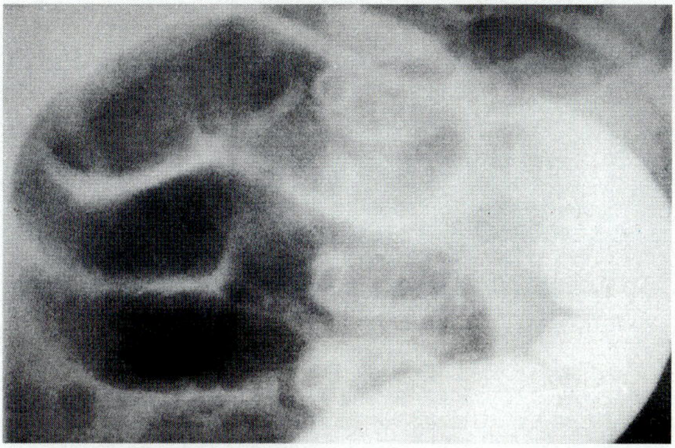

图 239　肠套叠
Intussusception

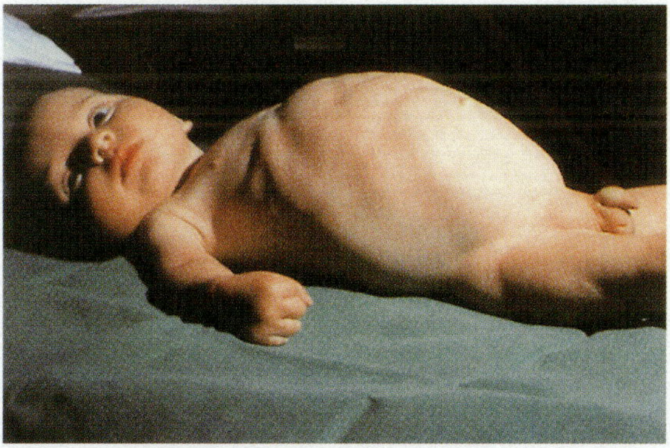

图 240　希施斯普龙病的腹胀（经由 Dr T. Lissauer 许可）
Distended abdomen in Hirschsprung's disease (courtesy of Dr T. Lissauer)

鼻后孔闭锁

发病率 罕见畸形，后鼻孔缺如或狭窄。

临床特征 新生儿双侧鼻后孔闭锁会引起发绀和呼吸道阻塞。单侧鼻后孔闭锁会引起单侧鼻液溢出，并且经常到儿童晚期才会做出诊断。

治疗 双侧鼻后孔闭锁时需要紧急建立经口气道。膜状鼻后孔闭锁可以进行外科切除，并在切除原位保留一小管（图 241），直到新孔上皮形成为止。

招风耳（横位耳甲）

发病率 通常是常染色体显性遗传。

临床特征 大的凸出的耳朵，一般是双侧的（图 242）。

病理学 对耳轮缺乏正常的折叠。如果耳朵凸出造成无法接受的外观异常，就需进行外科手术整形。

斜颈

病因学 通常急性发作，病因不明。慢性无痛性斜颈可能继发于胸骨乳突的纤维变性、宫内体位、颈半椎体畸形或双眼不平衡。在急性疼痛性斜颈或常见的歪颈（图 243）中，会突然出现颈部旋转受限，并伴有强烈的胸锁乳突肌疼痛，头部向患侧倾斜。

治疗 急性斜颈可以在数天内自行恢复，体位性斜颈会在数月内自行恢复。轻柔的理疗可能有所帮助。

Choanal atresia

Incidence

Rare anomaly with absence or narrowing of posterior nares.

Clinical features

Bilateral choanal atresia causes cyanosis and respiratory obstruction in the newborn. In unilateral choanal atresia, the condition causes unilateral rhinorrhoea and diagnosis is often not made until later in childhood.

Management

Urgent provision of an oral airway is needed in bilateral choanal atresia. The membranous posterior nares are then surgically excised and a small tube left in situ (Fig. 241) until the new orifice has epithelialized.

Bat ears

Incidence

Often autosomal dominant.

Clinical features

Large protruding ears, usually bilateral (Fig. 242).

Pathology

Defect in normal folding of the anti-helix. Surgery when protrusion of ears is cosmetically unacceptable.

Torticollis

Aetiology

Usually acute onset of unknown aetiology. Chronic painless torticollis may be secondary to sternomastoid fibrosis, intrauterine posture, cervical hemivertebrae, or ocular imbalance. In acute painful torticollis or the common wry-neck (Fig. 243), there is a sudden onset of limitation of neck rotation with an intensely painful sternomastoid muscle. The head is sometimes tilted towards the affected side.

Management

Spontaneous recovery occurs within days in acute torticollis or months in postural torticollis. Gentle physiotherapy may be helpful.

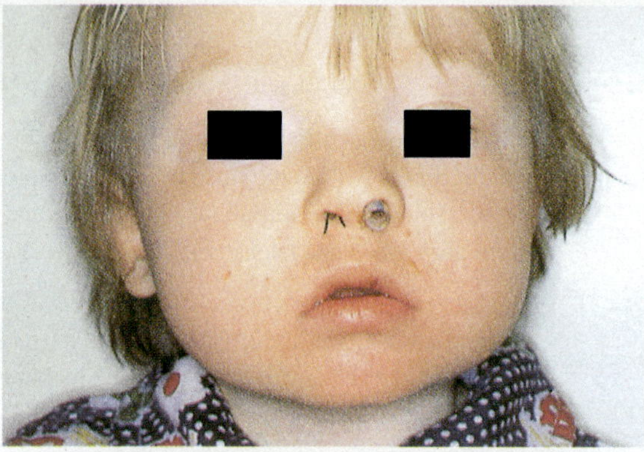

图 241 鼻后孔闭锁术后在鼻孔保留的小管
Choanal atresia with tube in nostril

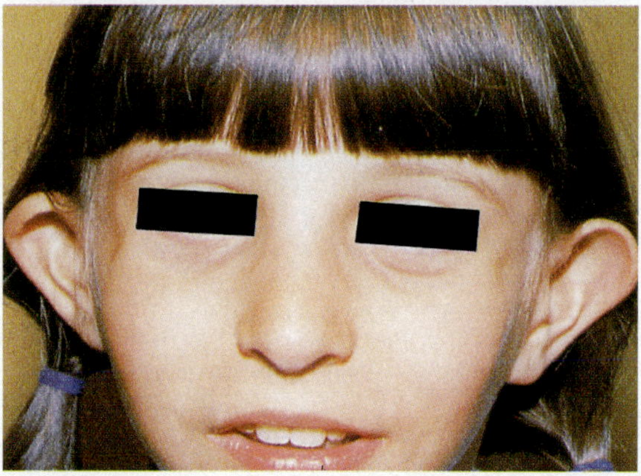

图 242 招风耳
Bat ears

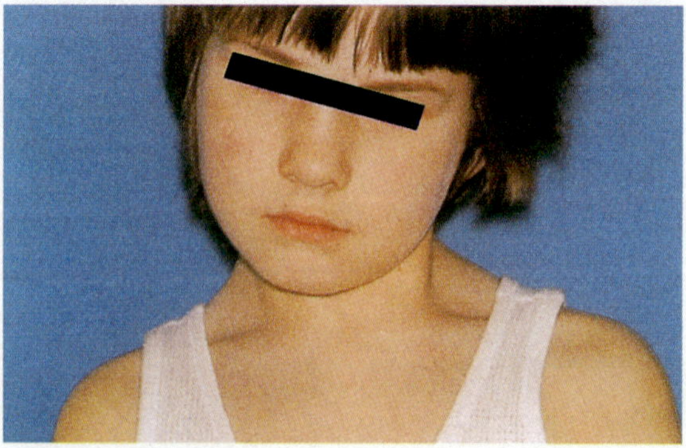

图 243 急性斜颈
Acute torticollis

烧伤和烫伤

临床特征

烫伤最常发生于刚学步的小孩，可能会因打翻水壶，沸腾的水烫伤脸部、颈部、肩膀和上肢（图244）。火焰灼伤常会发生于稍大一些的儿童。当衣服着火，烧伤可能会累及身体的广泛部位（图 245），并且经常是深度烧伤。

治疗

治疗要根据烧伤的广泛程度和严重度。所要采取的紧急措施包括合理减轻疼痛（尤其是浅表烫伤），保证呼吸道通畅，当有休克征象时用血浆增容剂进行复苏。如果烧伤的面积超过儿童体表面积的10%，那么就有必要进行静脉输液治疗。大量的液体、全血和蛋白会从烧伤部位丢失。一般要给予破伤风类毒素。为预防感染应对暴露的烧伤部位进行隔离护理，或局部使用抗生素进行封闭治疗，如在封闭敷料下涂以磺胺嘧啶银（图 246）。如果有特殊指征，就要全身应用抗生素。除了非常小的烫伤外，所有的烫伤都需要得到一组有经验的儿科监护医师、护士和整形外科医生团体的治疗。由于房屋着火而造成烧伤的儿童，因吸入烟雾，可能会导致严重的呼吸窘迫，即使没有皮肤烧伤征象，也需要转入医院进行观察。

病程和预后

浅表的烫伤当暴露于外界中会快速形成保护性焦痂。当新的上皮细胞形成后，焦痂会逐步脱落（图 247）。对于深部烧伤、广泛烧伤或为减轻挛缩则需要进行皮肤移植。

预防

儿童烧伤和烫伤应该通过对家庭和公众进行宣教以及对加热器和儿童衣物设计防护装置来预防。

Burns and scalds

Clinical features

The most common scald happens to the toddler who pulls boiling water onto the face, neck, shoulder and upper arm (Fig. 244). Flame burns tend to happen to older children. When clothes catch fire, burns may involve extensive areas of the body (Fig. 245) and are often deep.

Management

Treatment depends on the extent and severity of the burn. Emergency measures consist of appropriate pain relief (particularly for superficial scalds), ensuring an adequate airway, and resuscitation with plasma volume expanders when there are signs of shock. If burns involve more than 10% of the child's surface area, intravenous fluid therapy will be necessary. Large quantities of fluid, blood and protein are lost from burned areas. Tetanus toxoid should always be given. Infection should be prevented by barrier nursing of exposed burns or by the closed method with topical antibiotics such as silver sulphadiazine under occlusive dressings (Fig. 246). Systemic antibiotics are given if there are specific indications. All but the most minor scalds should be managed by a team of experienced paediatric intensivists, nurses and plastic surgeons. Children involved in house fires may develop severe respiratory distress due to smoke inhalation and should always be admitted to hospital for observation even if there are no signs of burns to the skin.

Course and prognosis

Superficial burns quickly form a protective eschar when left exposed. This eschar gradually lifts off when new epithelium has formed (Fig. 247). Skin grafts may be necessary for deep burns, extensive burns or to relieve tight contractures.

Prevention

Burns and scalds in children should be preventable by education of families and the public, and by safeguards in design of heating appliances and children's clothing.

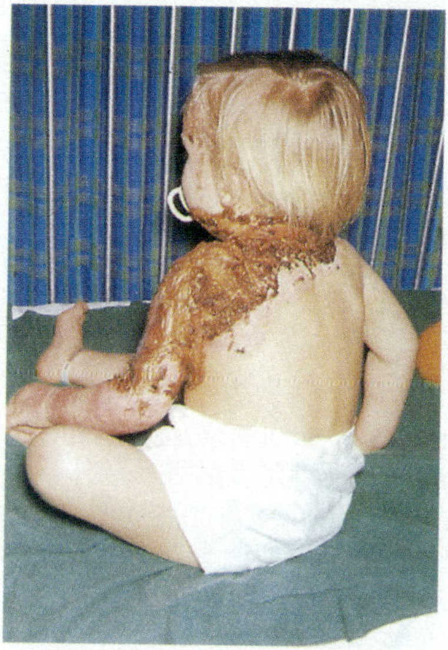

图 244 刚学步的小孩典型的热水烫伤
Typical hot water scald in toddler

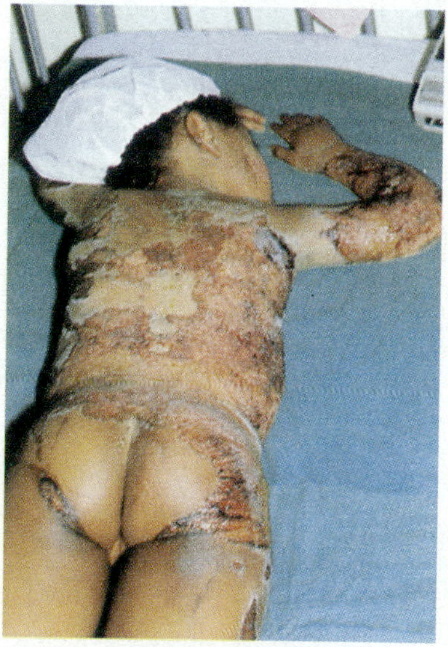

图 245 广泛的火焰烧伤
Extensive flame burns

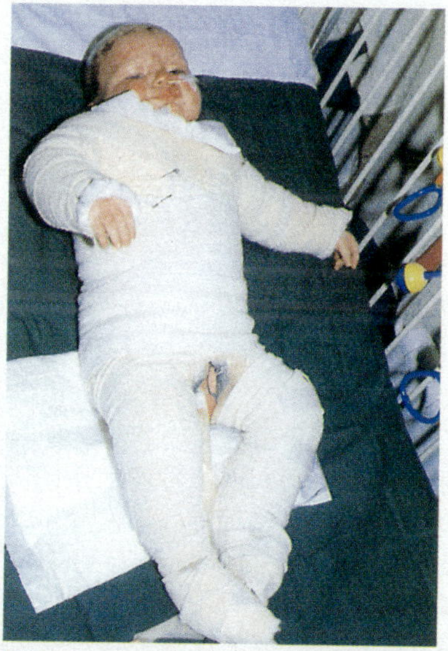

图 246 广泛的烧伤用封闭敷料疗法
Extensive burns treated by closed dressings

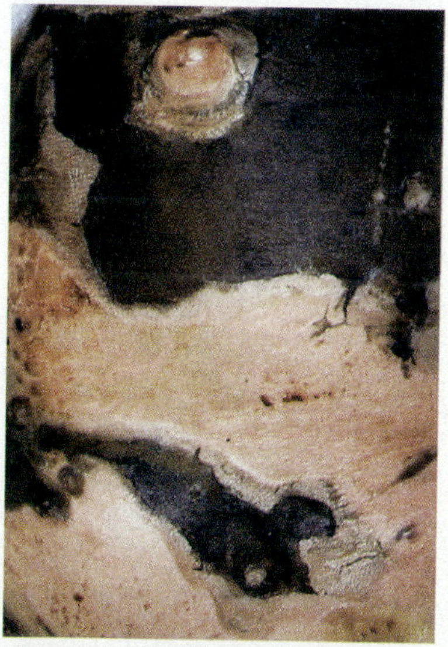

图 247 烫伤后新的上皮细胞形成
New epithelium forming after a scald

泌尿道感染（UTI）

发病率 很常见的感染，在女孩儿中的发病率为1%~2%。

临床特征 小婴儿可能有非特异性的症状，如体重不增、发烧、呕吐和易激惹。大一些的儿童可能会主诉排尿频繁、排尿困难和腰痛。

诊断 对于高度怀疑此病的患儿，必须获得足够的尿液样本进行尿液分析和培养。小婴儿经常需采用耻骨弓上抽吸术，因为清洁的中段尿可能被皮肤污染，使化验结果难以解释，尤其对于女孩儿。偶尔会用导尿标本，尤其是对于已患病或考虑紧急使用抗生素的孩子。

治疗 急性感染需用抗生素治疗。已证实的UTI需用超声检查肾尿道系统，有时需用放射性同位素扫描或排尿式膀胱尿道造影进行检查。至少50%的病例有潜在畸形，最常见的是膀胱输尿管反流（图248）。预防性使用抗生素可以预防肾脏瘢痕化。7岁以后很少会形成新的瘢痕。当有进行性肾瘢痕形成时或尽管采取了预防措施仍有反复发作的突破性感染进行时，有时需进行外科手术（输尿管再植术）。

肾尿道畸形

发病率 相对常见；大多数无症状，并且在功能上影响轻微。目前许多异常都是通过常规产前超声检查诊断出来的。

临床特征 重复输尿管通常没有症状，但是可能易于感染、梗阻或返流。在男婴后尿道瓣膜会引起尿流不畅，并且容易引起梗阻而导致肾功能衰竭。马蹄肾、骨盆肾和单侧肾发育不良一般都是无症状的，除非有感染发生。严重的肾尿道畸形，如：肾发育不全或干梅状腹综合征（图105）都可以通过产前常规超声检查发现异常。产前超声检查发现肾尿道轻度扩张很常见（图249），需要在出生后进一步检查，但偶尔由于发现梗阻性尿路病变需要外科手术治疗（图250）。

Urinary tract infection (UTI)

Incidence Very common infection; occurs in 1-2% of girls.

Clinical features Young infants may have non-specific symptoms of poor weight gain, fever, vomiting and irritability. Older children may complain of urinary frequency, dysuria and loin pain.

Diagnosis High index of suspicion; must obtain adequate urine sample for urinalysis and culture. Suprapubic aspirate is often necessary in young infants because skin contamination may make bag or clean-catch specimens difficult to interpret, particularly in girls. Occasionally catheter specimen, particularly if very unwell and antibiotic treatment is considered urgent.

Management Acute infection requires antibiotic therapy. Proven UTIs require investigation of the renal tract with ultrasound examination and sometimes, radioisotope scans or micturating cystourethrogram. At least 50% have an underlying abnormality, most commonly vesicoureteric reflux (Fig. 248). Prophylactic antibiotics may protect against renal scarring. New scars rarely develop after the age of 7 years. Surgery (ureteric reimplantation) is occasionally necessary when there is progression of renal scarring or recurrent breakthrough infections, despite prophylaxis.

Renal tract anomalies

Incidence Relatively common; most are asymptomatic and functionally insignificant. Many are now diagnosed on routine antenatal anomaly ultrasonography.

Clinical features Ureteric duplication is usually asymptomatic but may predispose to infection, obstruction or reflux. Posterior urethral valves in male infants cause poor urinary stream, and obstruction may cause renal failure. Horseshoe kidneys, pelvic kidneys, unilateral renal dysplasia are often asymptomatic unless there is infection. Severe anomalies of the renal tract such as renal agenesis or prune-belly (see Fig. 105) syndrome are usually diagnosed on routine antenatal anomaly ultrasound scans. Mild antenatally detected renal tract dilatation (Fig. 249) is common and needs investigation after birth, but only occasionally is due to an obstructive uropathy (Fig. 250) requiring surgery.

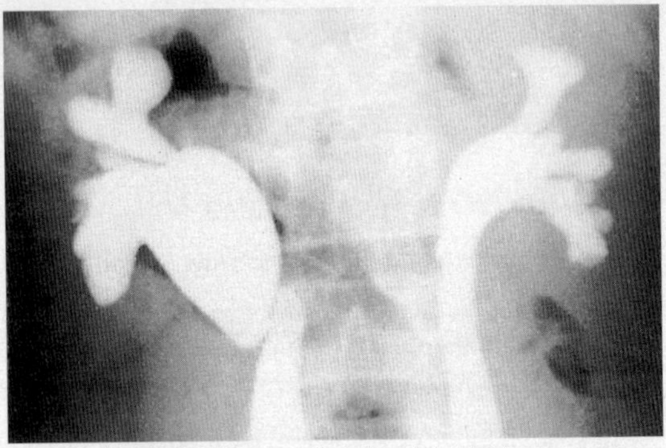

图 248 膀胱输尿管反流（双侧Ⅲ级）
Vesicoureteric reflux (bilateral grade III)

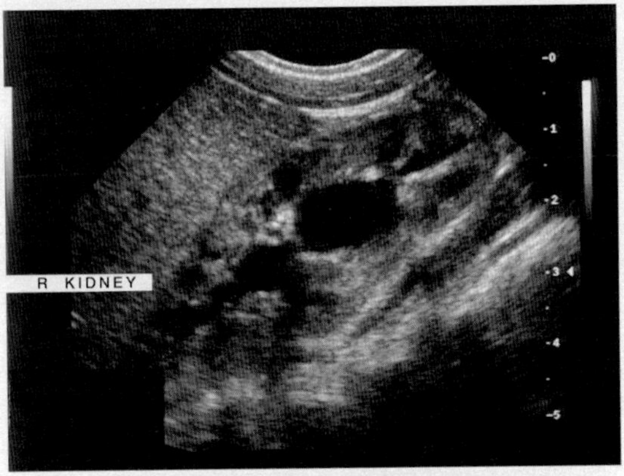

图 249 轻度的肾盂扩张
Minimal renal pelvic dilatation

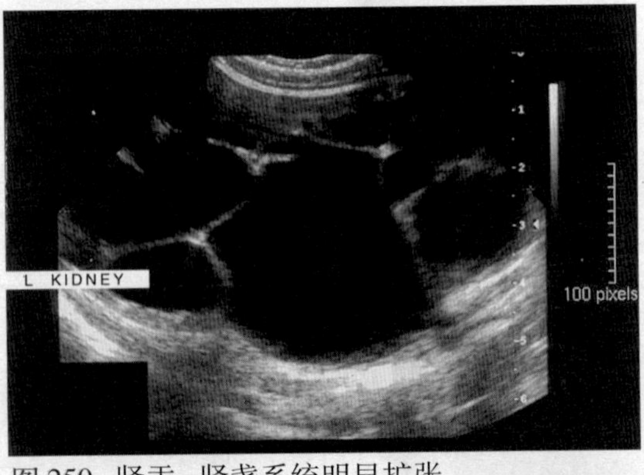

图 250 肾盂-肾盏系统明显扩张
Grossly dilated renal pelvi-calyceal system

肾病综合征

发病率 每 20 000 名儿童中就有 1 名。男孩儿更易患病。发病的高峰年龄是 1~5 岁。

病因学 原因未知，可能与免疫相关。

临床特征 眶周（图251）和全身水肿，腹痛和腹水。大量蛋白尿可能会导致低血容量和急性循环衰竭。有患肺炎球菌性腹膜炎的趋势。儿童肾组织活检的指征是高血压或血尿，在这些儿童中可能会发现更严重的潜在疾病。

治疗 卧床休息和高蛋白、限盐饮食直到出现利尿，一般在10~14天内开始口服皮质类固醇。出现低血容量可以给予血浆或无盐白蛋白。建议在复发时预防性应用青霉素并接种肺炎球菌疫苗。

病程和预后 大多数会有轻微损伤性病变，并且会在2年内完全痊愈。复发是很常见的，但是一般应用类固醇有效。对于频繁复发或应用类固醇有严重不良反应的儿童，硫唑嘌呤治疗也许会有帮助。

急性肾小球肾炎

发病率和病因学 不常见。可能继发于近期的链球菌或病毒感染。发病时可能伴随过敏性紫癜（图 252）。

临床特征 苍白，嗜睡，由于镜下血尿而呈现烟色尿，少尿和高血压。

治疗 卧床休息，治疗明显的高血压，注意体液平衡，直到症状自行改善为止。

病程和预后 大多数可以在几周内恢复，但是镜下血尿可能会存在数月。

Nephrotic syndrome

Incidence
1 in 20 000 children. Boys are more commonly affected. The peak age incidence is 1-5 years.

Aetiology
Cause unknown; immunological basis likely.

Clinical features
Periorbital (Fig. 251) and generalized oedema, abdominal pain and ascites. Gross proteinuria may lead to hypovolaemia and acute circulatory collapse. Prone to pneumococcal peritonitis. Renal biopsy is indicated in children with hypertension or haematuria, in whom a more serious underlying diagnosis is likely to be found.

Management
Bedrest and high protein, salt-restricted diet until diuresis occurs, usually within 10-14 days of starting oral corticosteroids. Hypovolaemia responds to infusion of plasma or salt-free albumin. Prophylactic penicillin during relapses and pneumoccal vaccination is recommended.

Course and prognosis
Majority have minimal change lesion and recover completely within 2 years. Relapses are common, but normally respond to steroids. Azothiaprine therapy is occasionally helpful in children who have frequent relapses or unacceptable side effects on steroids.

Acute glomerulonephritis

Incidence and aetiology
Uncommon. May be secondary to recent streptococcal or viral infection. May occur in association with Henoch-Schönlein purpura (Fig. 252).

Clinical features
Pallor, lethargy, smoky urine due to microscopic haematuria, oliguria and hypertension.

Management
Bed-rest, treatment of significant hypertension and careful fluid balance until spontaneous improvement occurs.

Course and prognosis
Most recover within a few weeks, but microscopic haematuria may persist for months.

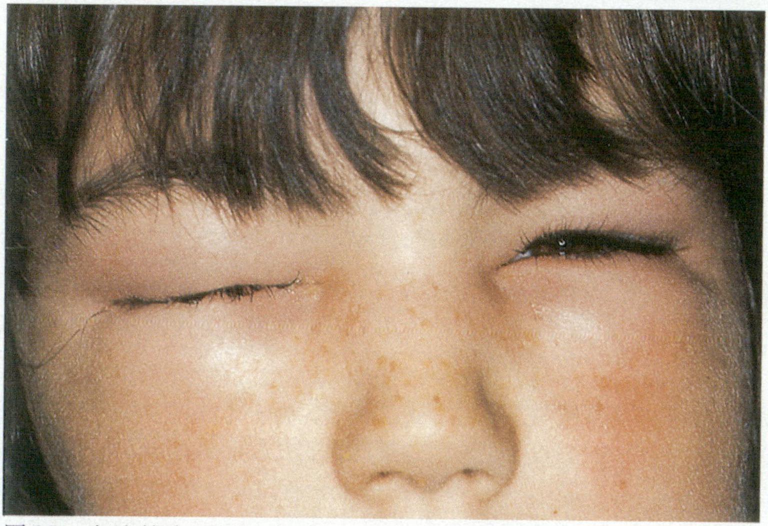

图 251 肾病综合征眶周水肿
Periorbital oedema in nephrotic syndrome

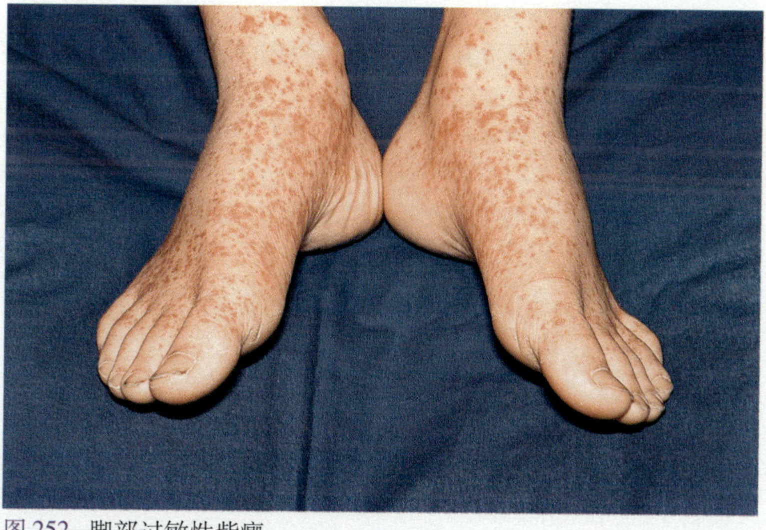

图 252 脚部过敏性紫癜
Henoch-Schönlein purpura on the feet

胃肠炎

发病率

是发展中国家小婴儿死亡最常见的原因，在这些国家中，断奶早和营养不良的现象较为常见。

病因学

轮状病毒感染是冬季小婴儿最常见的胃肠炎病因。大肠杆菌、沙门菌、志贺杆菌和弯曲杆菌都是较常见的致病菌。

临床特征

腹泻、呕吐和腹部绞痛。由于体液过多的丢失和水分摄入不足，因此最严重的并发症是脱水。轻度到中度脱水（达5%）的孩子会有口渴、嗜睡、眼窝下陷和皮肤弹性变差（图 253 和 254）。中度到重度脱水（5%~10%）的孩子可能会有心动过速和外周循环衰竭的征象。

治疗

认识到脱水并给予充分的水和电解质补充是很重要的。通常可反复给予口服葡萄糖电解质溶液，除非患儿有休克，这时有必要进行静脉治疗。

肠寄生虫

发病率

在发展中国家，是吸收不良、贫血和慢性腹泻常见的原因。

病因学和临床特征

兰伯贾第虫是一种原虫感染，可引起急性腹泻，有时会引起慢性吸收不良。人蛔虫（图255）会引起腹部绞痛和肠梗阻。钩虫是热带国家缺铁性贫血的常见原因。

治疗

给予合适的驱虫药进行治疗。

Gastroenteritis

Incidence

The most common cause of death in young infants in developing countries where early weaning and malnutrition are common.

Aetiology

Rotavirus infection is a common cause of gastroenteritis in infants in winter months. *Esherichia coli*, Salmonella, Shigella and Campylobacter are the common causes of bacterial gastroenteritis.

Clinical features

Diarrhoea, vomiting and colicky abdominal pain. The most serious complication is dehydration due to excessive water loss or inadequate fluid intake. In mild to moderate dehydration (up to 5%) the child is thirsty, lethargic, has sunken eyes and loss of skin turgor (Figs 253 and 254). In moderate to severe dehydration (5-10%) there may be tachycardia and signs of peripheral circulatory collapse.

Management

Recognition of dehydration and adequate fluid and electrolyte replacement is important. Frequent administration of an oral glucose electrolyte solution is usually possible, except when there is shock. Intravenous therapy will then be necessary.

Intestinal parasites

Incidence

Common cause of malabsorption, anaemia and chronic diarrhoea in developing countries.

Aetiology and clinical features

Giardia lamblia is a protozoal infestation which causes acute diarrhoea and sometimes chronic malabsorption. Ascaris *lumbricoides* (roundworm) (Fig. 255) causes colicky abdominal pain and gut obstruction. Ankylostoma (hookworm) is a common cause of iron deficiency anaemia in tropical countries.

Treatment

Appropriate anti-helminthic drug therapy.

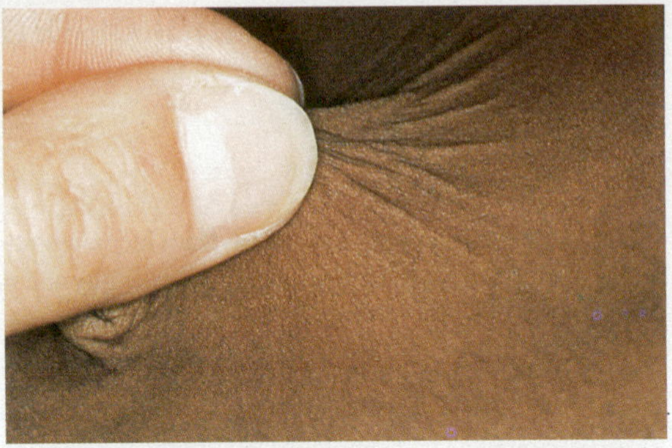

图 253　脱水的干燥皮肤
Dehydration with dry skin

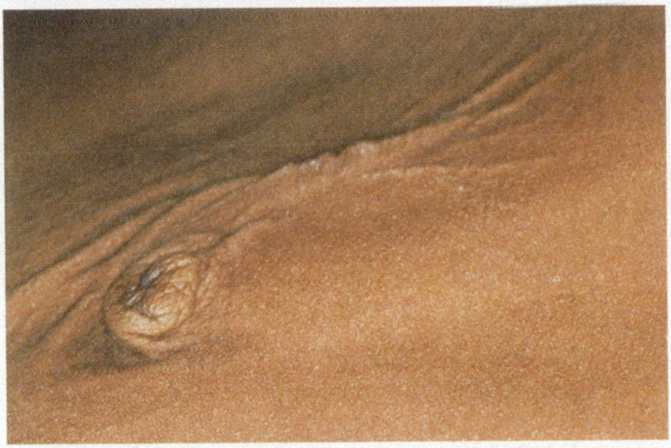

图 254　脱水的无弹性皮肤
Dehydration showing poor skin turgor after release

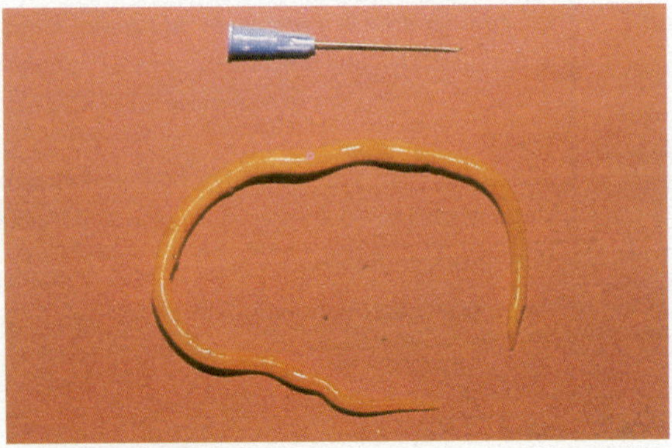

图 255　人蛔虫
Ascaris lumbricoides (roundworm)

腹部疾病

病因学 对谷蛋白敏感，谷蛋白不耐受。对食用小麦、黑麦、有时是大麦和燕麦永久性不耐受。

发病率 在英国，大约每 2000 名儿童中就有 1 名。

临床特征 大多数儿童在婴儿期就有症状（如在加用含有谷蛋白的固体食物后体重增长缓慢），但是体征比较隐蔽。呕吐、腹泻和腹胀都很常见；还会有食欲缺乏、易激惹的痛苦面容（图 256）、肌张力减退和臀部消瘦。有时生长发育迟滞是仅有的体征，可能直到青春期才能被诊断出来。

诊断 空肠活检，显示肠壁绒毛完全萎缩和黏膜固有层炎性浸润，具有确诊意义。可以在血液中发现抗麦醇溶蛋白的抗体。

治疗 诊断明确后给予无谷蛋白饮食，补充铁剂和维生素通常很有必要。有时也会有乳糖或牛奶蛋白不耐受。

病程和预后 可以通过无谷蛋白膳食使胃肠症状、情绪异常和生长不足得到改善。成年后，患小肠淋巴瘤的危险性增高。

炎性肠病

临床特征 腹痛，慢性腹泻，体重减轻，苍白，发热，嘴（图257）和肛门（图 258）溃疡，以及生长不足。

诊断 通常需要以钡餐灌肠和钡餐后追踪检查、结肠镜检查和活组织检查来鉴别克隆病（Crohn's disease）和溃疡性结肠炎。

治疗 克隆病可能难以治疗，但是口服类固醇、硫唑嘌呤、环孢菌素，或者基本的或整体的饮食调整，可以使症状减轻。在溃疡性结肠炎，如果类固醇治疗无效，可以最终选择结肠部分切除术。

Coeliac disease

Aetiology

Gluten sensitivity; gluten intolerance. Permanent intolerance of dietary wheat, rye and sometimes barley and oats.

Incidence

About 1 in 2000 in the UK.

Clinical features

Most children have signs in infancy (e.g. poor weight gain after introduction of gluten-containing solids), but signs are often insidious. Vomiting, diarrhoea and abdominal distension are common. Anorexia, irritability with miserable facies (Fig. 256), hypotonia and wasted buttocks occur. Sometimes failure to thrive or growth failure is the only sign and may not be diagnosed until adolescence.

Diagnosis

Jejunal biopsy, showing total villus atrophy and inflammatory infiltration of the lamina propria, is the definitive investigation. Anti-gliadin antibodies are often found in blood.

Management

Gluten-free diet. Supplementation with iron and vitamins is often necessary after diagnosis. Lactose or cow's milk protein intolerance sometimes occurs.

Course and prognosis

Gastrointestinal symptoms, mood disturbance and growth failure improve with a gluten-free diet. There is an increased risk of intestinal lymphoma in adult life.

Inflammatory bowel disorders

Clinical features

Abdominal pain, chronic diarrhoea, weight loss, pallor, fever, mouth (Fig. 257) and anal (Fig. 258) ulceration and growth failure.

Diagnosis

Barium meal and follow-through, colonoscopy and biopsy are usually required to differentiate between Crohn's disease and ulcerative colitis.

Management

Crohn's disease may be difficult to treat, but oral steroids, azothiaprine, cyclosporin or an elemental or polymeric diet may induce remission. Hemi-colectomy is ultimately necessary in ulcerative colitis if unresponsive to steroids.

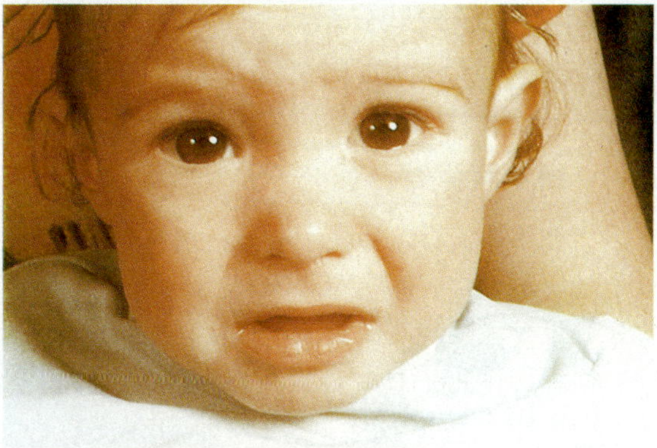

图 256 腹部疾病孩子的痛苦面容
Miserable facies of coeliac child

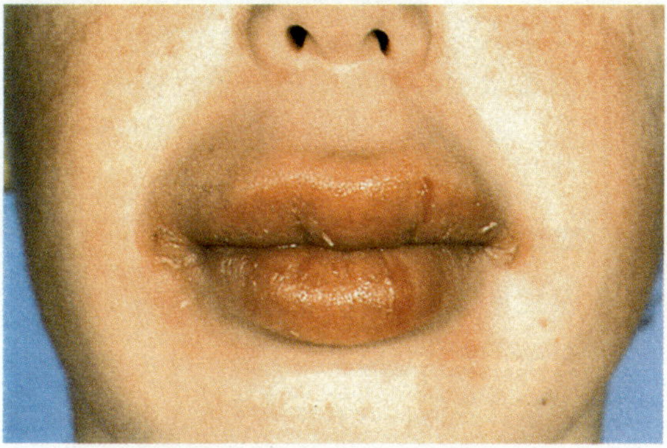

图 257 克隆病的嘴唇肿胀和口角炎
Swelling of lips and angular cheilitis in Crohn's disease

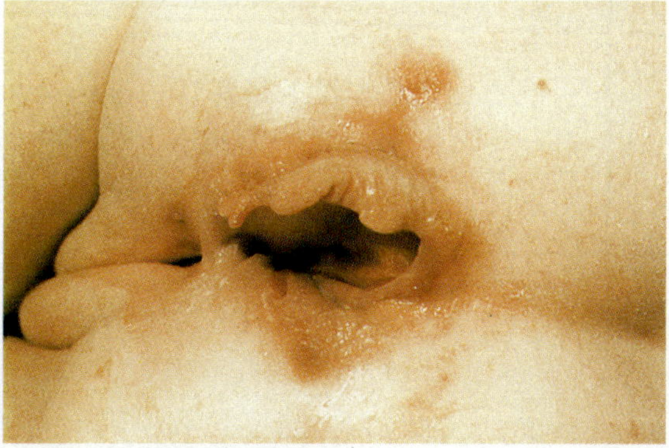

图 258 肛门皮赘和窦道
Anal tags and sinuses

细支气管炎

发病率 在冬季流行，多见于婴儿，通常是由呼吸道合胞病毒引起。

临床特征 鼻卡他症状，然后逐渐出现咳嗽、喘鸣、呼吸急促和喂养困难。孩子可能会有肺膨胀过度，引起桶状胸、发绀、肋骨下凹（图 259），偶尔会有心力衰竭。

治疗 必要时需进行吸氧支持治疗。通常需要鼻饲饮食或静脉补液。一般不需要用抗生素，但是如果怀疑有继发感染或对于十分虚弱的孩子可以应用抗生素。偶尔需治疗心力衰竭或给予机械通气。对于高危婴儿，如先天性心脏病患儿，给予抗病毒喷雾剂三氮唑核苷，可能会有所帮助。

哮喘

发病率 很常见，至少每 7 名儿童中就有 1 名。

病因学 过敏，尤其是房屋内尘螨，是儿童发病的重要原因。通常有哮喘、过敏或湿疹的家族史。

临床特征 轻度哮喘可能仅有慢性咳嗽，尤其是在夜间出现或由运动引起的哮喘。更严重的症状包括喘鸣和呼吸窘迫。治疗不充分的慢性哮喘患儿可能会导致胸廓畸形（图 260）和生长不足。

治疗 疾病发作严重程度的最好评估方法是监测呼吸峰流。急性支气管痉挛一般可给予吸入 β－拟交感神经药物或黄嘌呤进行治疗。通过吸入色甘酸钠或皮质类固醇来预防性治疗慢性哮喘很有帮助。

Bronchiolitis

Incidence

Commonly occurs in infants in winter epidemics; usually due to respiratory syncytial virus.

Clinical features

Coryzal symptoms, then gradual onset of cough, wheeze, tachypnoea and feeding difficulty. The child may develop over-inflation of the lungs, producing a barrel-shaped chest, cyanosis, subcostal recession (Fig. 259) and occasionally heart failure.

Management

Supportive care with added oxygen when necessary. Tube feeding or intravenous fluids are often required. Antibiotics are not usually indicated, but may be given if secondary infection is suspected or in a very ill child. Treatment of cardiac failure or mechanical ventilation is occasionally necessary. A nebulized antiviral agent, ribavirin, may be helpful in high-risk babies, such as those with congenital heart disease.

Asthma

Incidence

Very common; occurs in at least 1 in 7 children.

Aetiology

Allergens, particularly house dust mite, are always important in children. Often a family history of asthma, allergies or eczema.

Clinical features

Mild asthmatics may have only chronic cough, particularly nocturnal or exercise-induced. More severe symptoms include wheezing and respiratory distress. Children with chronic under-treated asthma may develop chest deformity (Fig. 260) and growth failure.

Management

Severity of attack best assessed by monitoring peak flow. Acute bronchospasm usually responds to inhaled beta-sympathomimetics or xanthines. Prophylaxis with inhaled sodium cromoglycate or corticosteroids is helpful in chronic asthma.

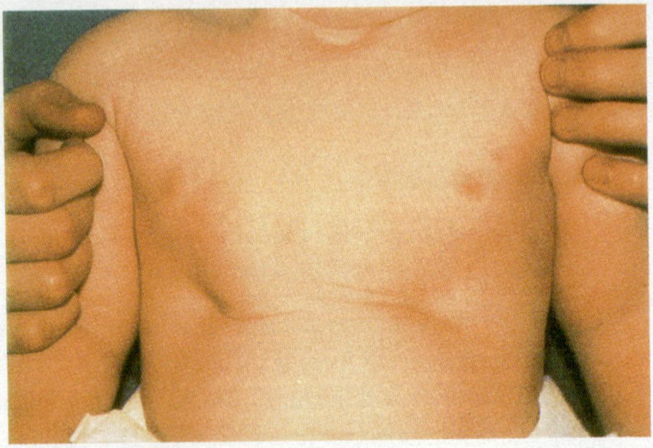

图 259　细支气管炎的胸部凹陷
Chest recession in bronchiolitis

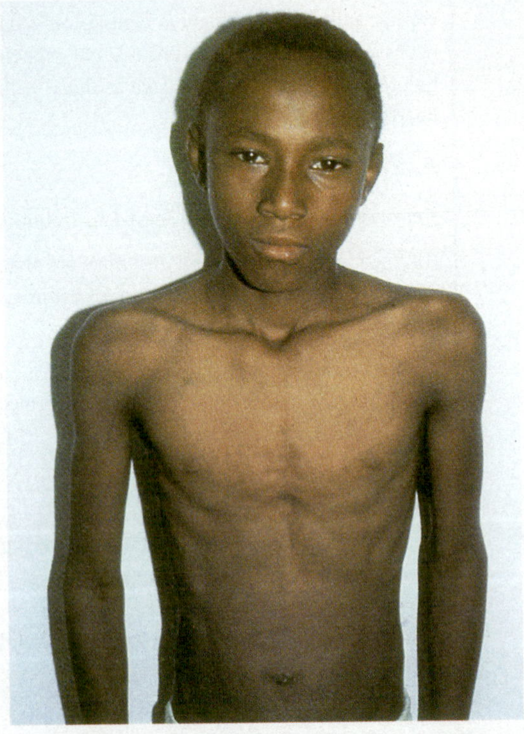

图 260　慢性哮喘的胸廓畸形
Chest deformity in a chronic asthmatic

肺炎

病因学 在婴儿期，支气管肺炎一般是由流感嗜血杆菌引起，或少数情况下由金黄色葡萄球菌引起。在大龄儿童肺炎球菌感染可引起大叶性肺炎（图 261）。支原体肺炎也很常见。

临床特征 发烧、呼吸急促、假性脑（脊）膜炎和喂养困难。婴儿常缺乏局部体征，所以胸部 X 线片对于任何患儿都很有必要。有时由于异物的吸入也会导致反复发作的肺部感染、喘鸣或肺局部空气滞留。

治疗 在致病菌和药敏结果被确定之前，先应用广谱抗生素。如果怀疑支原体感染应使用红霉素。

囊性纤维化病

发病率 在英国、美国和澳大利亚，该病是儿童慢性化脓性肺病和胰腺功能不全最常见的原因。常染色体隐性遗传疾病，在一般人群中的携带率为 1/20。每 1600 名出生存活儿中就有 1 名患有囊性纤维化病。

病因学 外分泌腺和黏液分泌腺异常，病因不明。杂合子携带者是无症状的，但是可通过遗传分析被检测到。

临床特征 胎粪性肠梗阻和新生儿肠梗阻。反复发生的肺部感染（图 262）。生长不足和吸收不良，可能出现杵状指（趾）。

诊断 发汗试验具有确诊性。有胰腺功能不全的新生儿在出生后的前几周内其血浆免疫反应性胰蛋白酶会升高。目前对受影响家庭通过采集绒毛膜绒毛样本进行 DNA 分析来作出产前诊断是可能的。

治疗 补充胰酶来改善吸收不良。用抗生素和体位性引流法快速积极地治疗肺部感染，也可以预防性应用抗生素。成年后长期存活率取决于肺部受累的严重程度。常常出现慢性胸部变形和由耐药性致病菌引起的感染。

Pneumonia

Aetiology

In infancy, bronchopneumonia is usually caused by *Haemophilus influenzae* or rarely by *Staphylococcus aureus*. Pneumococcal infection causes lobar pneumonia (Fig. 261) in older children. Mycoplasma pneumonia is also common.

Clinical features

Fever, tachypnoea, meningism and feeding difficulties. Localizing signs are often absent in infants, so chest X-ray is usually necessary in any ill child. Recurrent chest infections, wheeze or localized air-trapping is sometimes due to inhalation of a foreign body.

Management

Broad-spectrum antibiotics until specific organism and sensitivities identified. Erythromycin if Mycoplasma is suspected.

Cystic fibrosis

Incidence

The most common cause of suppurative chronic lung disease and pancreatic insufficiency in children in the UK, USA and Australia. Autosomal recessive inheritance; carrier rate in general population is 1 in 20. Cystic fibrosis affects 1 in 1600 live births.

Aetiology

Abnormality of exocrine and mucus-secreting glands; aetiology unknown. Heterozygote carriers are asymptomatic, but are detectable by genetic analysis.

Clinical features

Meconium ileus and neonatal gut obstruction. Recurrent chest infections (Fig. 262), failure to thrive and malabsorption. Clubbing of fingers and toes may occur.

Diagnosis

Sweat test is definitive diagnostic test. Elevated plasma immunoreactive trypsin in first few weeks of life in those with pancreatic insufficiency. Antenatal diagnosis is now possible in affected families using DNA analysis from chorionic villus sampling.

Management

Pancreatic supplements control malabsorption. Prompt and aggressive treatment of chest infections with antibiotics and postural drainage. Prophylactic antibiotics may be helpful. Long-term survival into adult life depends on severity of chest involvement. Chronic chest deformity and infections caused by antibiotic-resistant organisms frequently develop.

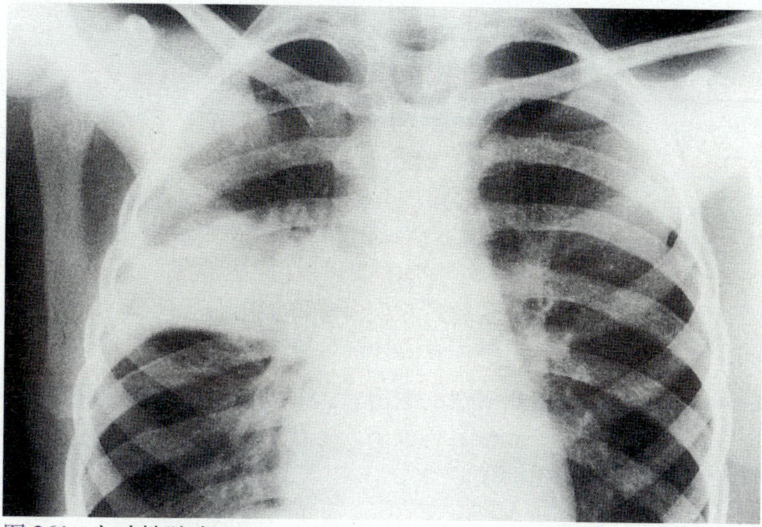

图 261 大叶性肺炎
Lobar pneumonia

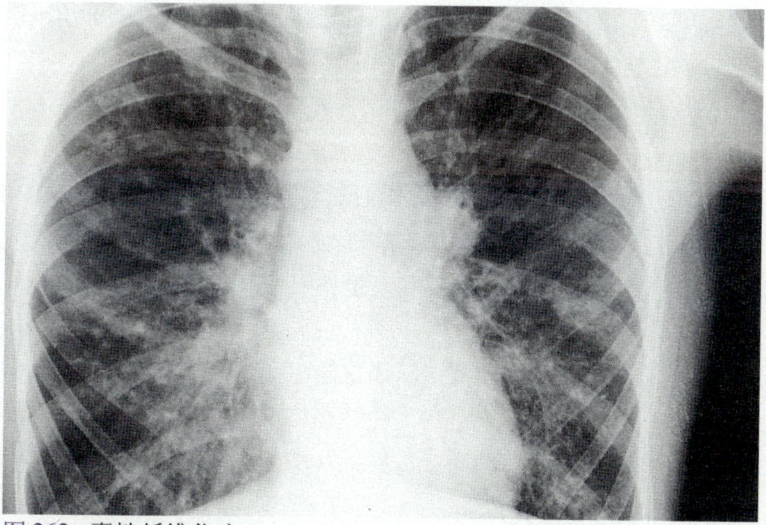

图 262 囊性纤维化病
Cystic fibrosis

先天性心脏病

发病率 常见，至少每300名出生存活儿中就有1名。

诊断 在常规性检查中经常会发现无症状性心脏杂音。发绀（图264）或心力衰竭一般提示有严重的心脏结构缺损。有些疾病会有杵状指（趾）（图263），如法洛四联症。超声心动图和心脏导管检查可以看到精确的心脏结构。胸部X光片和心电图对诊断也有帮助，但是很少通过它们来确诊。当有股动脉搏动不相同或延迟时，就要怀疑是否有主动脉缩窄。

治疗 要根据潜在的原因。大部分常见的畸形是室间隔缺损一般会自行关闭。一些更严重的缺损需进行外科手术治疗。

急性喉-气管-支气管炎（哮吼）

发病率 通常多发于4岁以下的孩子。一般由病毒感染引起。

临床特征 先有几天的鼻卡他症状，然后是特征性的犬吠样咳嗽和吸气性喘鸣（哮吼）。在夜间或当患儿焦虑不安或哭闹时，症状常常更为严重。

治疗 通常需要吸氧。布地奈德（一种皮质激素）喷雾剂和口服地塞米松可以减轻症状的严重程度。偶尔如果有严重的气道梗阻，则需要气管插管。

急性会厌炎

病因学和发病率 潜在的胎儿B型流感嗜血杆菌(Haemophilus influenzae type B, HiB)感染。但是在接种过HiB疫苗后就不常见。

临床特征 突发性的喘鸣和气道梗阻。

治疗 咽喉部检查是禁忌的，除非专门准备有气管插管（图265），即使这样插管往往也很困难。一般在48小时内静脉输入氨苄西林或头孢菌素来控制会厌部的水肿和炎症。

Congenital heart disease

Incidence
Common; at least 1 in 300 live births.

Diagnosis
Asymptomatic cardiac murmurs are often heard during routine examination. Cyanosis (Fig. 264) or heart failure usually indicate a serious structural defect. Clubbing of fingers (Fig. 263) and toes may develop in conditions such as Fallot's tetralogy. Echocardiogram and cardiac catheterization give precise detail of cardiac structure. Chest X-ray and electrocardiogram are helpful, but rarely diagnostic. Coarctation of aorta is suspected when there is inequality or delay of femoral pulses.

Management
Depends on underlying problem. Most common abnormality is ventricular septal defect which usually closes spontaneously. Surgery may be required for more serious defects.

Acute laryngo-tracheo-bronchitis (croup)

Incidence
Common under 4 years of age. Usually a viral illness.

Clinical features
Coryzal symptoms for a few days, then a characteristic barking cough and inspiratory stridor (croup). Symptoms often worse at night or when child is anxious or crying.

Management
Oxygen is often needed. Nebulized budesonide and oral dexamethasone reduce severity of symptoms. Occasionally, tracheal intubation may be required if there is severe airway obstruction.

Acute epiglottitis

Aetiology and incidence
Potentially fatal *Haemophilus influenzae* type B infection. Uncommon after HiB vaccination.

Clinical features
Sudden onset of stridor, toxicity and airways obstruction.

Management
Examination of throat is contraindicated unless there is immediate expert provision for tracheal intubation (Fig. 265) which is often difficult. Intravenous ampicillin or a cephalosporin usually controls oedema and inflammation of epiglottis within 48 h.

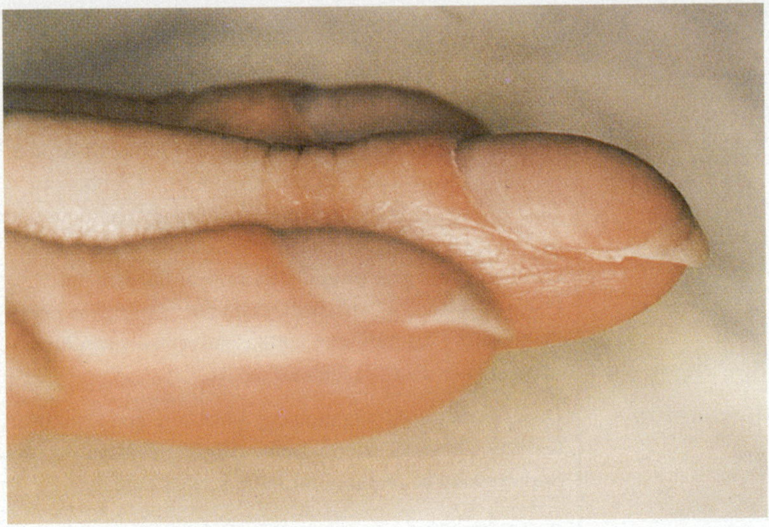

图 263　发绀性心脏病的杵状指
Finger clubbing in cyanotic heart disease

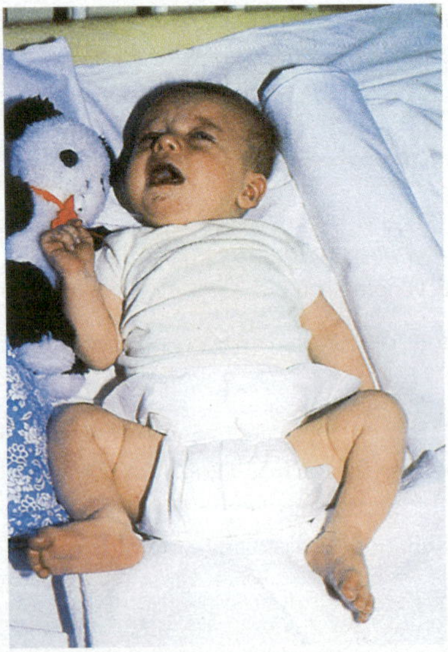

图 264　发绀性先心病
Cyanotic congenital heart disease

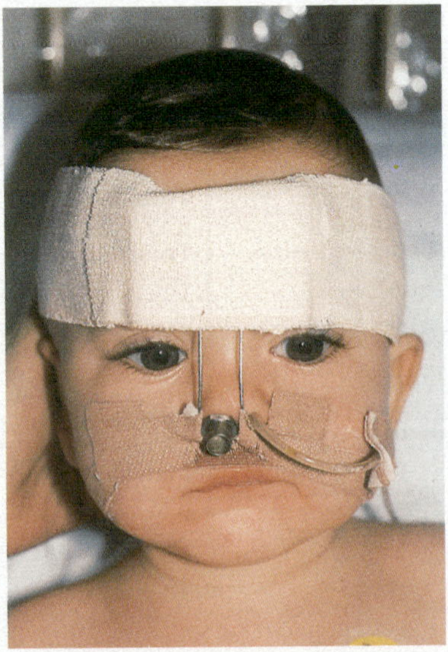

图 265　急性会厌炎进行鼻插管
Nasal intubation for acute epiglottitis

先天性异常

急性青光眼

由于眼睛前房角内液体引流障碍而导致的先天性眼内压升高。患儿的眼睛变得很大（牛眼），并且角膜会变得浑浊不清（图 266）。对于眼科医师而言，予以减压或手术治疗是十分紧急的。

白内障

一般都是先天性的，有时也有家族遗传性。白内障会继发于风疹性胚胎畸形、半乳糖血症和糖尿病发生。可以看见晶状体浑浊（图 267）。还经常表现有其他眼部异常，如眼球震颤或视觉障碍。治疗依赖于原因和视觉干预的可能性。生后前几个月内进行早期手术治疗可以减少以后发生弱视的危险。

小眼

通常伴随于先天性风疹的发育异常。如果睑裂较短，可以进行外科手术来改善外观。

上睑下垂

通常是家族性遗传，并且多为单侧。在大多数病例中，双眼的视力未受影响。如果上睑下垂严重且眼睑盖住瞳孔，缩短上睑提肌可改善外观，或可改善视力。

眼组织缺损

虹膜的发育异常（图268）。通常是家族性遗传。视力一般不受影响，除非有视网膜异常。

Congenital anomalies

Acute glaucoma

Congenital condition producing increased pressure inside eye from lack of drainage at angle of anterior chamber. The eye becomes large (buphthalmos) and the cornea becomes cloudy (Fig. 266). Urgent referral to ophthalmologist for decompression and surgery.

Cataract

Usually congenital and sometimes familial. Secondary cataracts occur in rubella embryopathy, galactosaemia and diabetes. Opacity in the lens (Fig. 267) is seen. Other ocular anomalies such as nystagmus or visual disturbance are often present. Management depends on cause and likelihood of interference with vision. Early surgery within the first months diminishes the risk of subsequent amblyopia.

Microphthalmos

Developmental anomaly often associated with congenital rubella. Surgery may improve appearance if the palpebral fissure is short.

Ptosis

Often familial and usually unilateral. In the majority of cases, binocular vision is unaffected. Shortening of the levator palpebrae superioris may improve the cosmetic appearance, or improve vision if ptosis is severe and the eyelid covers the pupil.

Coloboma

Developmental anomaly of the iris (Fig. 268). Often familial. Vision is usually unaffected, unless there is a retinal anomaly.

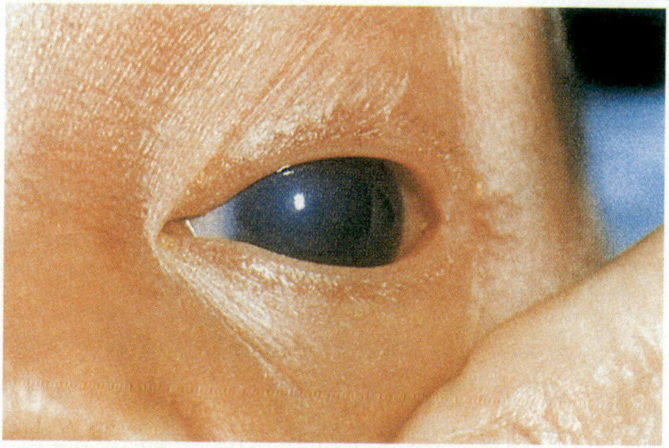

图 266 先天性青光眼浑浊不清的大角膜
Cloudy large cornea in congenital glaucoma

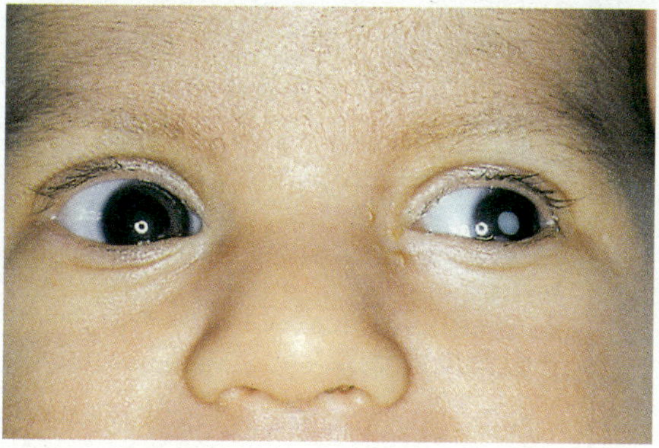

图 267 白内障
Cataract

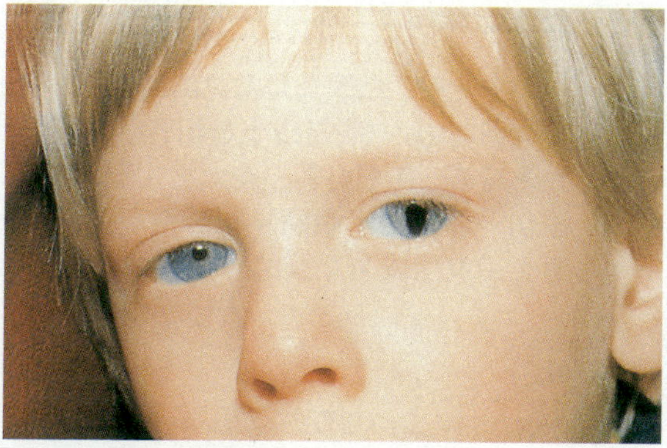

图 268 眼组织缺损
Coloboma

斜视

发病率 常见于儿童早期。所有固定性斜视和在生后5～6个月出现的持续性斜视都需要仔细的评估。

临床特征 一般较为明显（图269）。在一些不太明显的病例中，对称的角膜反射或遮闭试验都有助于诊断。内眦赘皮可能会引起类似斜视的外观。

治疗和预后 在斜眼中，如果斜视不被察觉或未能早期治疗，那么视力抑制（弱视）可能是永久性的。校正屈光不正和非斜视眼的遮挡是必须的。有时也需要进行外科手术。

恶性肿瘤

发病率和遗传特性 视网膜母细胞瘤是儿童最常见的眼内恶性肿瘤。有时具有常染色体显性遗传特性。

临床特征 患侧眼睛瞳孔混浊、斜视或视力较差。若肿瘤累及眼眶，会发生眼球突出，尤其在转移的神经母细胞瘤。

治疗 视网膜母细胞瘤的治疗包括手术治疗和放疗。肿瘤转移较罕见，且长期预后较好。

外眦角皮样囊肿

一般发生于眼眶周围，通常位于睑裂的上外侧。外科手术对于改善外观通常是有必要的，因为囊肿体积会逐渐增大。

感染和外伤

在新生儿期，结膜炎是常见的。反复发生的轻微结膜炎（图270）一般是由于鼻泪管引流不畅而引起，会在生后第一年中好转。在大龄儿童，疼痛的角膜上皮擦伤一般是由于眼睛异物所引起。结膜出血可能在出生后发生或与直接的外伤有关（图 271）。

Strabismus (squint)

Incidence

Common in early childhood. All fixed squints and any squint persisting after 5-6 months of age require careful evaluation.

Clinical features

Usually obvious (Fig. 269). Symmetrical corneal reflection or occlusion testing may assist diagnosis in less obvious cases. Epicanthic folds may give rise to a false appearance of squint.

Management and prognosis

Suppression of vision (amblyopia) in the deviated eye may be permanent if squint is not detected and treated early. Correction of refractive error and occlusion of the non-squinting eye are mandatory. Surgery is sometimes necessary.

Malignancy

Incidence and inheritance

Retinoblastoma is the most common malignant intraocular tumour in childhood. Sometimes autosomal dominant inheritance.

Clinical features

Opacity of pupil, squint or poor vision in affected eye. Proptosis occurs with tumours involving the orbit, particularly metastatic neuroblastoma.

Management

Treatment of retinoblastoma includes surgery and radiotherapy. Metastases are rare and long-term prognosis is good.

External angular dermoid cyst

Commonly found around the orbit, usually above and lateral to the palpebral fissure. Surgery is usually necessary to improve appearance, because the cysts gradually increase in size.

Infection and trauma

Conjunctivitis is common in neonatal period. Recurrent mild conjunctivitis (Fig. 270) is usually due to non-patency of the nasolacrimal duct which resolves in the first year of life. In older children, painful corneal abrasions are usually caused by foreign bodies in the eye. Conjunctival haemorrhage may occur after birth or in association with direct trauma (Fig. 271).

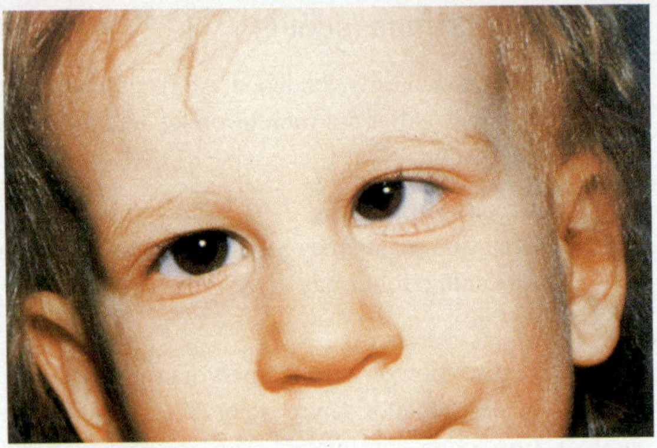

图 269　斜视
Squint

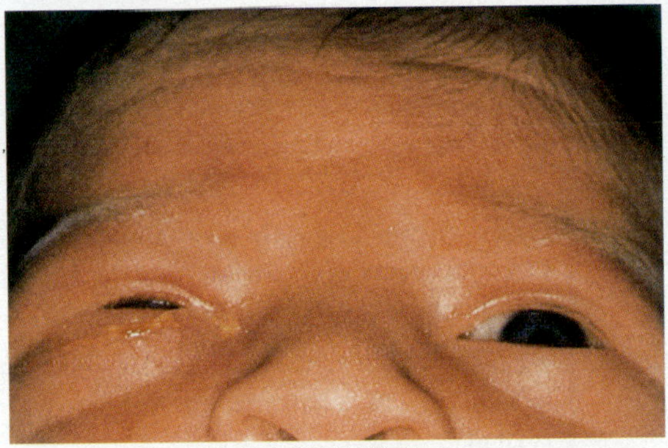

图 270　反复发生的轻微结膜炎
Recurrent minor conjunctivitis

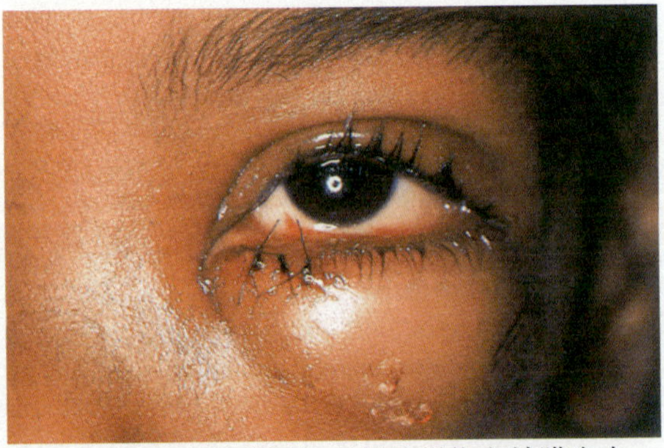

图 271　外伤性眼睛损伤引起的裂伤和结膜出血
Traumatic eye lesion with laceration and conjunctival haemorrhage

非意外伤害（NAI）

病因学

非意外伤害或儿童虐待一般发生于当父母或其他照顾儿童的成年人伤害了依赖性强且需要照顾的儿童时。儿童虐待也可能表现为更微妙的身体或情感方面的需求被忽视或剥夺的形式。

临床特征

通常都假定有一个意外伤害史。当病史和损伤有所不符、互相矛盾或反复发生时，就应该对病史有所怀疑。经常可发现无法解释的骨折或瘀伤，尤其是多发性或不同年龄段的。粗暴操作或直接撞击会引起肋骨或长骨的骨折。抓握和摇晃婴儿可能会留下指痕样瘀青、后侧肋骨骨折、视网膜和颅内出血。婴儿可能会由于摇晃婴儿综合征而导致严重的长期神经发育障碍。烟蒂烫伤（图272）会留下不连续的打孔样损伤。鞭痕（图273）在大龄儿童中较为多见。当将婴儿放入滚烫的水中，就会发生臀部和脚部的浸泡灼伤（图 274）。有时会很清楚地发现人的咬痕（图275）。仔细测量牙痕的大小将有助于确定是成人还是儿童引起了咬伤。

治疗

如果怀疑是非意外伤害，社会就会有义务去保护儿童。除了对损伤进行医学上的治疗外，还需要对家庭状况和可能的原因进行多学科的评估，排除其他的诊断。通过仔细监督和给予情感上的支持，许多孩子可以继续由他们的父母进行照料。少数情况下，孩子由他人照管可能会更安全。

Non-accidental injury (NAI)

Aetiology

Non-accidental injury (NAI) or child abuse usually occurs when parents or other adults caring for children injure the dependent but demanding child. Child abuse may also take the more subtle form of physical or emotional neglect or deprivation.

Clinical features

There is often a history of supposed accident. Suspicion should be aroused when history and injury are conflicting, inconsistent or repeated. Unexplained fractures or bruises, particularly multiple or of varying age, are often found. Rough handling or direct hitting may cause fractures of ribs or long bones. Gripping and shaking an infant may leave finger-mark bruises, posterior rib fractures, retinal and intracranial haemorrhage. Babies may suffer serious long-term neurodevelopmental disability as a result of shaken baby syndrome. Cigarette burns (Fig. 272) leave discrete punched out lesions. Whip marks (Fig. 273) are more common in older children. Dip-burns to the buttocks and feet (Fig. 274) occur when an infant is lowered into scalding water. Human bite marks (Fig. 275) are sometimes clearly seen. Careful measurement of the size of the teeth marks will determine whether an adult or child has inflicted the bite injury.

Management

If non-accidental injury is suspected, society has a responsibility to protect the child. In addition to medical treatment of the injuries, this will involve multi-disciplinary assessment of the family situation and possible contributing factors, and exclusion of alternative diagnoses. With careful supervision and sympathetic support, many children can continue to be cared for by their parents. Occasionally, the child may be safer in the care of others.

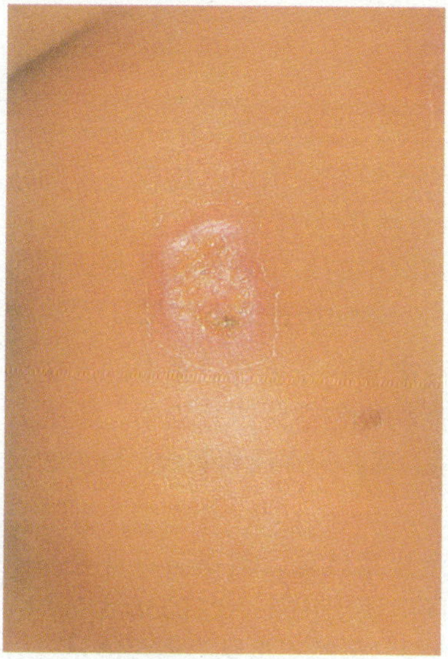

图 272 烟蒂烫伤
Cigarette burn

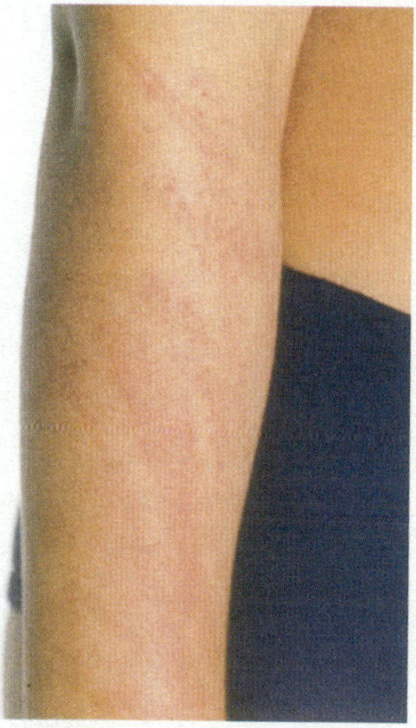

图 273 鞭痕
Whip marks

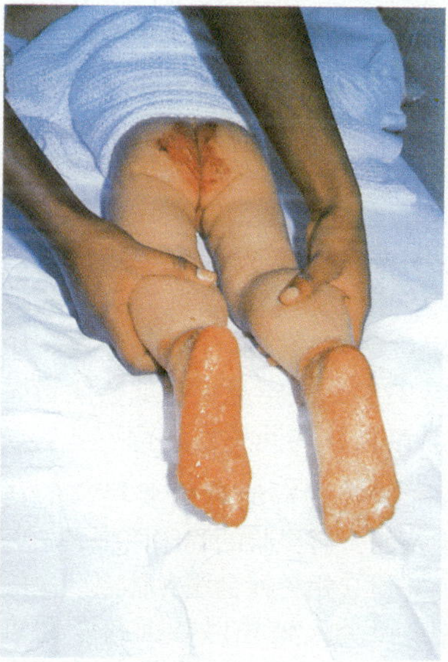

图 274 浸泡灼伤
Dip-burns

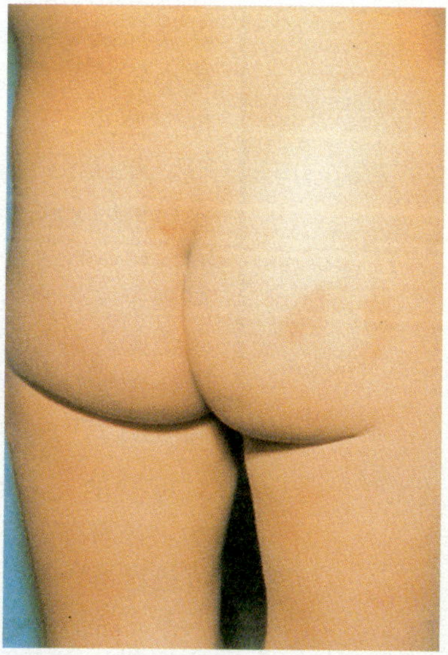

图 275 人的咬痕
Human bite marks

23 儿童性虐待 (CSA)

最近对儿童性虐待的认识有所增加。仅仅一小部分病例与突然的或暴力性伤害有关。在大多数病例中，儿童会遭受到家庭中的某位成员或儿童认识的某个人的虐待。因此，急性伤害并不常见。

症状

相信一个提供可疑受虐史的儿童是很重要的。儿童可能会有许多小的症状，包括阴道分泌物、阴道流血、尿道感染、腹痛、或会阴疼痛和刺激。行为的改变可能非常明显。

体征

大多数病例没有显示异常体征，但是会有重要的诊断线索，即使它们仅出现于10%~30%的病例中。会阴区瘀青和处女膜撕裂，虽然不常见，但可能是暴力虐待的诊断证据。大多数病例的阴道分泌物（图276）并不是由于性传播感染引起，但是极少数病例在通过细菌培养之后被诊断为淋病。其他感染，如生殖器疣（图277）可以通过性接触而被传染，但是因为人乳头瘤病毒还可以通过其他途径进行传播，所以仅凭这点就确定是儿童性虐待是很困难的，尤其在小年龄儿童。一名婴儿可能在正常的阴道分娩过程中感染了母亲的乳头瘤病毒，而母亲是无症状的，并且该损伤在儿童可能需要2年的时间来发展。无论何时只要有阴道流血或疼痛，就应该进行仔细的检查，看是否存在阴道或肛门裂口的体征。有时候很难定义正常的界限，所以要经常请教有经验的临床医师对可疑的情况进行评估。其他的一些疾病如硬化萎缩性苔癣（图 278），或罕见疾病如会阴银屑病（图 279），可能会被误认为儿童性虐待

治疗

对可疑的儿童性虐待病例进行治疗需要很高的技术。必须有一名高年资的、有经验的临床医师，由警方进行适当的咨询，并建立相关社会服务体系。一般需要长期的家庭治疗和个人辅导以帮助孩子和家庭。偶尔需要采取法律程序来保护儿童的利益。

Recognized with increasing frequency recently. Only a minority of cases are associated with a sudden or violent attack. In most cases, the children have been abused by somebody in the family or known to the child; therefore, acute injury is uncommon.

Presentation

It is important that a child who gives a suspicious history of abuse is believed. Children may present with many minor symptoms including vaginal discharge, vaginal bleeding, urinary tract infection, abdominal pain, or perineal soreness and irritation. A change in behaviour may be extremely significant.

Physical signs

The majority show no abnormal physical signs, but there are important pointers to the diagnosis even though they occur in only 10-30% of cases. Visible bruising in the perineal region and a torn hymen, although uncommon, may be diagnostic of violent abuse. Most vaginal discharge (Fig. 276) is not due to sexually transmitted infection, but occasionally gonorrhoea may be diagnosed on culture. Other infections, such as genital warts (Fig. 277) can be transmitted by sexual contact, but proving that this was due to child sexual abuse is difficult because there may be other methods of transmission of the human papilloma virus, particularly in very young children. An infant can become infected with papilloma virus during birth by normal vaginal delivery of an asymptomatic but infected mother, and the lesions in the child may take up to 2 years to develop. Whenever there is vulval bleeding or soreness, a careful inspection should be made to see if there are signs such as gaping vagina or anus. The limits of normality are difficult to define: always ask an experienced clinician to make an assessment if in doubt. Other medical conditions, lichen sclerosis et atrophicus (Fig. 278) or rare conditions such as vulval psoriasis (Fig. 279), may be mistaken for child sexual abuse.

Management

The management of suspected child sexual abuse requires great skill. A senior and experienced clinician must be involved and appropriate consultations made with police and social services. Long-term family therapy or individual counselling are often needed to support children and families. Occasionally, legal steps may need to be taken to protect the child.

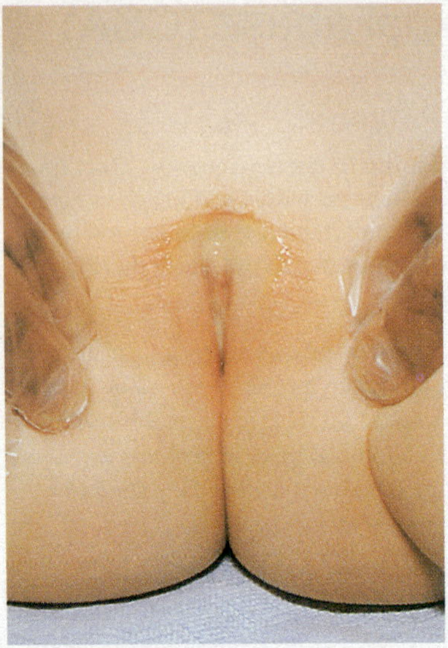

图 276 阴道分泌物
Vaginal discharge

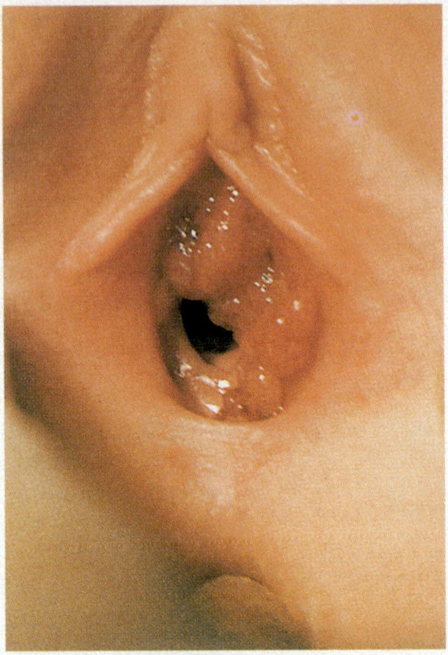

图 277 生殖器疣
Genital warts

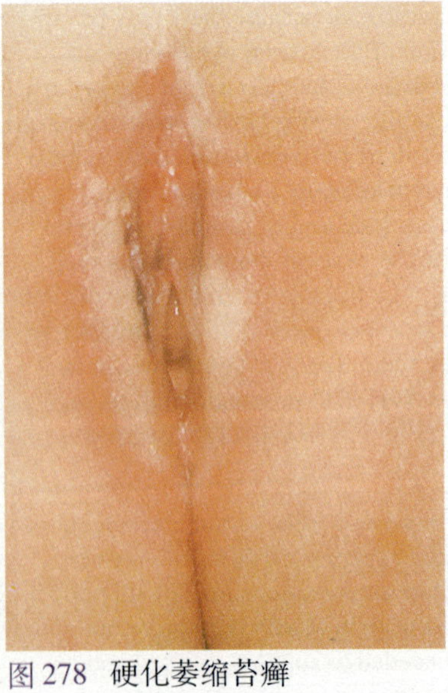

图 278 硬化萎缩苔癣
Lichen sclerosus et atrophicus

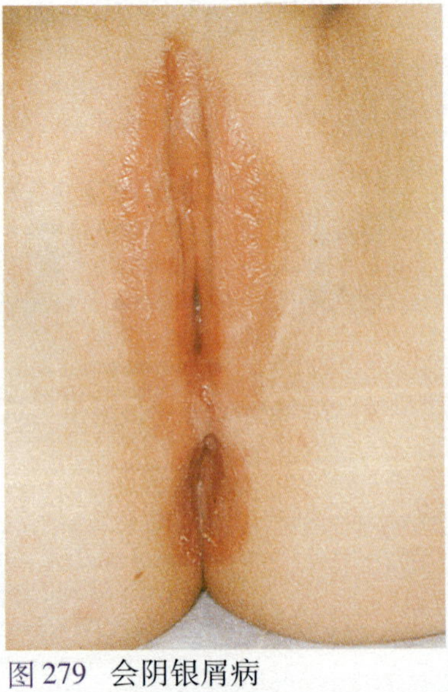

图 279 会阴银屑病
Vulval psoriasis

犯罪和失败感经常会伴随于低出生体重儿。早产儿的外观、行为和疾病可能很难被父母接受和理解。讨论和解释婴儿的情况和治疗方法，包括现代新生儿病房那些令人恐惧的设备，都会有助于减轻一些家属的不安，即使是在较早阶段还不能对治疗结果做出准确预测的情况下。对于情况良好的低出生体重儿没有必要入院，只要可能的情况下应尽量避免其进入新生儿专用病房，因为这样常常会导致其与家庭成员的分离。应该鼓励对有家庭成员开放探视，包括兄弟姐妹（图280和281）；一些积极参与照料婴儿的活动也是可能的，并且总是令人满意。这包括对所有的（除了病情非常严重的）早产儿进行护理、拥抱、换尿布、洗澡、喂养等服务。甚至如果发生婴儿死亡，父母通常也应得到最好的支持，允许他们参与最后的决定，并且和婴儿度过生命中最后一刻。通过理解和良好的情感支持，可以克服许多问题和父母忧虑焦急的情绪。

对于我们所有人，入院是令人苦恼的，但是对于孩子这却更糟糕。5岁以下的孩子可能不仅会受到病痛的惊吓，而且还可能因为离开家庭而感到悲伤。所以让某些孩子认识的人留在医院陪伴他们是很重要的，最好是父母中的一个。父母、兄弟姐妹和其他亲属留在医院经常会增加工作人员的工作量，因为他们会很自然地希望询问有关对孩子进行的检查和治疗的问题。尽管这样，他们的存在会帮助医护人员更好地照看患儿，并且使住院对孩子而言变得不那么可怕。对于有母亲陪伴在医院的孩子，噩梦、依赖性强和反复发生的遗尿等不良影响都更加少见。游戏让孩子能够忍受住院的心理压力（图282），并且也可通过游戏来暴露患儿的生理和心理问题。对于患有长期慢性疾病的孩子，尤为重要的是应该帮助他们学校作业，以缩小他们与正常儿童生活的差距，并提高教育程度。

Guilt and a sense of failure often accompany the birth of a low birth weight infant. The appearance, behaviour and illness of a preterm infant may be difficult for the parents to accept and understand. Discussion and explanation of the infant's condition and management, including the awesome equipment of the modern neonatal unit, will help to alleviate some of the uncertainty faced by the family, even though an accurate prediction of outcome cannot be made in the early stages. Unnecessary admission of well, low birth weight infants to a specialized neonatal unit should be avoided whenever possible, as such admission always results in separation for some members of the family. Open visiting for all family members, including siblings (Figs 280 and 281) should be encouraged, and some contribution towards active participation in the infant's care is usually possible and is always satisfying. This may include nursing, cuddling, nappy changing, bathing and feeding all but the most ill preterm infant. Even in the event of the death of the baby, parents are often best supported by allowing them to participate in the final decisions and moments of the infant's life. With understanding and good support, many problems and parental anxieties can be overcome.

Admission to hospital is distressing for all of us, but it is worse for children. A child under 5 years may not only be frightened by the illness and painful procedures, but also may be even more upset by separation from the family. It is very important that someone already known to the child should stay with them in hospital; preferably this should be one of the parents. Parents, siblings and other relatives on the ward often add to the work of the staff because they naturally expect to ask questions about the tests and treatment that is happening to their child. Even so, their presence helps the staff to care for the ill child better, and makes the stay in hospital much less frightening for the child. After-effects, such as nightmares, clinging and a recurrence of enuresis, are less common in children whose mothers stay with them in hospital. Play allows children to bear the strain of the admission (Fig. 282) and often reveals information about their physical and emotional problems. It is very important that in a long chronic illness there should be help with schoolwork to minimize disruption to the child's daily life and educational progress.

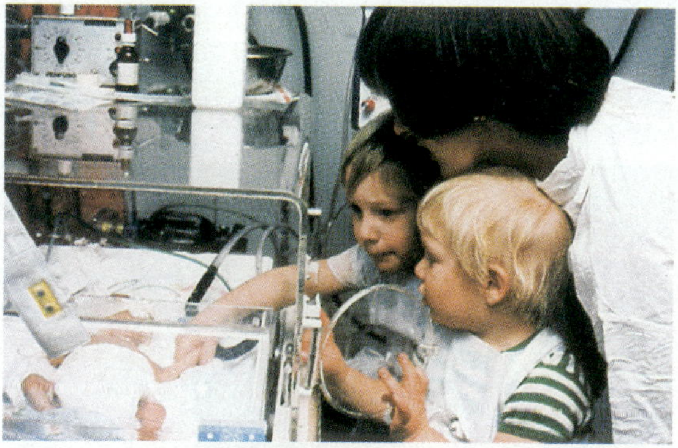

图 280　兄弟姐妹探视婴儿室
Siblings visiting neonatal nursery

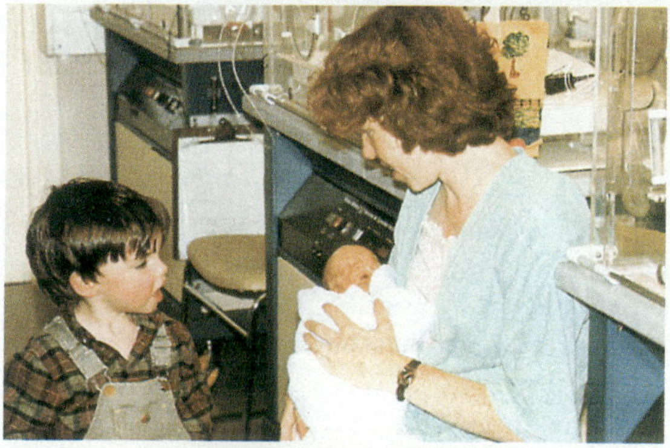

图 281　让哥哥看望婴儿
Showing the baby to her brother

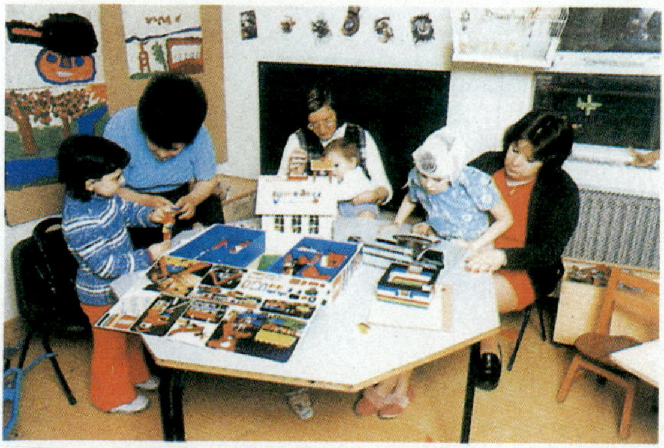

图 282　医院里父母和孩子一起游戏
Hospital playgroup with children and parents

问题

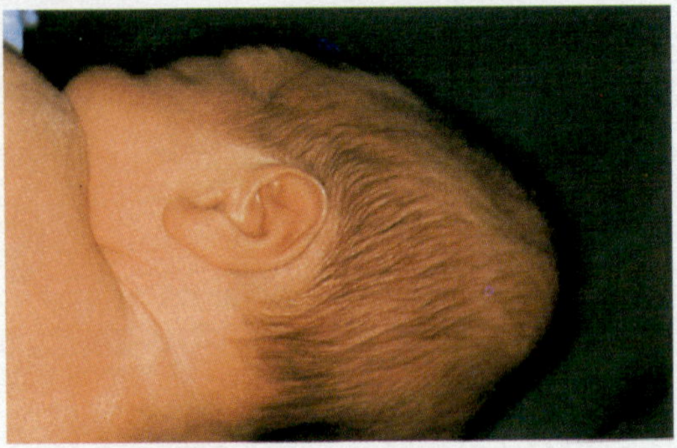

1．2天大的新生儿的头部。

a. 有什么鉴别诊断？

b. 如何作出特异性诊断？

c. 这种情况有什么样的意义和自然病史？

Head of a 2-day-old infant.

a. What is the differential diagnosis?

b. How can a specific diagnosis be made?

c. What is the significance and natural history of the conditions?

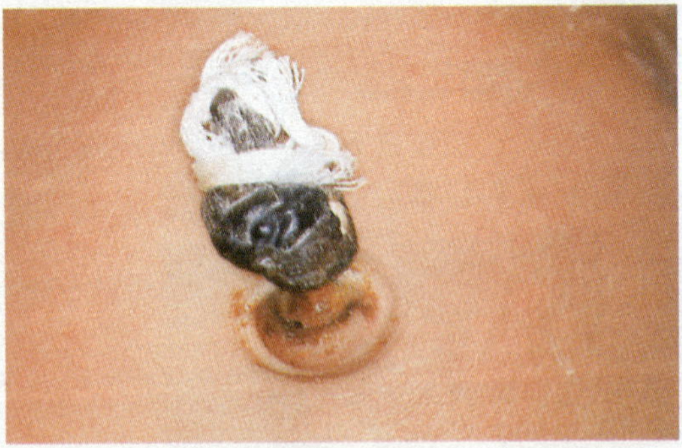

2．5天大的新生儿的脐带。

a. 是什么诊断？

b. 对这种情况有何处理方法？

Umbilical cord of a 5-day-old infant.

a. What is the diagnosis?

b. What is the management of this condition?

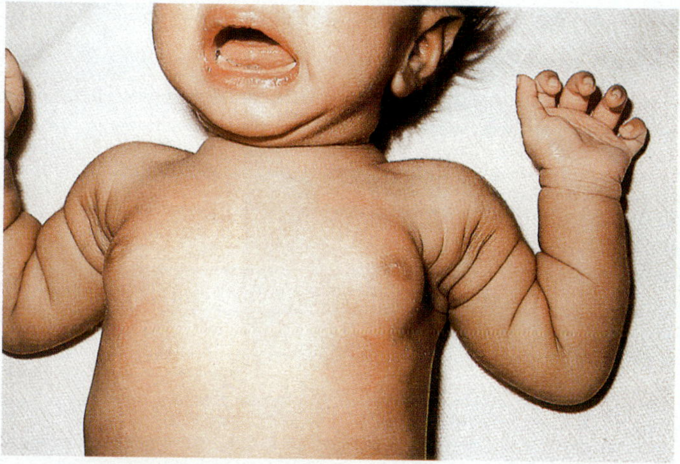

3．3天大的健康男婴的胸部。

a. 是什么诊断？

b. 描述一下其他伴随情况。

c. 怎样对家长进行解释？

Chest of a healthy 3-day-old male infant.

a. What is the diagnosis?

b. Describe other associated conditions.

c. What explanation should be given to the parents?

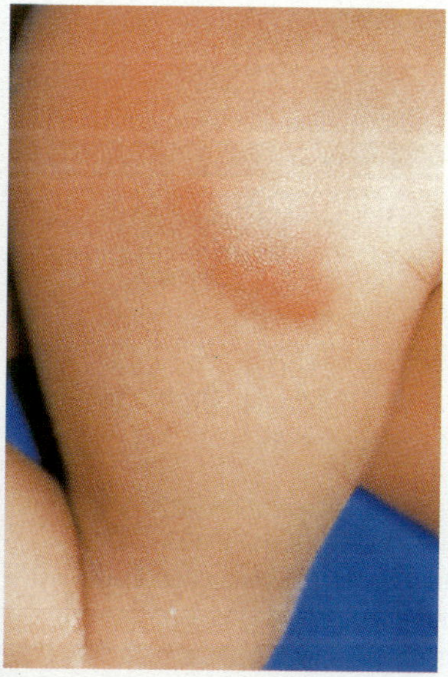

4．4周大的健康婴儿的大腿。

a. 有什么鉴别诊断？

b. 它们在临床上如何区分？

c. 描述相应的治疗方法。

Thigh of a healthy thriving 4-week-old infant.

a. What is the differential diagnosis?

b. How can they be differentiated clinically?

c. Describe the management of both conditions.

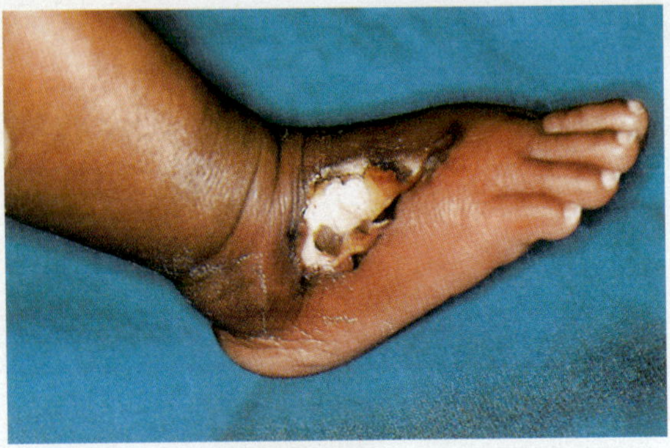

5．6周大早产儿的脚部溃疡。

a. 溃疡最可能的原因是什么?

b. 如何控制长期的损害?

Ulceration of foot of a 6-week-old preterm infant.

a. What is the most likely cause of the ulceration?

b. How may long-term damage be limited?

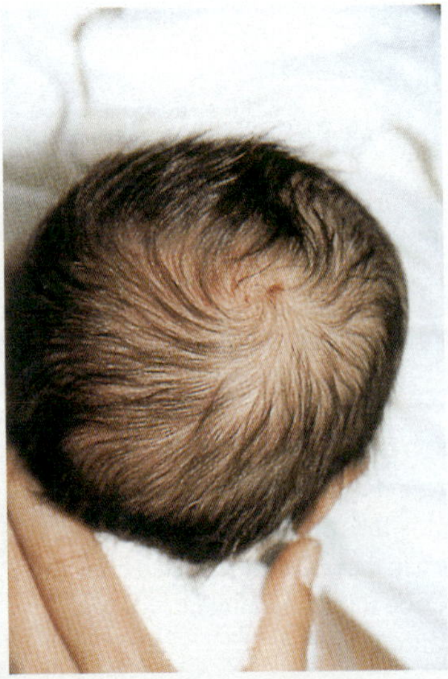

6．新生儿头皮损伤。

a. 有什么鉴别诊断?

b. 列举能引起类似损伤的三种操作。

c. 描述这些操作的目的。

Lesion on scalp of newborn infant.

a. What is the differential diagnosis?

b. Name three procedures that may cause a similar lesion.

c. What is the purpose of the procedures?

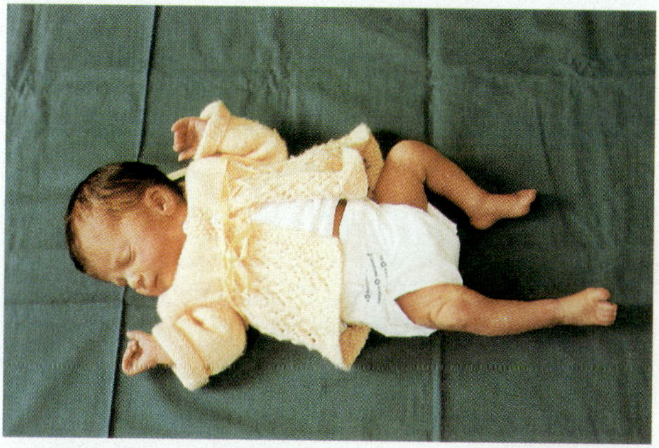

7. 新生儿的头部转向右侧。

a. 这是什么新生儿反射?

b. 列举至少4个其他的新生儿反射。

c. 新生儿反射的相关意义是什么?

Newborn infant with head turned towards the right.

a. Which neonatal reflex is being demonstrated?

b. Name at least four other neonatal reflexes.

c. What is the relevance of neonatal reflexes?

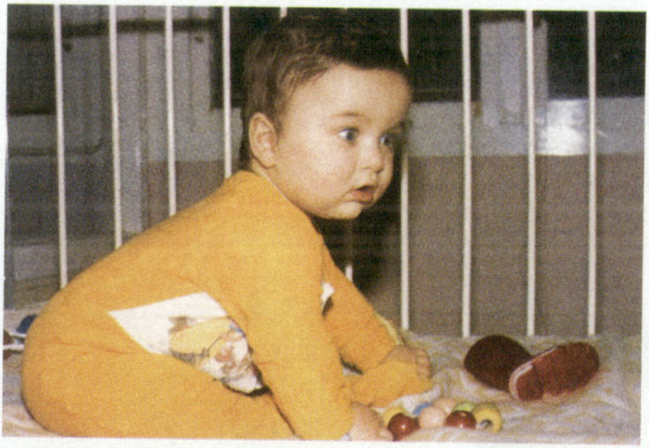

8. 婴儿三脚架式的坐位。

a. 该婴儿的年龄是多大?

b. 在这个年龄段的婴儿还应该具有什么样其他标志性的运动?

Infant sitting in tripod position.

a. What is the age of the infant?

b. What other motor milestones should be achieved by this age?

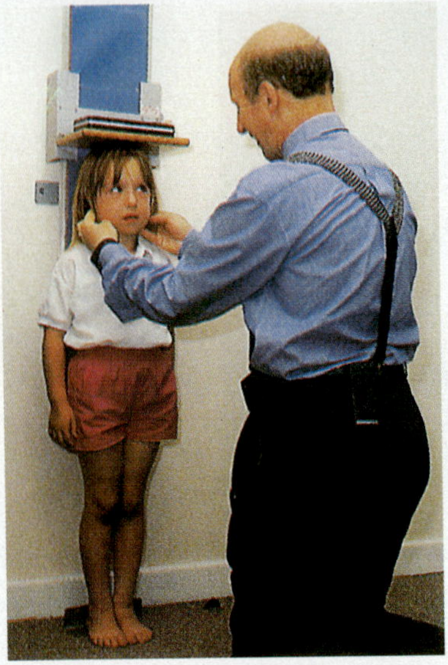

9. 一名站立着的5岁儿童。
a. 这位儿科医师在干什么?
b. 这种仪器的名称是什么?
c. 怎样对小婴儿进行该项检查?

5-year-old child in the standing position.
a. What is the paediatrician doing?
b. What is the instrument called?
c. How is the test applied in younger infants?

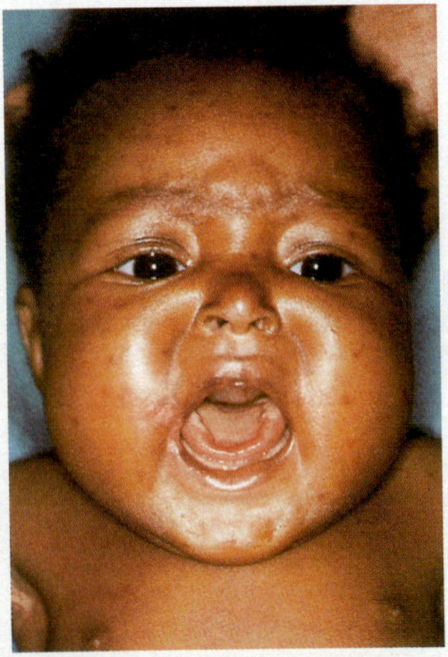

10. 一个易激惹、倦怠且食欲差的婴儿的面部。
a. 显示出什么样的特征?
b. 诊断和原因是什么?
c. 治疗方案是什么?

Face of an irritable, listless infant with poor appetite.
a. What features are shown?
b. What is the diagnosis and cause?
c. What is the treatment?

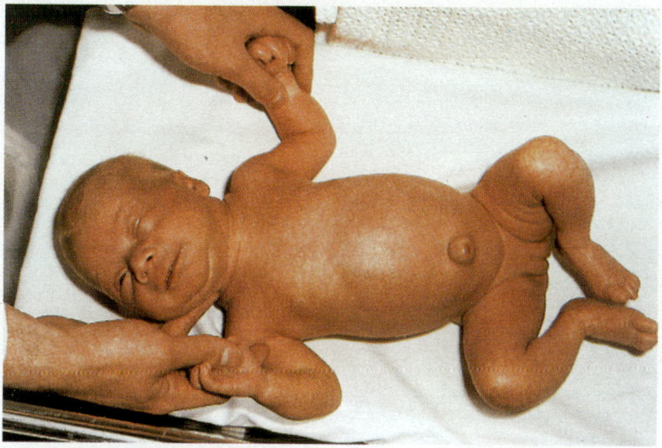

11．一个3周大的婴儿。

a. 显示出哪一种临床体征？

b. 可能的诊断是什么？

c. 列举其他相关的症状和体征。

d. 这种情况的预后如何？

A 3-week-old infant.

a. Which clinical signs are shown?

b. What is the underlying diagnosis?

c. Name other associated signs and symptoms.

d. What is the prognosis of this condition?

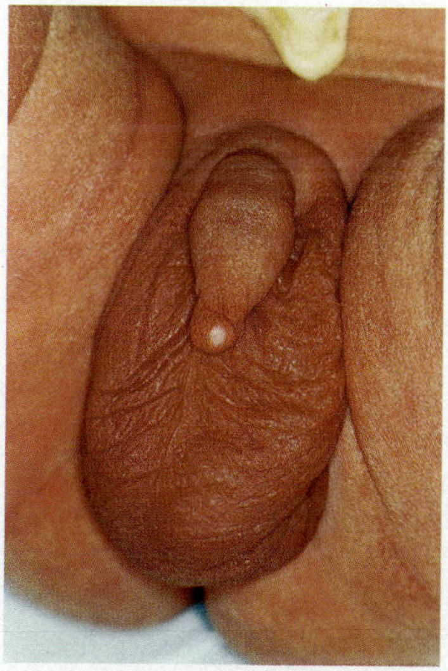

12．新生儿男婴阴茎包皮上的小的白色皮损。

a. 诊断是什么？

b. 可能的病理学是什么？

c. 哪里也可能有类似的皮损出现？

Small white lesion on prepuce of a newborn male infant.

a. What is the diagnosis?

b. What is the underlying pathology?

c. Where may similar lesions occur?

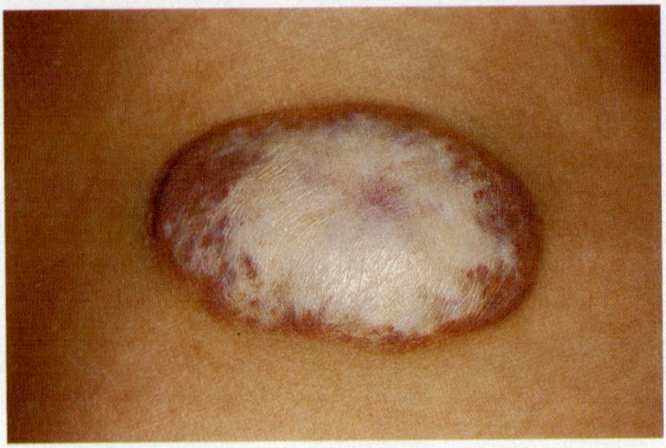

13. 2 岁儿童的皮损，皮损是在生后几周出现，呈现鲜红色大约有 18 个月。

a. 诊断是什么？

b. 这种类型的皮损自然病程是什么？

c. 有什么并发症？

Skin lesion on a child now aged 2 years. The lesion developed a few weeks after birth and was bright red for about 18 months.

a. What is the diagnosis?

b. What is the natural course of this type of lesion?

c. What are the complications?

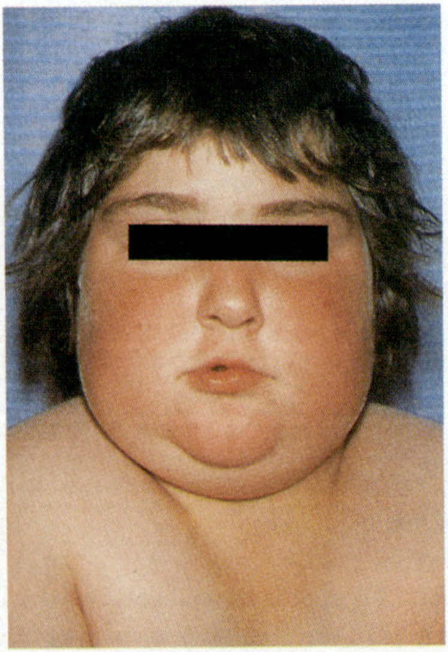

14. 10 岁男孩的脸。

a. 鉴别诊断是什么？

b. 有助于支持诊断的其他临床特征是什么？

c. 哪一项生化检查有助于诊断？

Face of a 10-year-old boy.

a. What is the differential diagnosis?

b. Which other clinical features would be helpful to support the diagnosis?

c. Which biochemical investigations will assist in diagnosis?

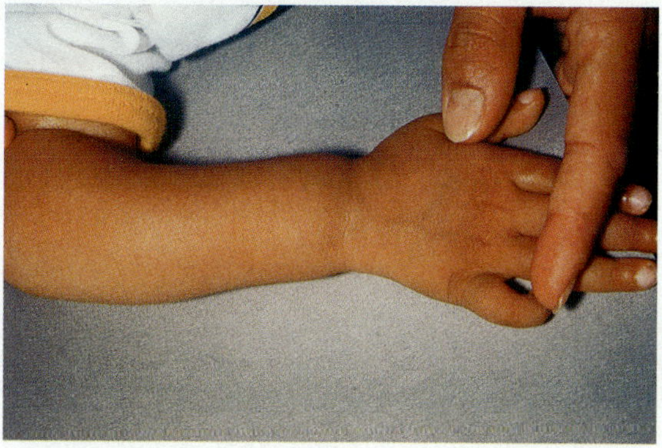

15．3 岁儿童的手和前臂。

a. 诊断是什么？

b. 列举其他临床体征。

c. 经典的生化学和放射学改变是什么？

Hands and forearm of a 3-year-old child.

a. What is the diagnosis?

b. Name other clinical signs.

c. What are the classic biochemical and radiological changes?

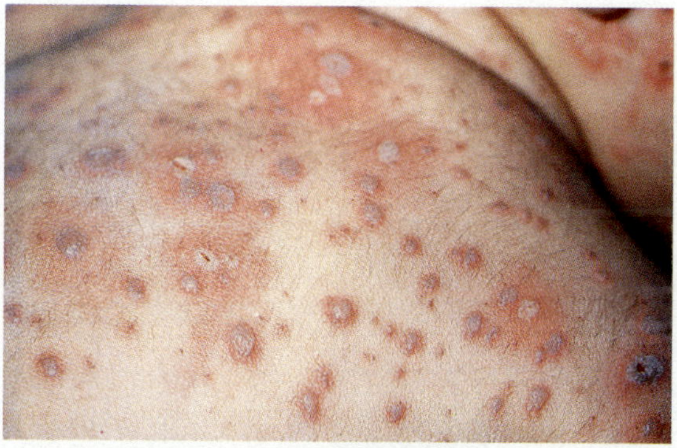

16．在其他方面健康的 5 岁男孩身上发痒的皮疹。

a. 诊断是什么？

b. 这种感染的潜伏期是多长？

c. 对于怀孕 39 周的孩子的母亲应该给予什么建议？

Itchy rash in an otherwise healthy 5-year-old child.

a. What is the diagnosis?

b. What is the incubation period of this infection?

c. What advice should be given to the child's mother who is 39 weeks' pregnant?

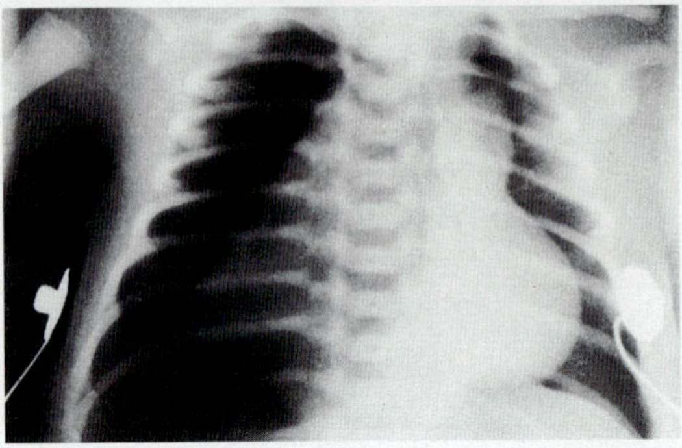

17. 具有呼吸窘迫的出生4小时的婴儿其胸部X线片。

a. 诊断是什么?

b. 列举相关临床体征。

c. 诱发该病的原因是什么?

d. 应该怎样对这种情况进行处理?

Chest X-ray of a 4-hour-old infant with respiratory distress.

a. What is the diagnosis?

b. Name associated clinical signs.

c. What are the predisposing conditions?

d. How should this condition be managed?

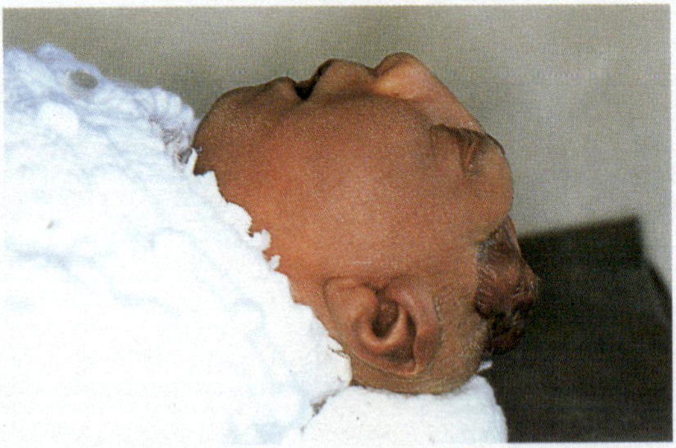

18. 生后数小时死亡的新生儿。

a. 诊断是什么?

b. 列举其他相关的异常体征。

c. 这种疾病的预后和治疗是什么?

Newborn infant who died a few hours after birth.

a. What is the diagnosis?

b. Name other associated anomalies.

c. What is the prognosis and management of this condition?

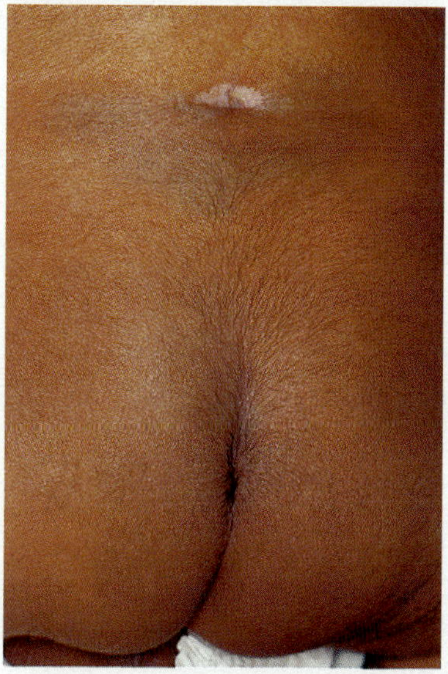

19．一个新生儿的背部。
a. 诊断是什么？
b. 如何进行确诊？
c. 该病在以后出生的孩子中再发危险是多少？
d. 如何降低该病发生的危险？

Back of a newborn infant.
a. What is the diagnosis?
b. How can the diagnosis be confirmed?
c. What is the recurrence risk in future pregnancies?
d. How can the risk be reduced?

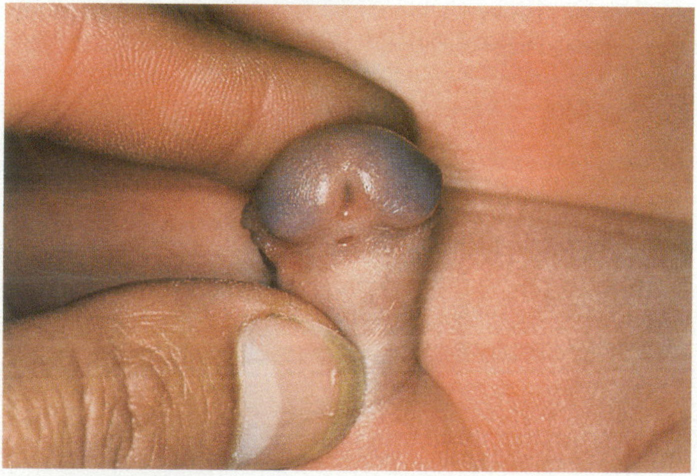

20．新生儿的阴茎。
a. 诊断是什么？
b. 相关疾病是什么？
c. 这种疾病的治疗方法是什么？

Phallus of a newborn infant.
a. What is the diagnosis?
b. What are associated conditions?
c. What is the management of this condition?

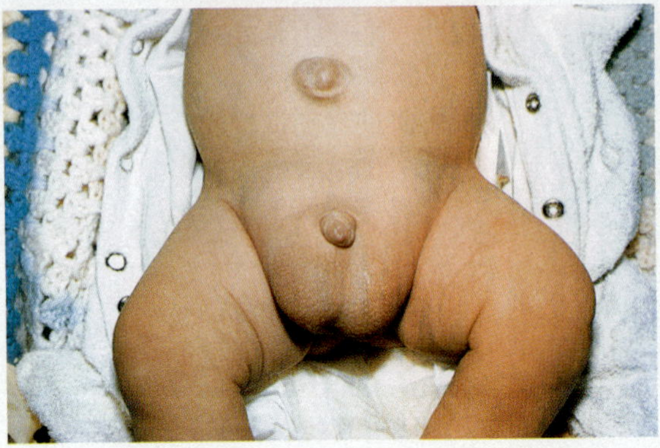

21．6个月大婴儿的腹部和外生殖器。
a. 诊断是什么？
b. 诱病因素是什么？
c. 对这些疾病的治疗方法是什么？

Abdomen and genitalia of a 6-month-old infant.
a. What are the diagnoses?
b. What are predisposing factors?
c. What is management of these conditions?

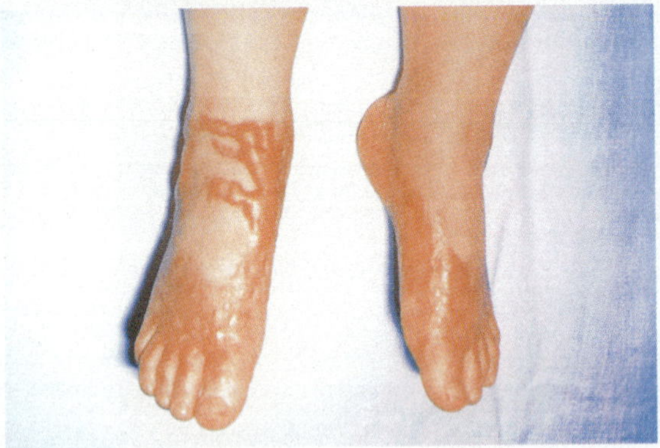

22．3岁男孩的脚部。
a. 诊断是什么？
b. 诱病因素是什么？
c. 怎样治疗这种疾病？

Feet of a 3-year-old child.
a. What is the diagnosis?
b. What are predisposing factors?
c. How can this condition be treated?

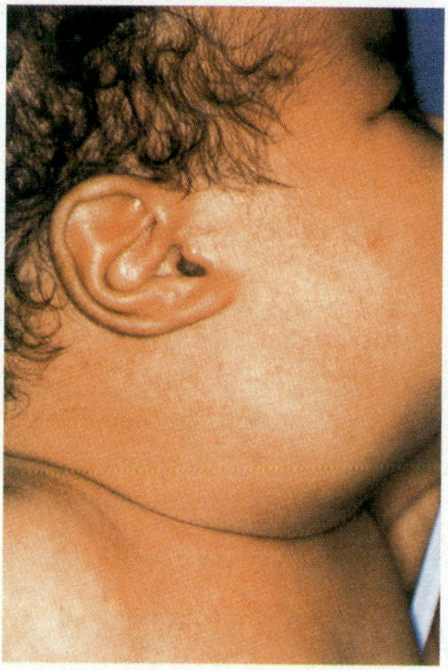

23．6个月大的婴儿颈部肿胀。
a. 鉴别诊断是什么？
b. 有助于确定诊断的其他临床体征是什么？
c. 对这些疾病的治疗方法是什么？

Neck swelling in a 6-month-old infant.
a. What is the differential diagnosis?
b. Which other clinical signs help to confirm the diagnosis?
c. What is the management of these conditions?

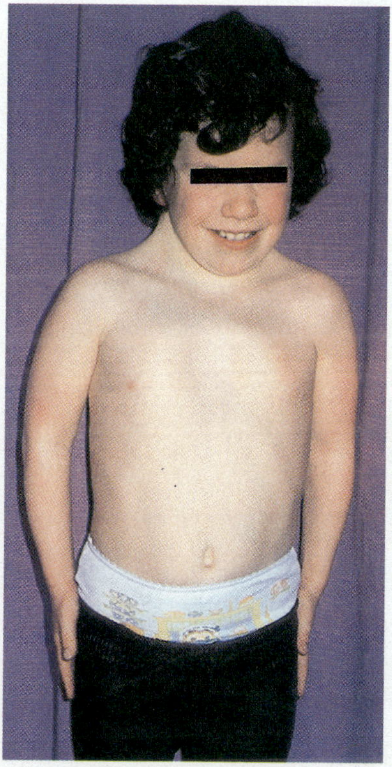

24．矮小的14岁女孩。
a. 描述其所显示的临床特征。
b. 诊断是什么？
c. 列举相关的问题。
d. 该疾病的治疗方法是什么？

A 14-year-old girl with short stature.
a. Describe the clinical features shown.
b. What is the diagnosis?
c. Name associated problems.
d. What is the management of the condition?

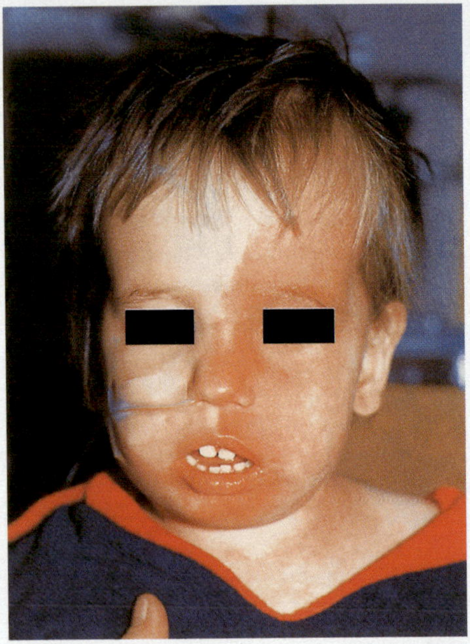

25. 学习困难的 4 岁男孩。
a. 诊断是什么?
b. 列举有关这种疾病的其他特征。
c. 哪些检查有助于诊断?

This is a 4-year-old boy with learning difficulties.
a. What is the diagnosis?
b. Name other associated features of this condition.
c. Which investigations will be helpful?

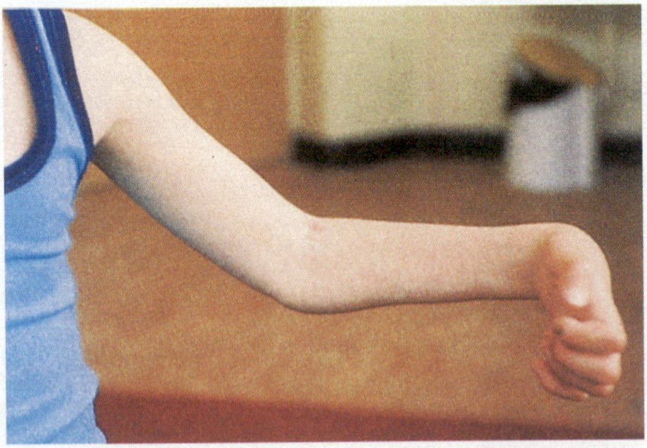

26. 9 岁男孩在数月前曾有肘部骨折。
a. 诊断是什么?
b. 这种情况的病因是什么?

This 9-year-old boy had a fracture of the elbow some months previously.
a. What is the diagnosis?
b. What is the aetiology of the condition?

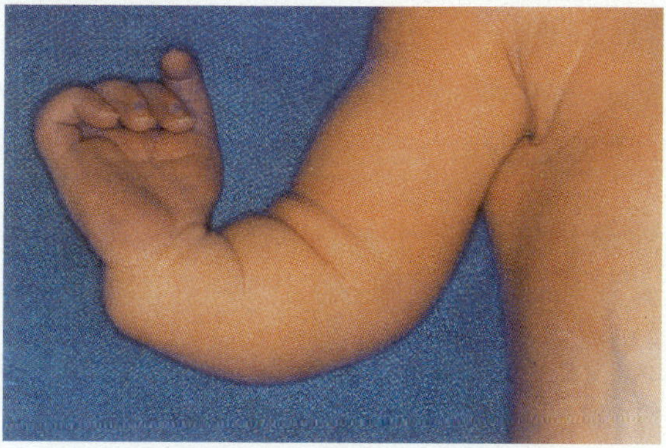

27．小婴儿的前臂和手。
a. 显示出什么特征？
b. 什么检查有助于诊断？

This is the forearm and hand of a young infant.
a. What features are shown?
b. Which investigations will be helpful?

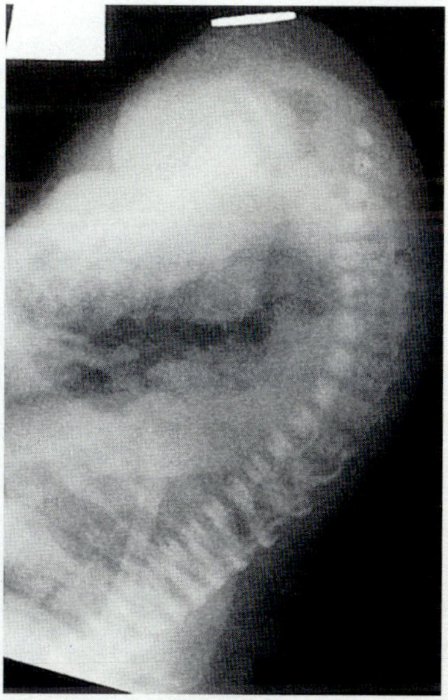

28．新生儿的腹部X线片。
a. 诊断是什么？
b. 这个婴儿的情况是怎样的？
c. 列举其他相关的问题。

Abdominal X-ray of a newborn infant.
a. What is the diagnosis?
b. How would this infant present?
c. Name other associated problems.

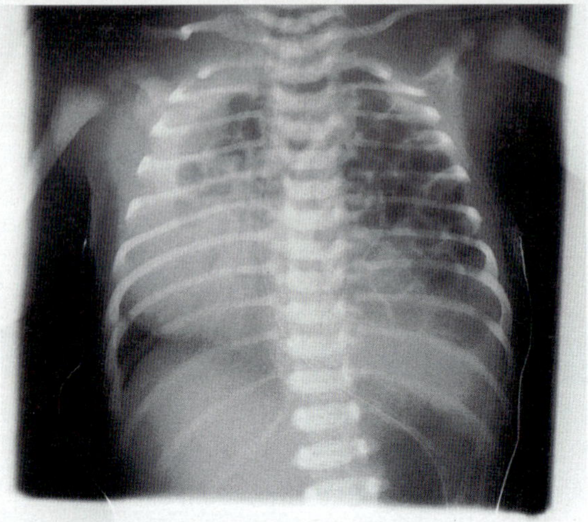

29．生后即有呼吸窘迫的新生儿的胸部 X 线片。
a. 诊断是什么？
b. 对于这种情况应该采取什么紧急措施？
c. 预后如何？

Chest X-ray of a neonate with respiratory distress soon after birth.
a. What is the diagnosis?
b. What is the emergency treatment of this condition?
c. What is the prognosis?

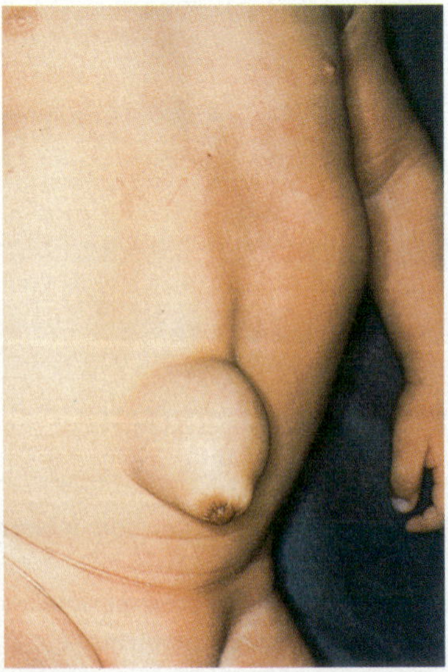

30．3 个月大早产儿的腹部。
a. 描述一下所显示的临床特征。
b. 怎样治疗？
c. 预后如何？

Abdomen of 3-month-old ex-preterm infant.
a. Describe the clinical features shown.
b. What is the treatment?
c. What is the prognosis?

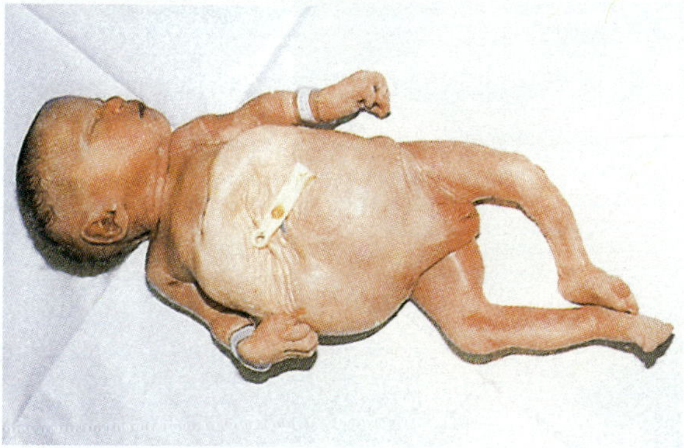

31．复苏失败的新生儿。
a. 诊断是什么？
b. 描述一下临床特征。
c. 死亡的可能原因是什么？
d. 如何对该病进行产前诊断？

Newborn infant who could not be resuscitated at birth.
a. What is the diagnosis?
b. Describe the clinical features.
c. What is the likely cause of death?
d. How can this condition be diagnosed antenatally?

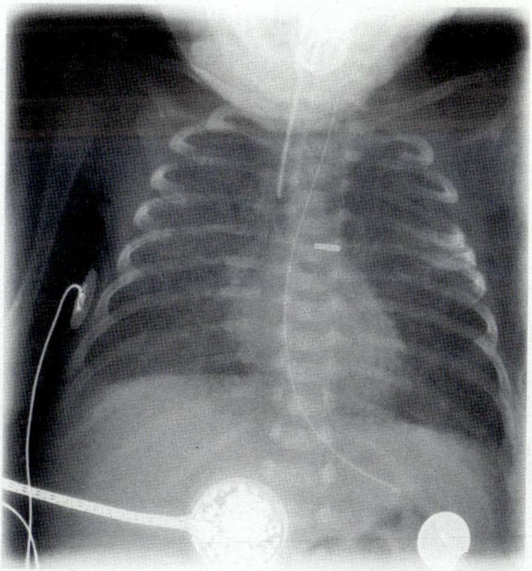

32．需要长期氧疗的早产儿胸部X线片。
a. 诊断是什么？
b. 进行了什么手术操作？
c. 长期预后如何？

Chest X-ray of ex-preterm infant who required long term oxygen therapy.
a. What is the diagnosis?
b. What operative procedure has been performed?
c. What is the long term prognosis?

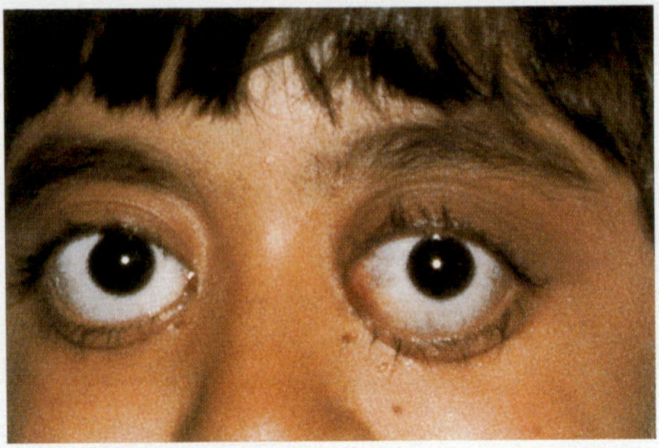

33. 12 岁男孩的眼睛。
a. 显示出什么样的临床体征?
b. 鉴别诊断是什么?

Eyes of a 12-year-old boy.
a. What clinical sign is shown?
b. What is the differential diagnosis?

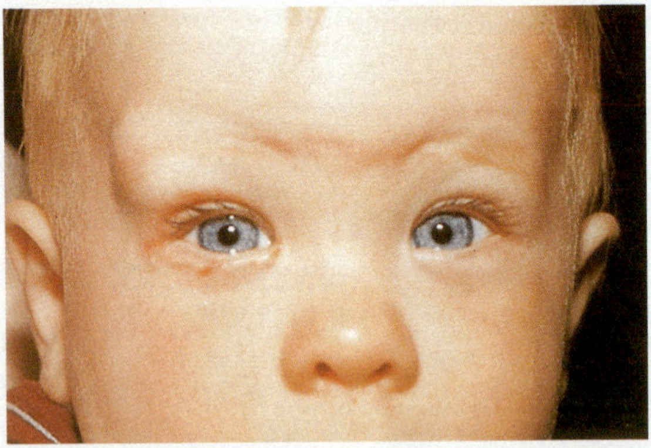

34. 9 个月大婴儿的脸。
a. 诊断是什么?
b. 病因是什么?
c. 治疗和预后如何?

Face of a 9-month-old infant.
a. What is the diagnosis?
b. What is the aetiology?
c. What is the prognosis and management?

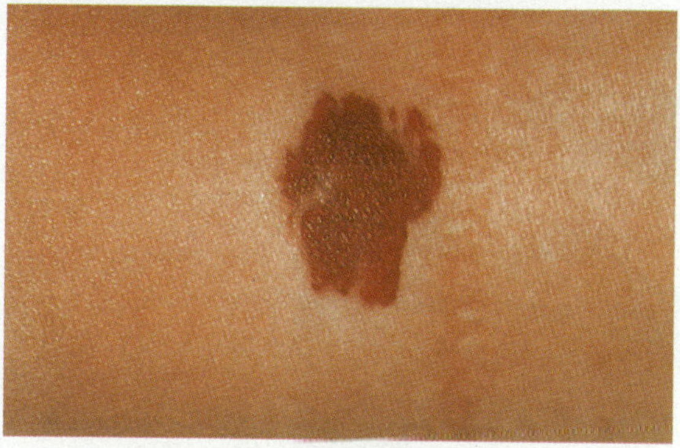

35. 9 个月大儿童的皮肤损伤。
a. 诊断是什么?
b. 描述这种皮损的临床过程。
c. 并发症是什么?
d. 合并症是什么?

Skin lesion on a 9-month-old child.
a. What is the diagnosis?
b. Describe the clinical course of this type of lesion.
c. What are the complications?
d. What are the associations?

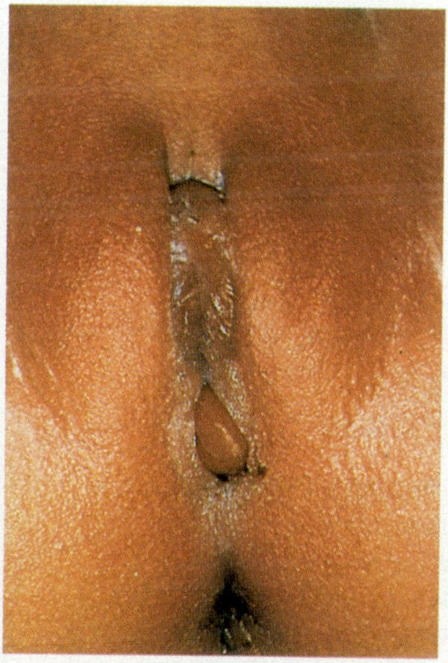

36. 4 天大女婴的会阴。
a. 诊断是什么?
b. 这种情况的原因和临床意义是什么?

Perineum of a 4-day-old female infant.
a. What is the diagnosis?
b. What is the cause and significance of this condition?

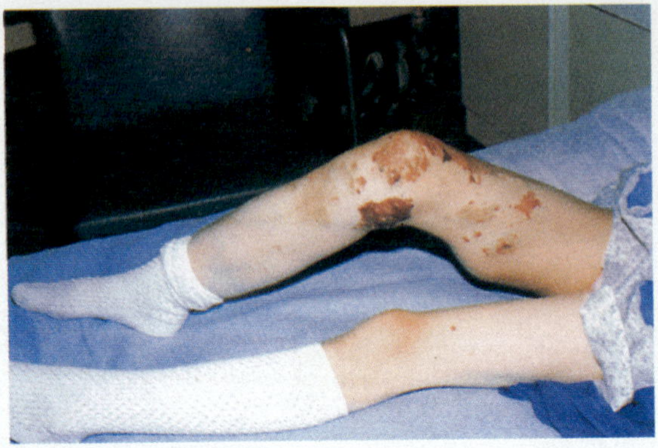

37. 10岁女孩的腿。

a. 描述一下所显示的临床特征。

b. 诊断是什么?

c. 可能的病理情况与合并症是什么?

d. 该病的遗传模式是什么?

Legs of a 10-year-old girl.

a. Describe the clinical features shown.

b. What is the diagnosis?

c. What are the underlying pathology and associations?

d. What is the mode of inheritance?

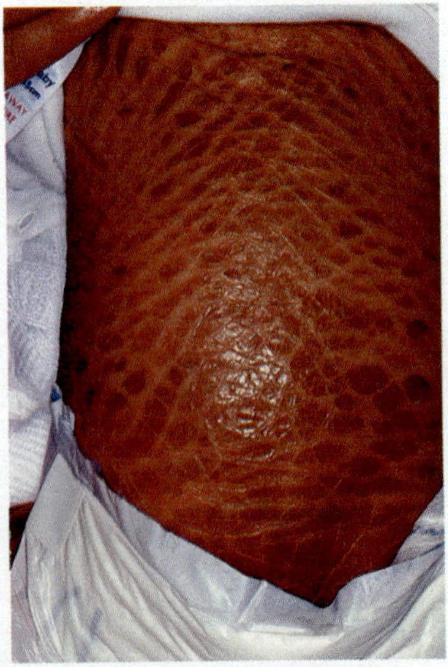

38. 出生时有火棉胶样皮肤的孩子2岁时的背部。

a. 诊断是什么?

b. 如何治疗?

c. 预后如何?

Back of a 2-year-old child who had collodion skin at birth.

a. What is the diagnosis?

b. What is the treatment?

c. What is the prognosis?

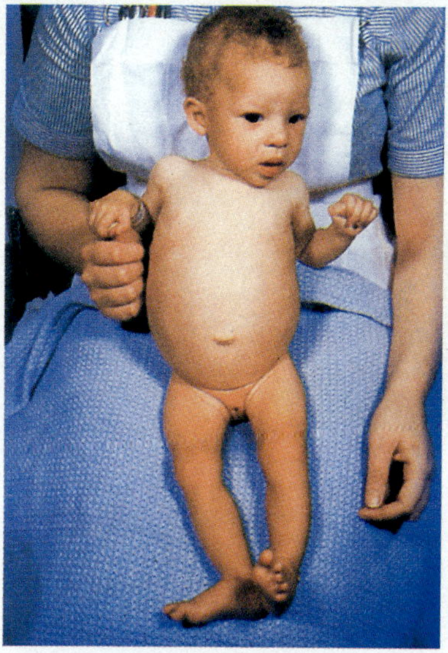

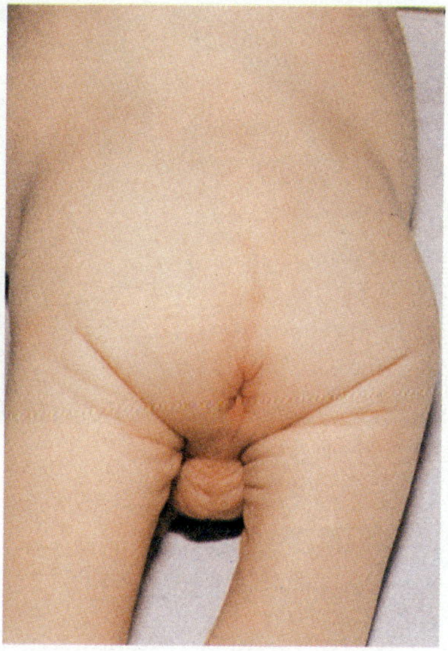

39．一名食欲差、体重增长缓慢的 12 个月婴儿。

a. 最可能的诊断是什么?

b. 潜在的原因是什么?

c. 可能有什么样的其他临床体征和症状?

A12-month-old infant with poor appetite and poor weight gain.

a. What is the most likely diagnosis?

b. What is the underlying cause?

c. What other clinical signs and symptoms may occur?

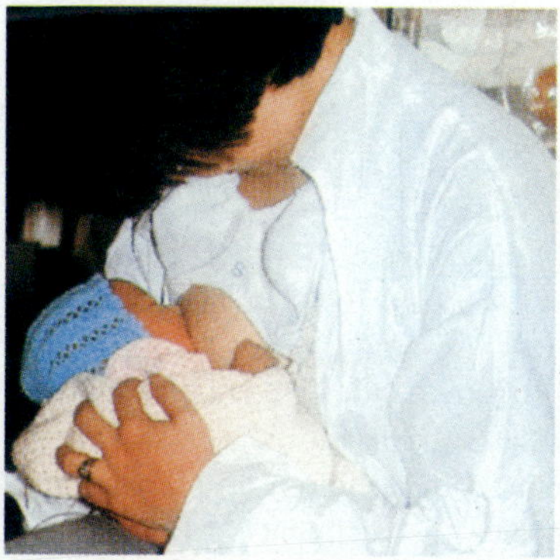

40．母乳喂养。

a. 母乳喂养的优点是什么?

b. 有哪些禁忌证?

Breast-feeding.

a. What are the benefits of breast-feeding?

b. Are there any contraindications?

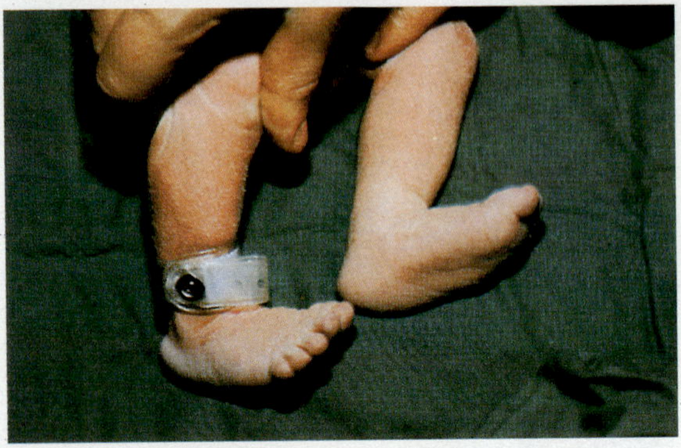

41．新生儿的脚。

a. 描述一下脚部异常。

b. 鉴别诊断是什么?

c. 列举其他相关的临床特征。

Feet of a newborn infant.

a. Describe the foot abnormality.

b. What is the differential diagnosis?

c. Name other associated clinical features.

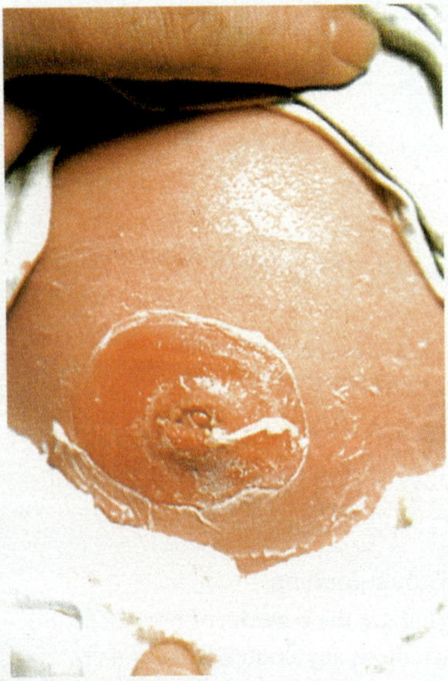

42．10天大婴儿的腹部。

a. 诊断是什么?

b. 这种疾病的病因是什么?

c. 如何治疗?

Abdomen of a 10-day-old infant.

a. What is the diagnosis?

b. What is the aetiology of this condition?

c. What is the treatment?

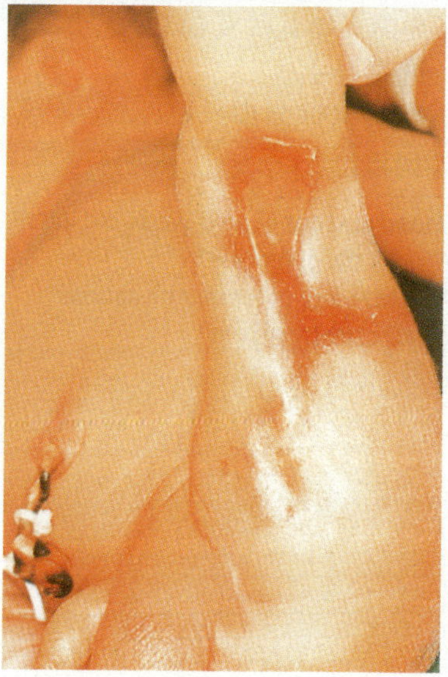

43．新生儿的腿部，其母亲在孕早期有瘙痒性皮疹。

a. 诊断是什么？

b. 如何在孕晚期治疗这种疾病？

Leg of a newborn infant whose mother had an itchy rash in early pregnancy.

a. What is the diagnosis?

b. How is this condition treated in late pregnancy?

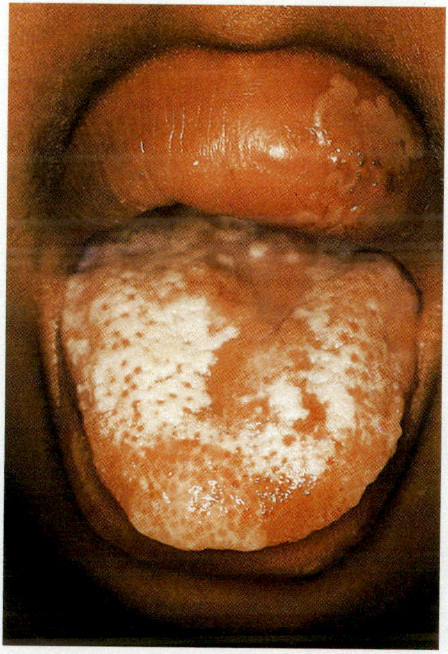

44．一位有广泛的淋巴结肿大和生长缓慢的 8 岁孩子。

a. 诊断是什么？

b. 可能的原因是什么？

An 8-year-old child with generalized lymphadenopathy and poor growth.

a. What is the diagnosis?

b. What are the underlying causes?

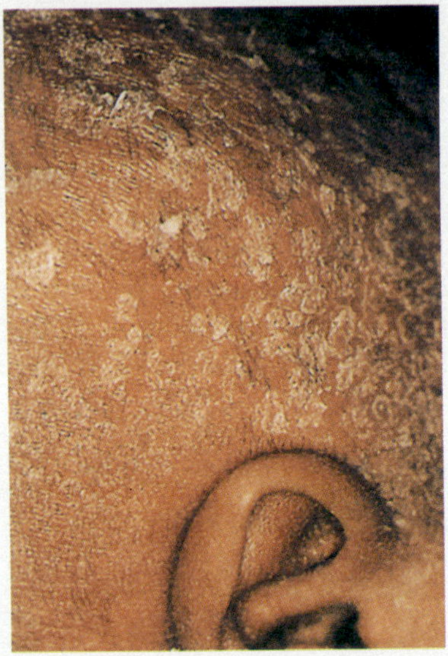

45．8周大婴儿的头部和耳朵。

a. 诊断是什么?

b. 有没有其他表现?

c. 如何治疗?

Head and ear of an 8-week-old infant.

a. What is the diagnosis?

b. Are there any other manifestations?

c. What is the treatment?

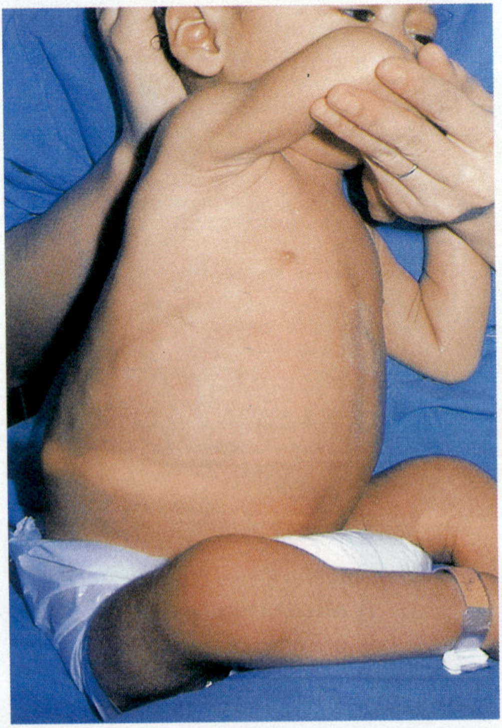

46．母乳喂养的10个月大婴儿的胸部。

a. 诊断是什么?

b. 这种情况的一般处理方法是什么?

c. 有没有其他的可能原因?

Chest of a breast-fed 10-month-old infant.

a. What is the diagnosis?

b. What is the usual management of this condition?

c. Are there any other underlying causes?

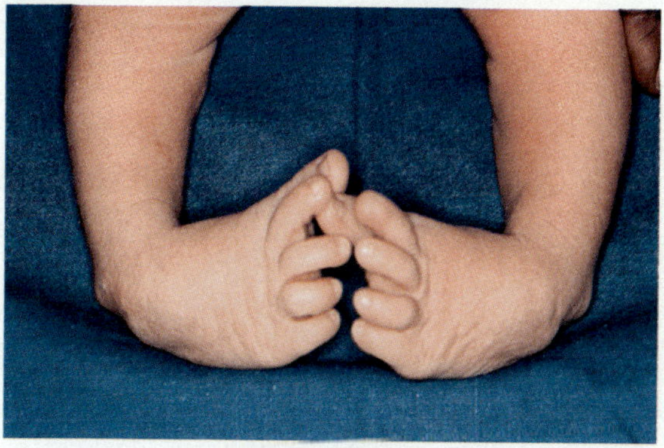

47．一位羊水过少的母亲所生新生儿的脚。
a. 这种情况的原因是什么？
b. 如何处理？
c. 有没有其他相关异常？

Feet of a newborn infant born to a mother with oligohydramnios.
a. What is the cause of this condition?
b. What is the management?
c. Are there any other associated anomalies?

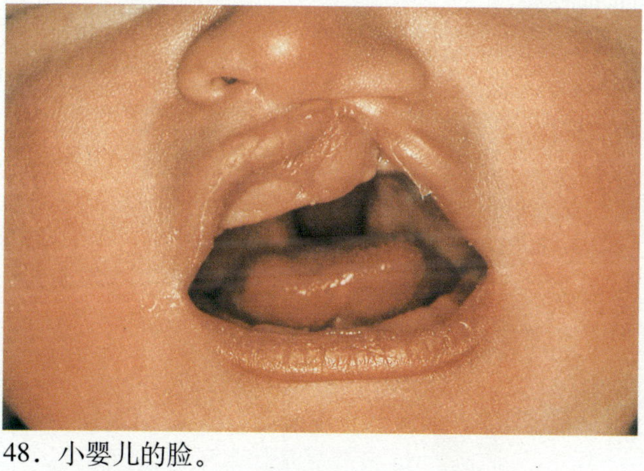

48．小婴儿的脸。
a. 这种疾病相关的并发症是什么？
b. 该病在以后出生的孩子中再发率是多少？

Face of a young infant.
a. What are the complications associated with this condition?
b. What is the risk of recurrence in future pregnancies?

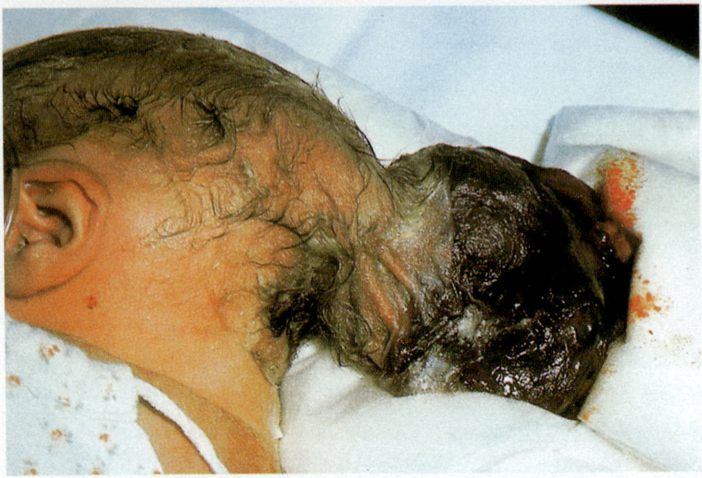

49．新生儿的头部和颈部。

a. 诊断是什么？

b. 并发症是什么？

c. 该病在以后出生的孩子中再发率是多少？

Head and neck of a newborn infant.

a. What is thc diagnosis?

b. What are the complications?

c. What is the recurrence risk in future pregnancies?

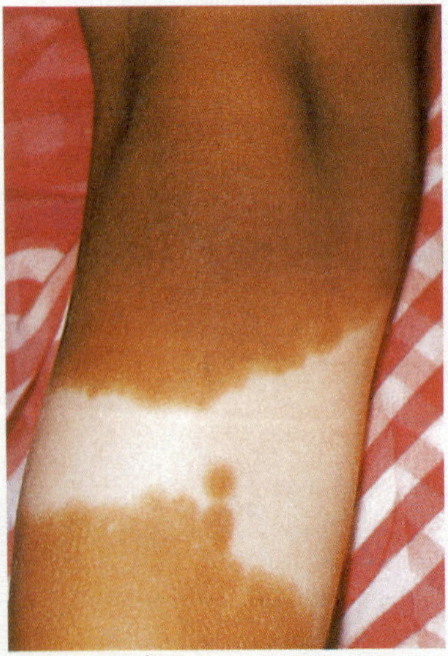

50．5 岁孩子的肢体。

a. 诊断是什么？

b. 合并症是什么？

c. 如何治疗？

Limb of a 5-year-old child.

a. What is the diagnosis?

b. What are the associations?

c. What is the management?

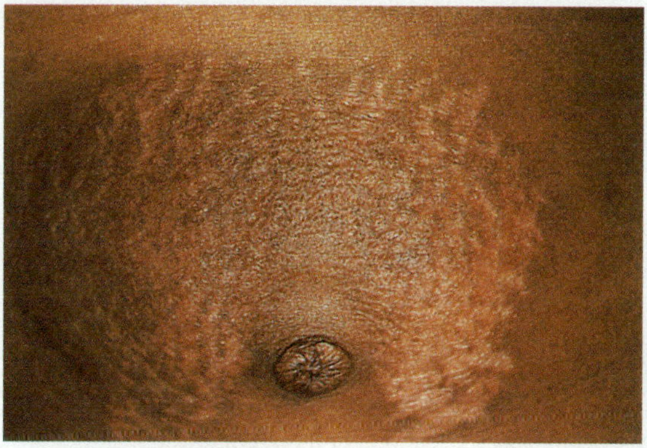

51．10 岁男孩的腹部。

a. 临床体征是什么？

b. 列举 2 个可能的原因和其他相关的临床特征。

Abdomen of a 10-year-old boy.

a. What is the clinical sign?

b. Name two underlying causes and other associated clinical features.

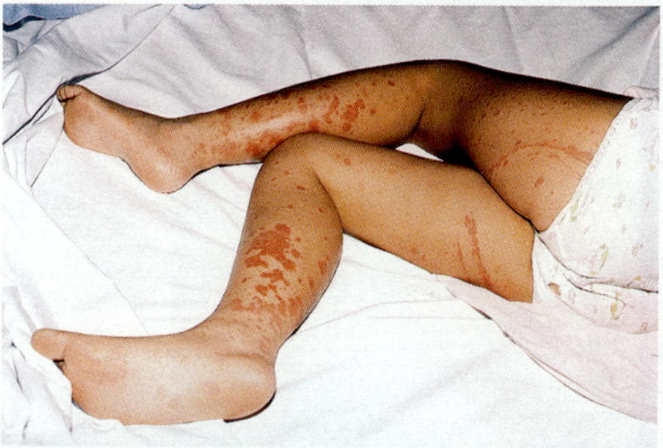

52．一名走路困难的 6 岁孩子。

a. 诊断是什么？

b. 什么检查有助于诊断？

c. 预后如何？

This 6-year-old child presented with difficulty in walking.

a. What is the diagnosis?

b. Which investigations will be helpful?

c. What is the prognosis?

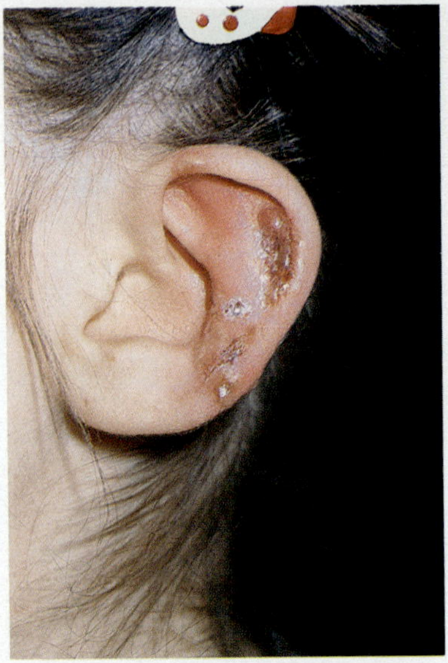

53．一名 8 岁孩子的耳朵，有不明原因的发热和腹痛。

a. 鉴别诊断是什么？

b. 这些情况可能的严重并发症是什么？

Ear of an 8-year-old child with a pyrexia of unknown origin and abdominal pain.

a. What is the differential diagnosis?

b. What are the potentially serious complications of these conditions?

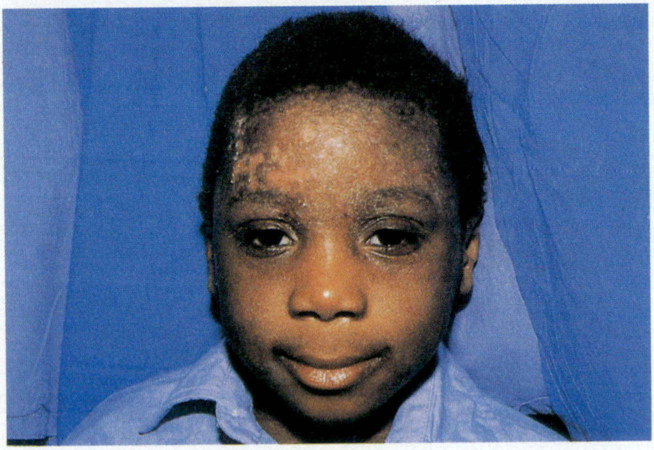

54．一名患有哮喘的 8 岁男孩。

a. 诊断是什么？

b. 还经常累及其他什么部位？

c. 这种疾病的并发症是什么？

This 8-year-old boy has asthma.

a. What is the diagnosis?

b. Which other sites are commonly affected?

c. What are the complications of this condition?

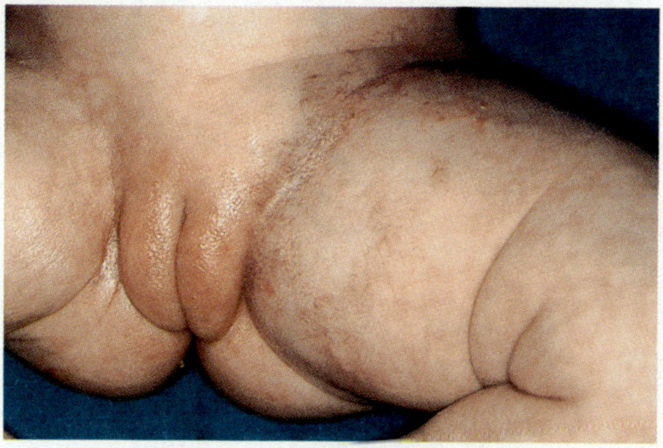

55. 一名喂养困难的4周大婴儿的大腿。

a. 鉴别诊断是什么?

b. 什么检查有助于诊断?

c. 如何治疗?

Thigh of a 4-week-old infant with poor feeding.

a. What is the differential diagnosis?

b. Which investigations will be helpful?

c. What is the treatment of this condition?

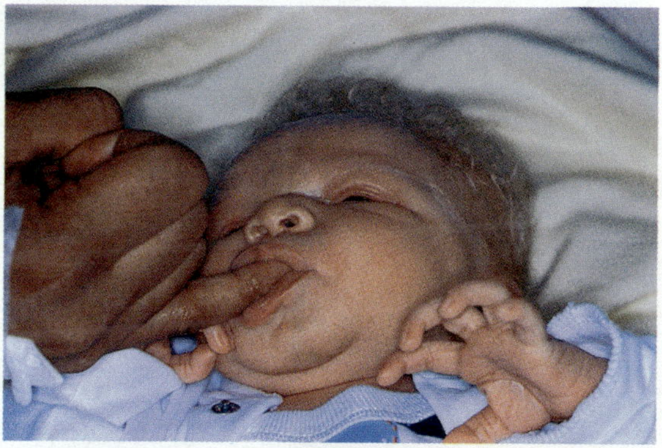

56. 非洲父母所生的孩子。

a. 诊断是什么?

b. 相关的疾病是什么?

c. 如何治疗?

Child born to African parents.

a. What is the diagnosis?

b. What are the associated conditions?

c. What is the management of this condition?

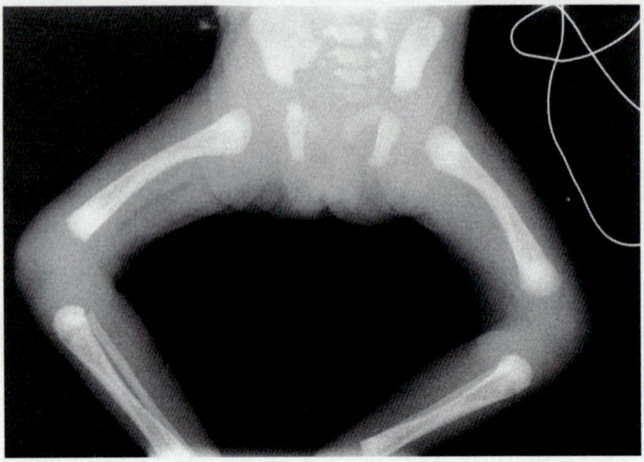

57．一名宫内生长迟缓和血小板减少的新生儿X线片。

a. 描述一下骨骼的异常。

b. 诊断是什么?

c. 列举其他临床合并症。

X-ray of a newborn with intra-uterine growth retardation and thrombocytopenia.

a. Describe the bony abnormality.

b. What is the diagnosis?

c. Name other clinical associations.

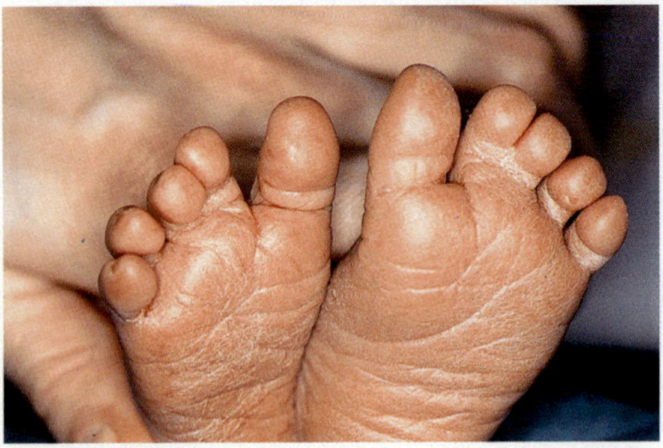

58. 新生儿的脚。

a. 诊断是什么?

b. 这种疾病的意义是什么?

Feet of a newborn infant.

a. What is the diagnosis?

b. What is the significance of this condition?

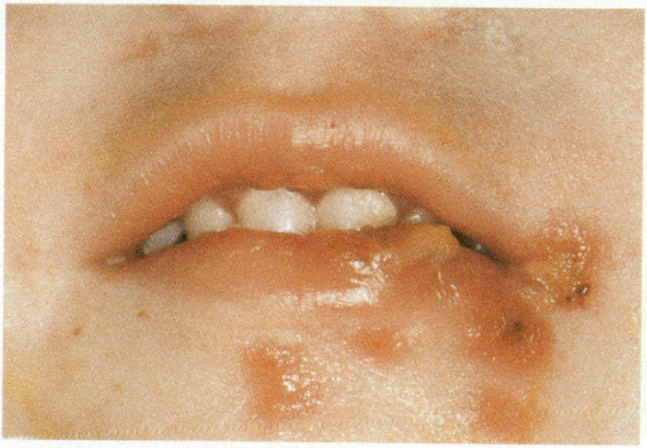

59．2岁大孩子的口唇。

a. 这种疾病的症状是什么？

b. 诊断是什么？

c. 描述一下临床病程和并发症。

Mouth of a 2-year-old child.

a. What are the symptoms of this condition?

b. What is the diagnosis?

c. Describe the clinical course and complications.

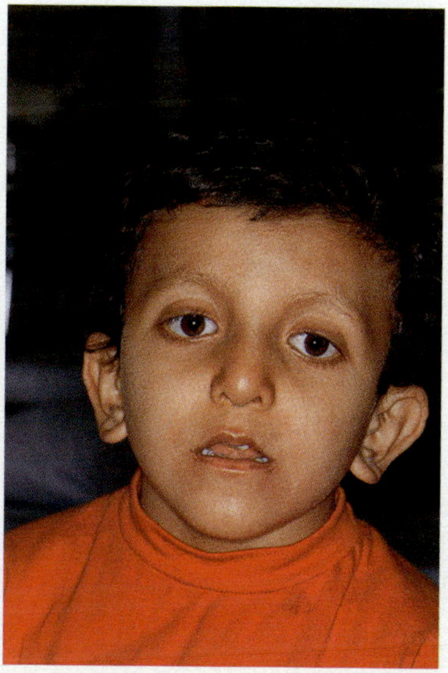

60．一名有心脏杂音的4岁男孩。

a. 诊断是什么？

b. 临床体征是什么？

c. 潜在的心脏疾病是什么？

d. 该病的遗传模式是什么？

A 4-year-old boy with a heart murmur.

a. What is the diagnosis?

b. What are the clinical signs?

c. What is the underlying cardiac condition?

d. What is the mode of inheritance?

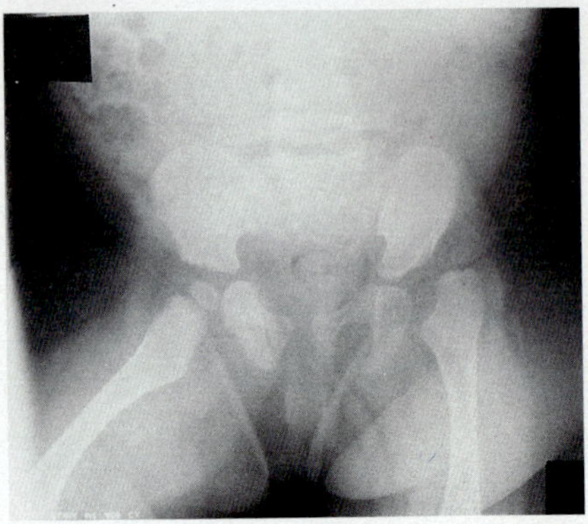

61．一名有异常步态的 16 个月大孩子的骨盆 X 线片。
a. 诊断是什么？
b. 引起这种疾病的原因是什么？
c. 如何治疗这种疾病？

X-ray of the pelvis of a 16-month-old child with an abnormal gait.
a. What is the diagnosis?
b. What are predisposing factors?
c. How is the condition treated?

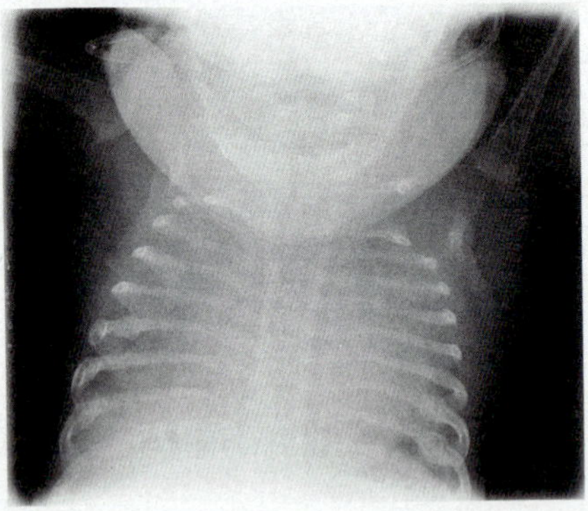

62．25 孕周出生的 3 个月大婴儿的胸部 X 线片。
a. 有什么异常放射学体征？
b. 引起这些疾病的原因是什么？
c. 怎样降低这些疾病发生的危险？

Chest X-ray of 3-month-old infant born at 25 weeks' gestation.
a. What are the abnormal radiological signs?
b. What are the causes of these conditions?
c. How can the risk of these conditions be reduced?

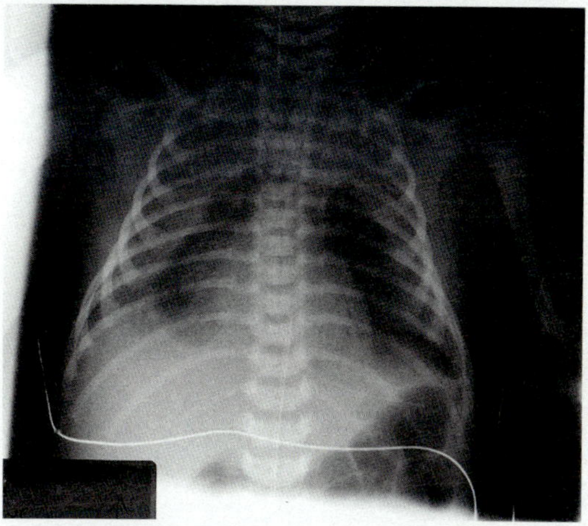

63．有严重呼吸窘迫的足月儿的胸部 X 线片。
a. 诊断是什么？
b. 引起这种疾病的原因是什么？
c. 如何治疗这种疾病？

Chest X-ray of a term infant with severe respiratory distress.
a. What is the diagnosis?
b. What are predisposing conditions?
c. What is the management of this condition?

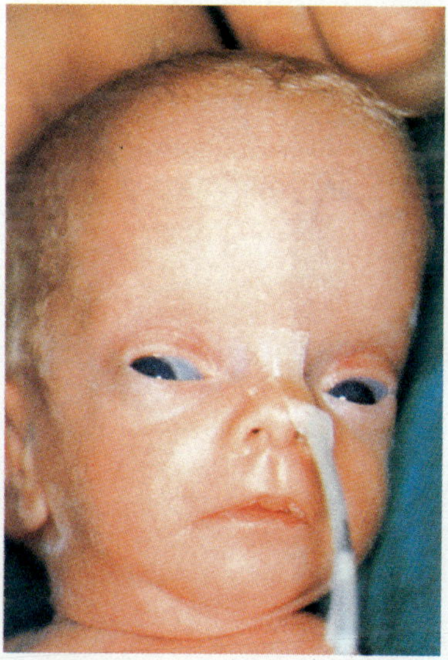

64．一名 3 个月大的早产儿。
a. 所显示的临床体征是什么？
b. 什么检查有助于诊断？
c. 如何治疗这种疾病？

A 3-month-old ex-preterm infant.
a. Which clinical signs are shown?
b. Which investigations may be helpful?
c. What is the management of this condition?

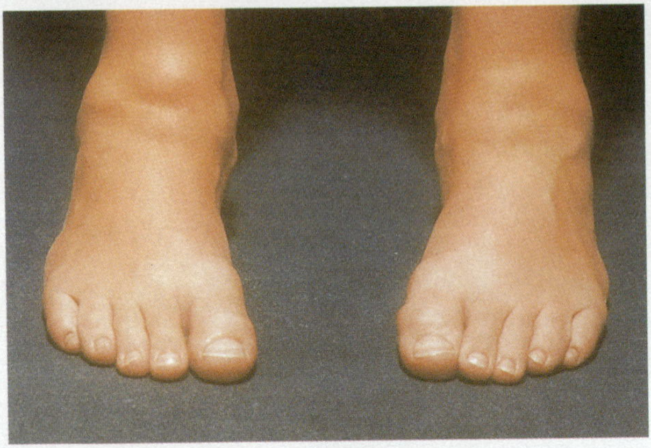

65．一名行走困难的 8 岁孩子。

a. 鉴别诊断是什么?

b. 什么检查有助于诊断?

c. 如何治疗?

This 8-year-old has difficulty in walking.

a. What is the differential diagnosis?

b. Which investigations will be helpful?

c. What is the management?

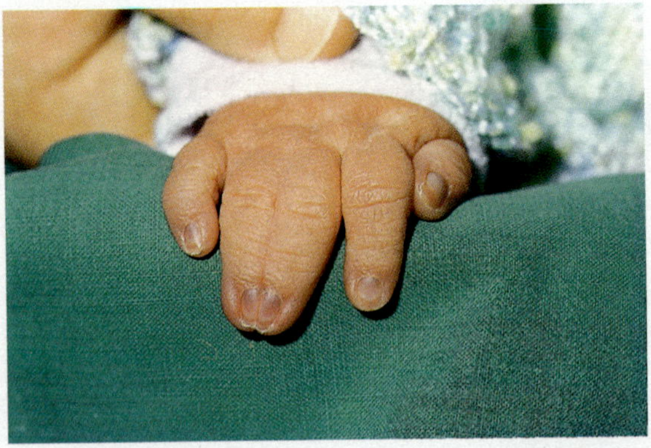

66．小婴儿的手。

a. 诊断是什么?

b. 如何处理这种情况?

Hand of a young infant.

a. What is the diagnosis?

b. What is the management of this condition?

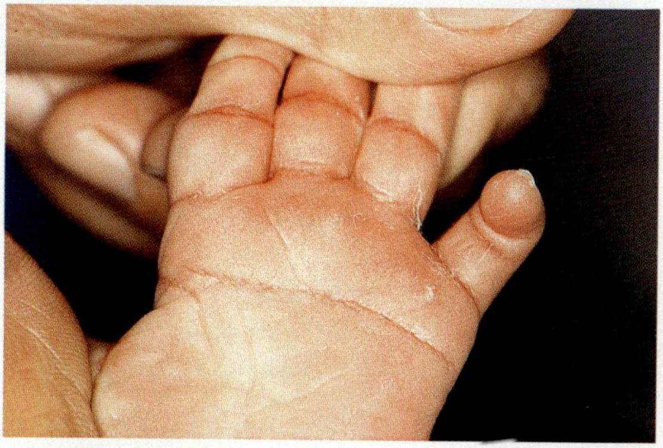

67．新生儿的手。

a. 临床体征是什么？

b. 这种体征的临床意义是什么？

c. 其他相关的临床特征是什么？

Hand of newborn infant.

a. What is the clinical sign?

b. What is the clinical significance of this sign?

c. What are other associated clinical features?

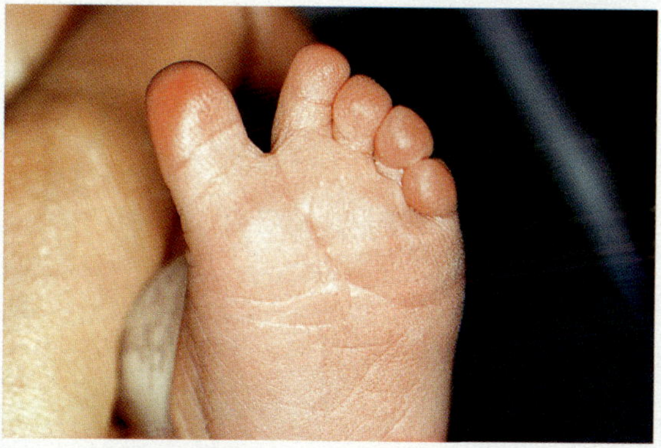

68．小婴儿的脚。

a. 临床体征是什么？

b. 在有这种体征的儿童中哪种疾病最常见？

Foot of a young infant.

a. What is the clinical sign?

b. Which diseases are more common in children with this condition?

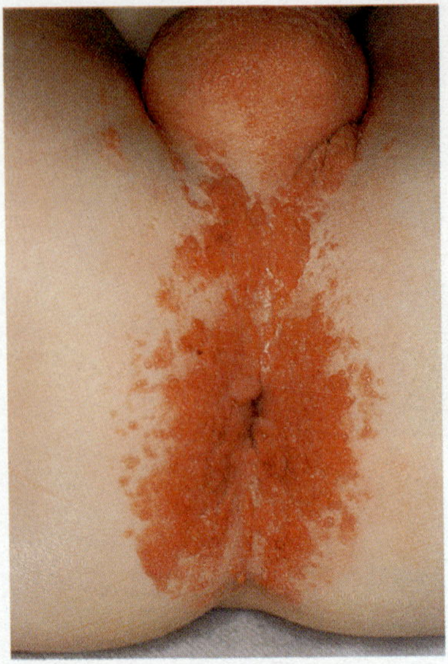

69．3 岁男婴的肛门和会阴。
a. 这种损伤是什么？
b. 这种损伤是怎样形成的？
c. 什么检查有助于诊断？

Anus and perineum of a 3-year-old male infant.
a. What are the lesions?
b. How are these lesions acquired?
c. Which investigations will be helpful?

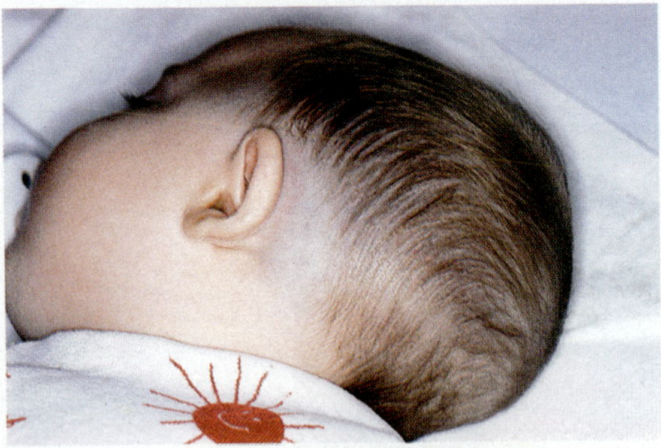

70．一名右耳后有青肿的 10 个月大婴儿。
a. 诊断是什么？
b. 如何处理这种情况？

10-month-old infant with a bluish swelling behind the right ear.
a. What is the diagnosis?
b. What is the management of this condition?

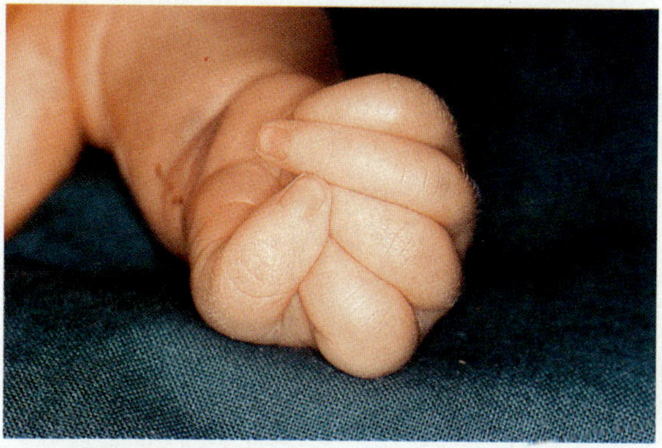

71．出生体重为1850g的足月新生儿的手。
a. 诊断是什么？
b. 这种疾病的其他临床特征是什么？
c. 患有这种疾病的婴儿预期寿命是多少？

Hand of a term newborn infant of birth weight 1850 g.
a. What is the diagnosis?
b. What are other clinical features of this condition?
c. What is the life expectancy of infants with this condition?

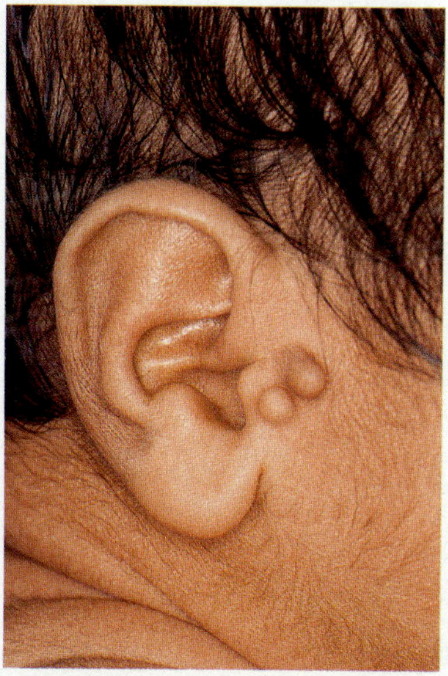

72．小婴儿的耳朵。
a. 诊断是什么？
b. 应该进行哪些检查？
c. 该病的遗传模式是什么？

Ear of a young infant.
a. What is the diagnosis?
b. Which investigations should be undertaken?
c. What is the inheritance of this condition?

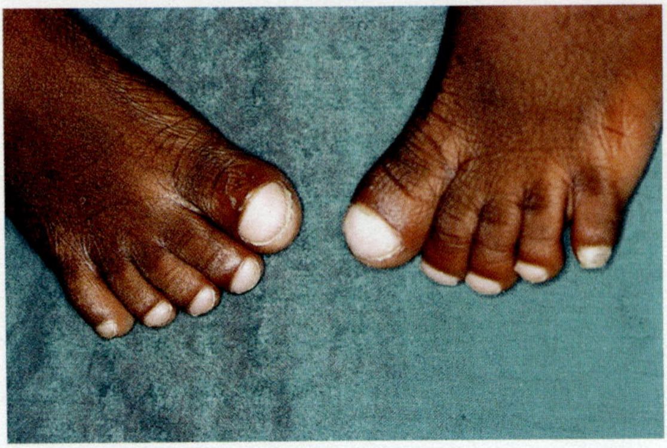

73．一名生长停滞的4岁孩子的脚趾。

a. 诊断是什么?

b. 可能的原因是什么?

c. 什么检查有助于诊断?

Toes of a 4-year-old child with failure to thrive.

a. What is the diagnosis?

b. What are the underlying causes?

c. Which investigations will be helpful?

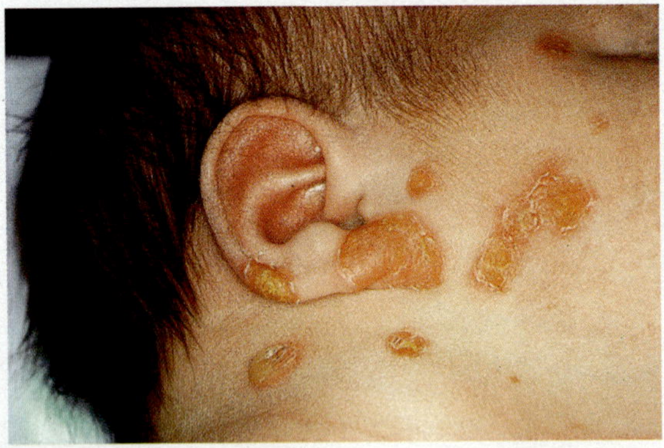

74．6周大婴儿的脸部。

a. 是什么样的损伤?

b. 可能的原因是什么?

c. 如何治疗这种疾病?

Face of a 6-week-old infant.

a. What are the lesions?

b. What is the underlying cause?

c. What is the management of this condition?

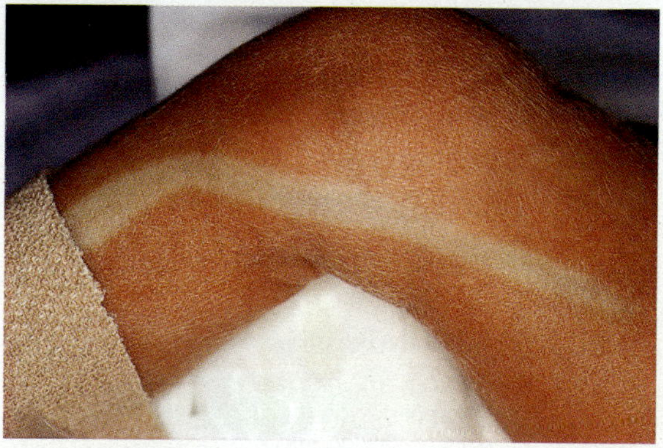

75．一名患病的早产儿的腿，其脚上有静脉输液。
a. 诊断是什么？
b. 对于这种并发症如何治疗？

Leg of a sick preterm infant with an intravenous infusion in the foot.
a. What is the diagnosis?
b. What is the management of this complication?

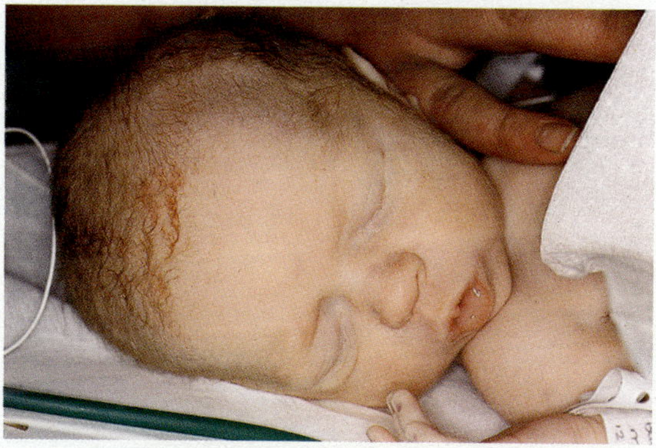

76．Hb 为 3.5g/dl 的新生儿。
a. 鉴别诊断是什么？
b. 什么检查有助于诊断？

Newborn infant with Hb 3.5 g/dl.
a. What is the differential diagnosis?
b. Which investigations will be helpful?

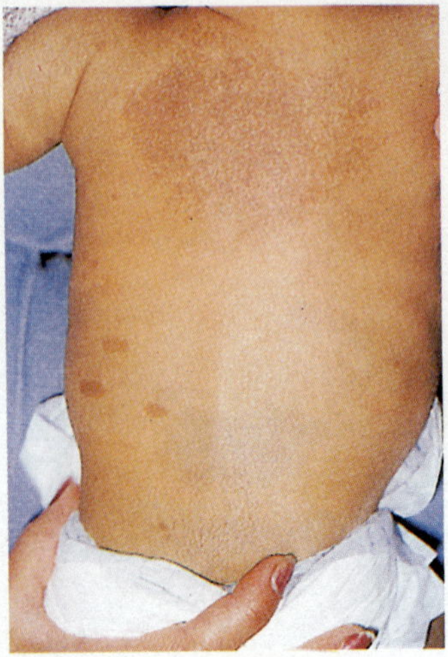

77. 一名患有癫痫的18个月大孩子的躯干部。

a. 皮肤上所显示的临床体征是什么？

b. 诊断是什么？

c. 该病的遗传模式是什么？

Trunk of an 18-month-old child with seizures.

a. What are the clinical signs shown on the skin?

b. What is the diagnosis?

c. What is the inheritance of this condition?

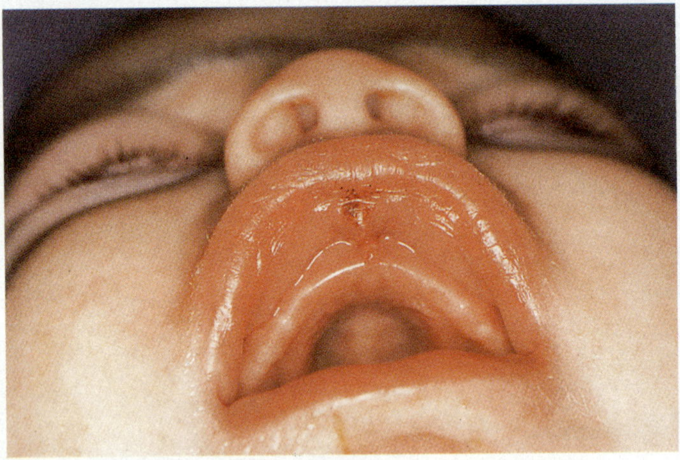

78. 一名易激惹的小婴儿的嘴。

a. 诊断是什么？

b. 可能的原因是什么？

c. 如何处理？

Mouth of an irritable young infant.

a. What is the diagnosis?

b. What is the underlying cause?

c. What is the management?

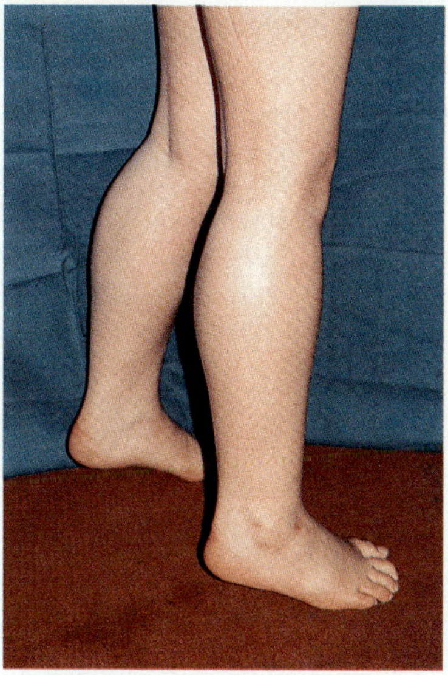

79．一名跑步困难的7岁男孩的腿。
a. 临床体征是什么？
b. 诊断是什么？
c. 在该病中还会出现什么样的其他症状和体征？
d. 如何确诊？

Legs of a 7-year-old boy who has difficulty running.
a. What is the clinical sign?
b. What is the diagnosis?
c. What other signs and symptoms occur in this condition?
d. How can the diagnosis be confirmed?

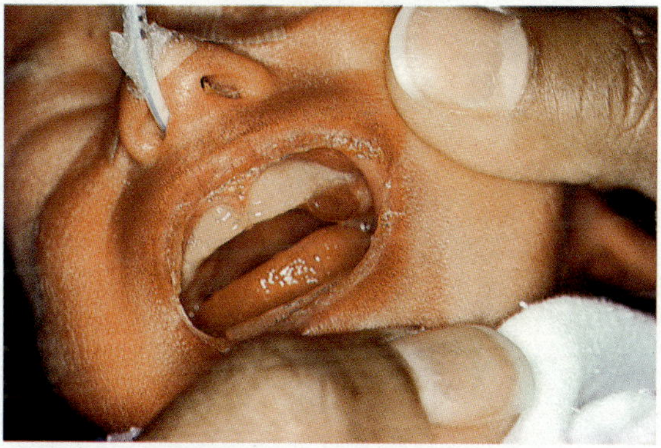

80．新生儿的嘴。
a. 诊断是什么？
b. 会有什么症状发生？
c. 如何治疗该病？

Mouth of a newborn infant.
a. What is the diagnosis?
b. What symptoms will occur?
c. What is the management of this condition?

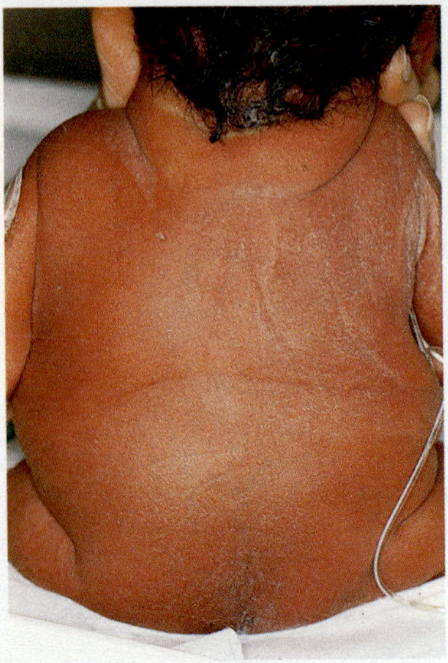

81. 新生儿的背部。
a. 临床体征是什么?
b. 鉴别诊断是什么?
c. 哪些检查有助于诊断?

Back of a newborn infant.
a. What are the clinical signs?
b. What are the differential diagnoses?
c. Which investigations will be helpful?

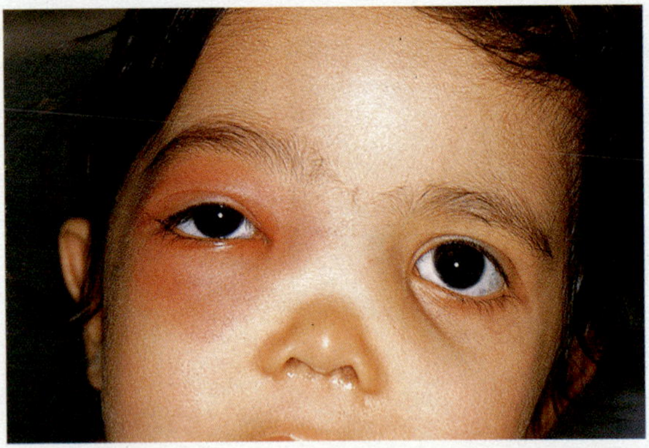

82. 2岁孩子的脸。
a. 诊断是什么?
b. 如何治疗这种疾病?
c. 可能会发生什么并发症?

Face of a 2-year-old child.
a. What is the diagnosis?
b. What is the treatment of this condition?
c. What complications may occur?

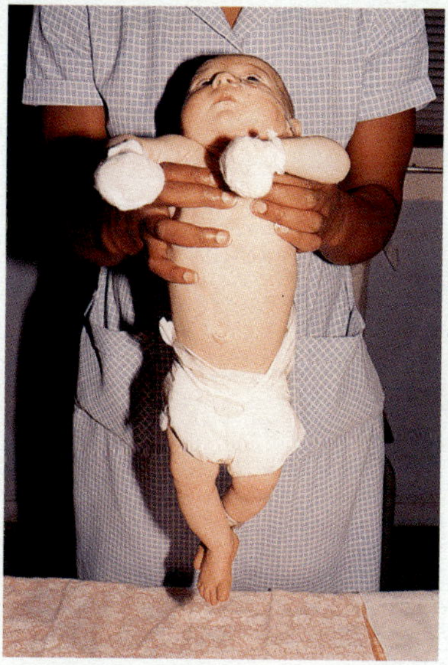

83．一名4个月大的婴儿。
a. 所显示的临床体征是什么？
b. 可能的诊断是什么？
c. 发生该病的病因是什么？

A 4-month-old infant.
a. What is the clinical sign shown?
b. What is the likely diagnosis?
c. What is the aetiology of this condition?

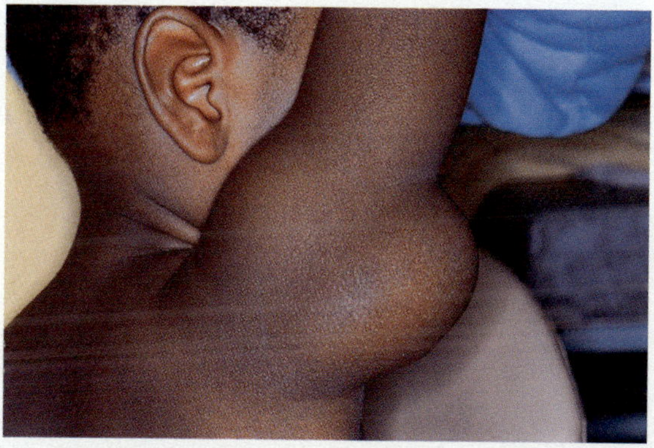

84．2岁孩子手臂下方的无痛性肿块。
a. 鉴别诊断是什么？
b. 如何治疗这种疾病？
c. 复发的危险是多少？

Painless swelling under the arm of a 2-year-old child.
a. What is the differential diagnosis?
b. What is the management of this condition?
c. What is the recurrence risk?

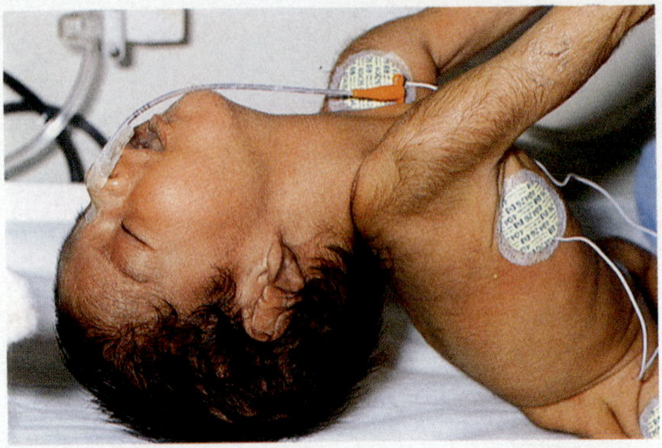

85．握着新生儿的前臂，将其从仰卧位拉起。

a. 所显示的临床体征是什么?

b. 鉴别诊断是什么?

c. 什么检查有助于诊断?

Newborn infant being pulled up by forearms.

a. What clinical sign is shown?

b. What is the differential diagnosis?

c. Which investigations will be helpful?

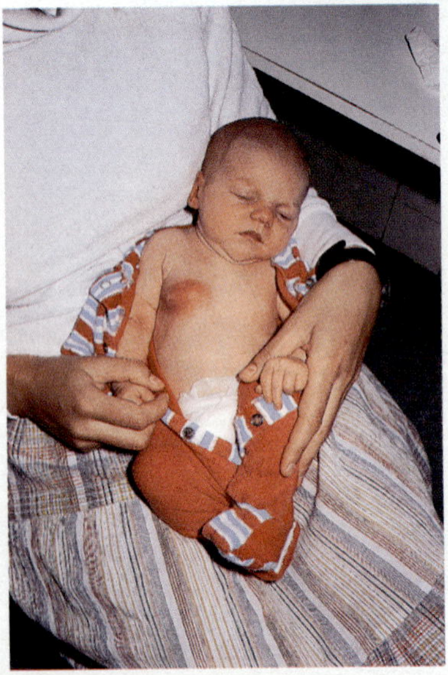

86．3 天大新生儿的胸部。

a. 诊断是什么?

b. 如何治疗?

c. 预后如何?

Chest of a 3-day-old neonate.

a. What is the diagnosis?

b. What is the treatment?

c. What is the prognosis?

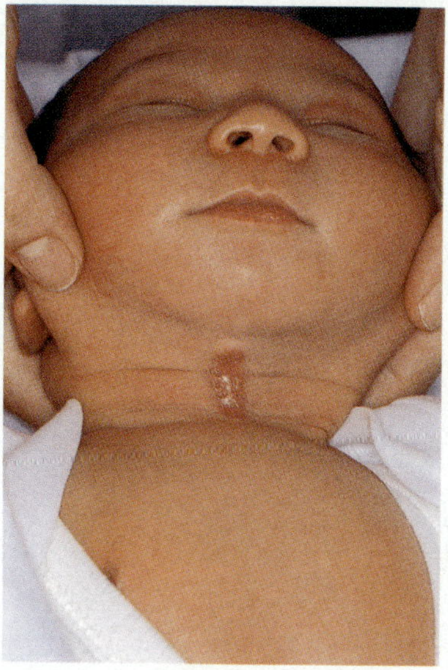

87. 新生儿的颈部。
a. 诊断是什么?
b. 什么检查有助于诊断?

Neck of a newborn term infant.
a. What is the diagnosis?
b. Which investigations will be helpful?

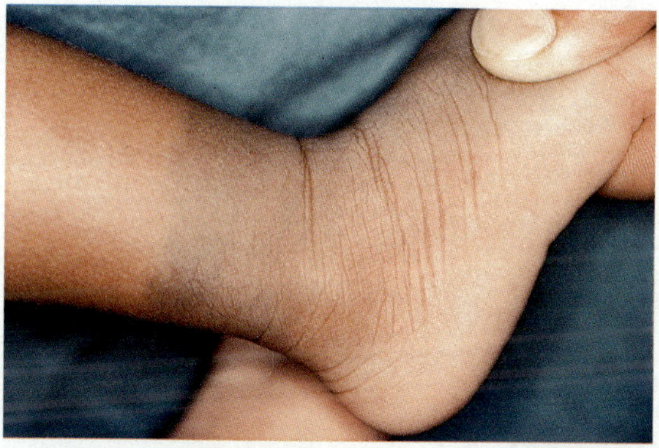

88. 4 个月大婴儿的脚。
a. 诊断是什么?
b. 这种皮损最常见于什么部位?
c. 病程和预后如何?

Foot of a 4-month-old infant.
a. What is the diagnosis?
b. Where is the lesion most commonly seen?
c. What is the course and prognosis?

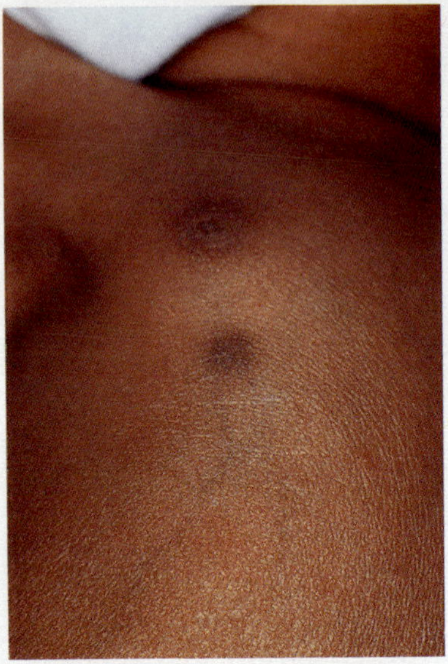

89．新生男婴的胸部和腋窝。
a. 诊断是什么？
b. 如何治疗该病？

Chest and axilla of a newborn male infant.
a. What is the diagnosis?
b. What is the management of this condtion?

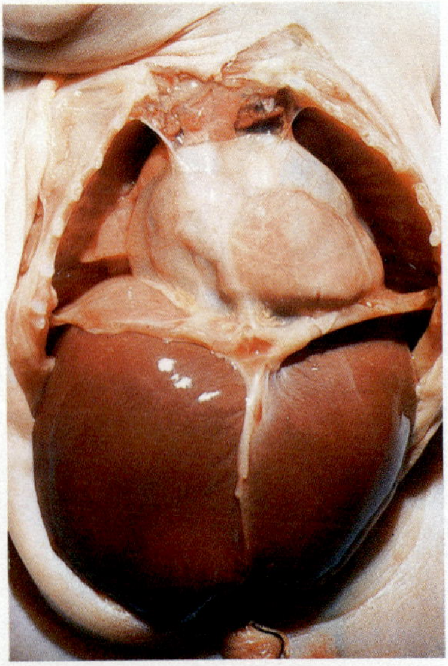

90．对出生时 Hb 为 2g/dl 的苍白、水肿的新生儿死后所进行的尸体检查。
a. 这是什么腹部脏器？
b. 鉴别诊断是什么？
c. 对怀疑须进行产前诊断的母亲要进行什么检查？

Postmortem examination of a pale, hydropic neonate born with Hb 2 g/dl.
a. What is the abdominal organ?
b. What is the differential diagnosis?
c. What maternal investigations will raise suspicion of the diagnosis antenatally?

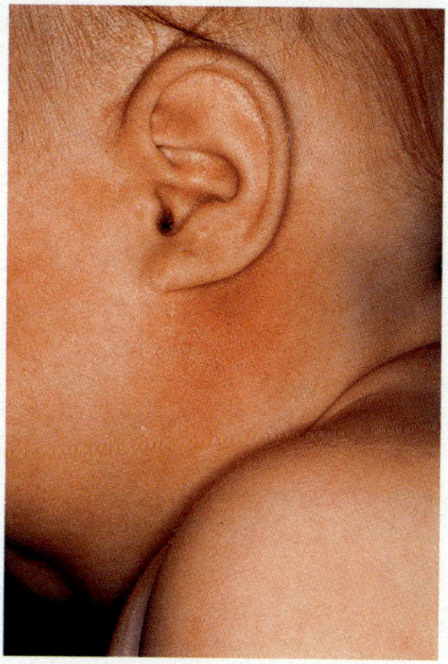

91．一名颈部有疼痛性肿胀的2岁孩子。
a. 诊断是什么？
b. 常见致病菌是什么？
c. 如何治疗该病？

A 2-year-old child with a painful swelling in the neck.
a. What is the diagnosis?
b. Which organisms are commonly involved?
c. What is the management of the condition?

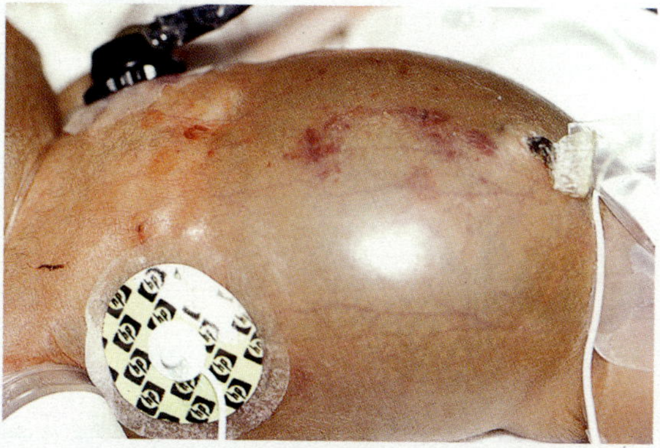

92．26孕周出生的3天大孩子的腹部。
a. 所显示的临床体征是什么？
b. 可能的诊断是什么？
c. 什么体征会有较差的预后？

Abdomen of a 3-day-old born at 26 weeks' gestation.
a. Which clinical signs are shown?
b. What is the likely diagnosis?
c. Which signs are associated with a poor prognosis?

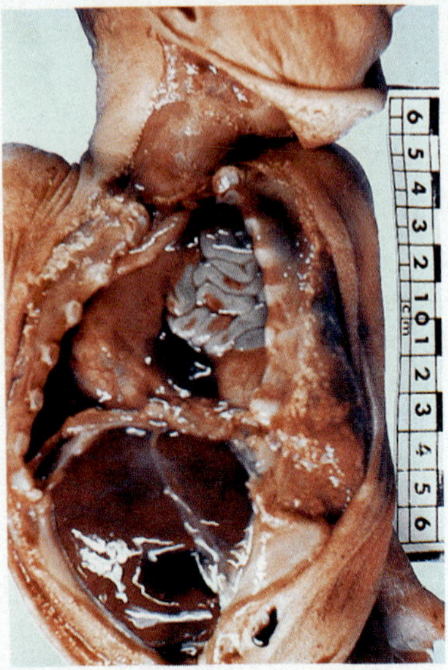

93. 无法复苏而死亡的新生儿的尸体解剖。

a. 诊断是什么?

b. 这种疾病会出现的临床体征是什么?

c. 怎样对这种疾病进行紧急处理?

Postmortem of a newborn infant who did not respond to resuscitation.

a. What is the diagnosis?

b. Which clinical signs occur in this condition?

c. What is the emergency treatment?

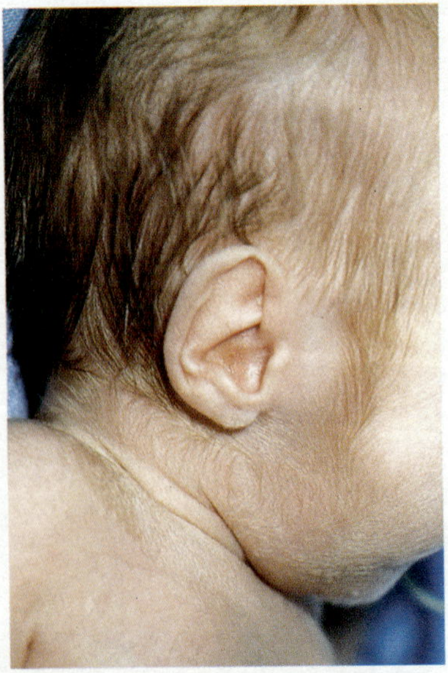

94. 耳前部有疼痛性肿胀的婴儿。

a. 诊断是什么?

b. 可能的原因是什么?

c. 如何治疗?

Painful swelling in front of the ear of a baby.

a. What is the diagnosis?

b. What are the underlying causes?

c. What is the treatment?

95．耳后皮肤变色的 5 岁孩子。
a. 诊断是什么？
b. 可能的原因是什么？
c. 如何治疗？

Discoloration behind the ear of a 5-year-old child.
a. What is the diagnosis?
b. What is the underlying cause?
c. What is the management?

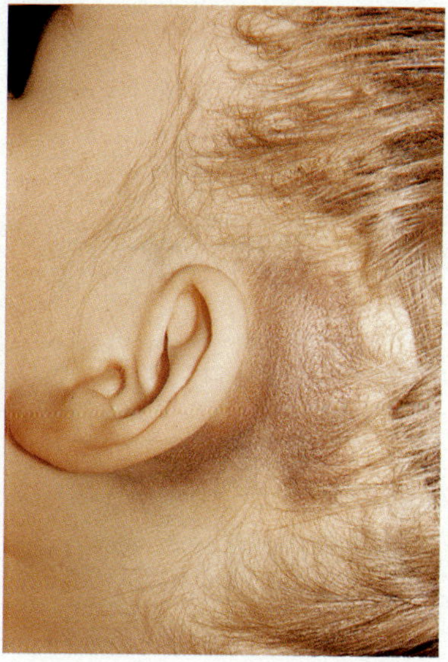

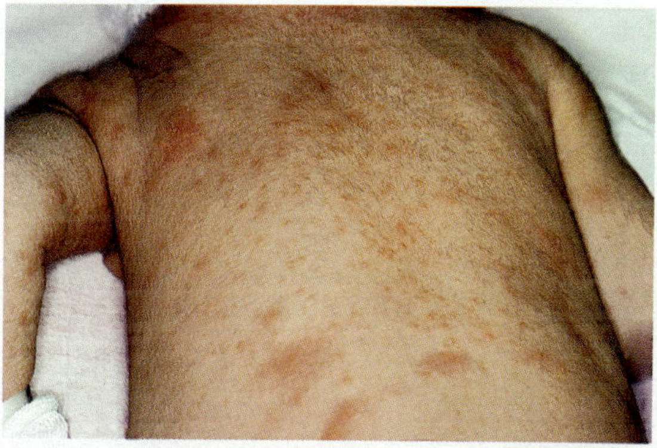

96．10 天大婴儿躯干部的红斑性皮疹。
a. 诊断是什么？
b. 这种疾病会出现什么症状？
c. 病程和预后如何？

Erythematous rash on the trunk of a 10-day-old infant.
a. What is the diagnosis?
b. What symptoms occur in this condition?
c. What is the course and prognosis?

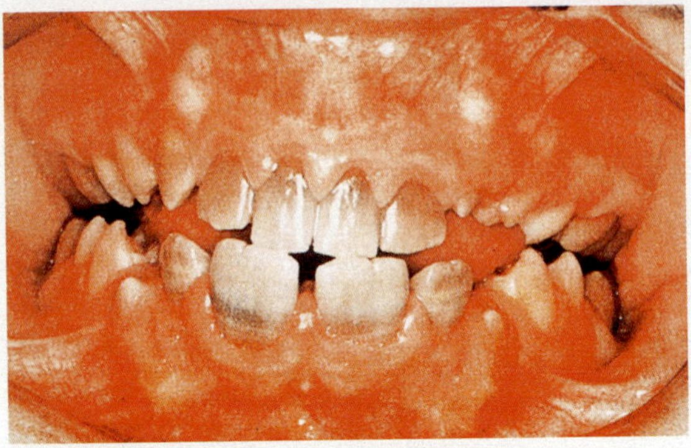

97．有慢性咳嗽的 12 岁孩子的牙齿。

a. 诊断是什么?

b. 其他哪些系统会被累及?

c. 怎样预防这种情况?

Teeth of a 12-year-old with a chronic cough.

a. What is the diagnosis?

b. Which other system will be affected?

c. How can the condition be prevented?

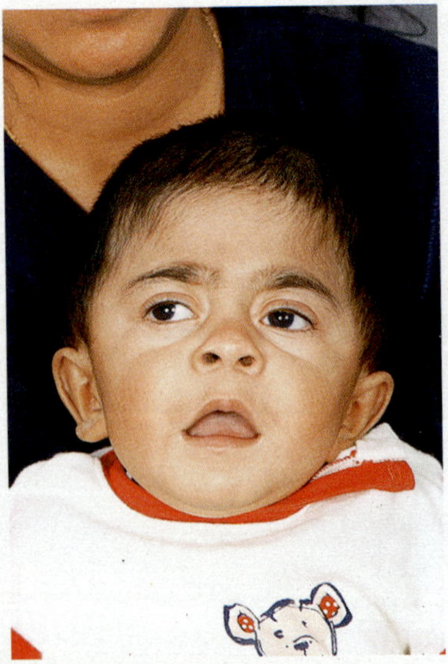

98．这是一个发育延缓的 12 个月大孩子。

a. 临床特征和鉴别诊断是什么?

b. 这种疾病会有什么放射学改变?

c. 怎样进行确诊?

This 12-month-old child has delayed development.

a. What are the clinical features and differential diagnosis?

b. Which radiological changes occur in this condition?

c. How can the diagnosis be confirmed?

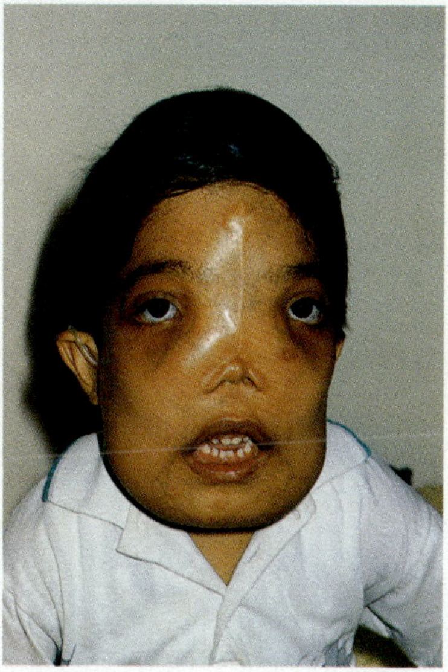

99．这是一个自从婴儿期便有头部快速生长的 8 岁男孩。

a. 诊断是什么？

b. 会发生什么症状和体征？

c. 该病的遗传模式是什么？

This is an 8-year-old boy with increasing head growth since infancy.

a. What is the diagnosis?

b. What signs and symptoms will he develop?

c. What is the inheritance of this condition?

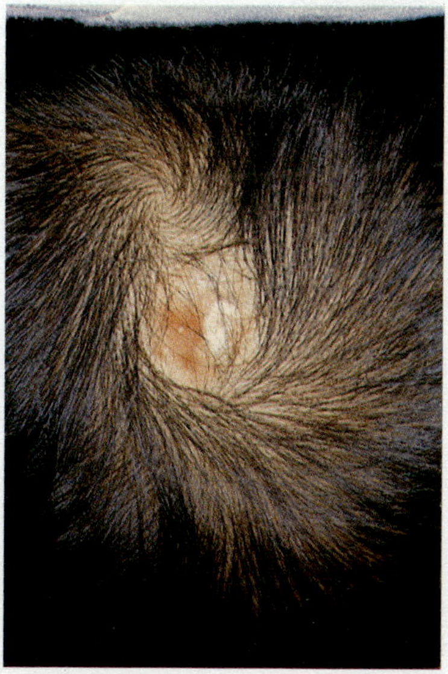

100．健康小婴儿的头皮。

a. 鉴别诊断是什么？

b. 怎样进行确诊？

c. 如何治疗？

Scalp of a healthy young infant.

a. What is the differential diagnosis?

b. How can the diagnosis be confirmed?

c. What is the management?

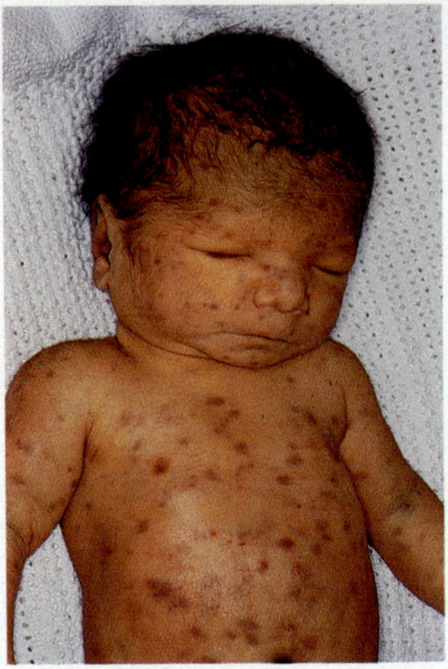

101．有贫血和血小板减少的新生儿。
a. 诊断是什么？
b. 相关的并发症是什么？
c. 什么检查有助于诊断？

Newborn infant with anaemia and thrombocytopenia.
a. What is the diagnosis?
b. What are associated complications?
c. Which investigations will be helpful?

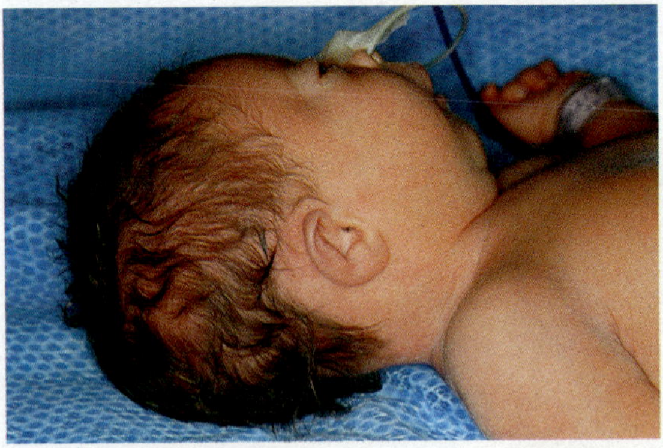

102．小婴儿的颈和头部。
a. 所显示的异常特征是什么？
b. 会发现什么样相关的异常？
c. 什么检查有助于对相关异常进行诊断？

Head and neck of a young infant.
a. What abnormal features are shown?
b. What associated abnormalities may be found?
c. What investigations will help to identify associated anomalies?

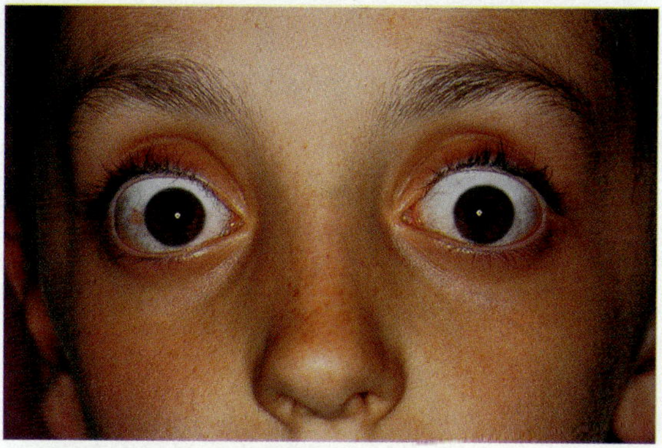

103．12 岁女孩的眼睛。

a. 临床体征是什么？

b. 可能会有哪些其他症状和体征？

c. 如何治疗该病？

Eyes of a 12-year-old girl.

a. What is the clinical sign?

b. Which other signs and symptoms may be present?

c. What is the treatment of this condition?

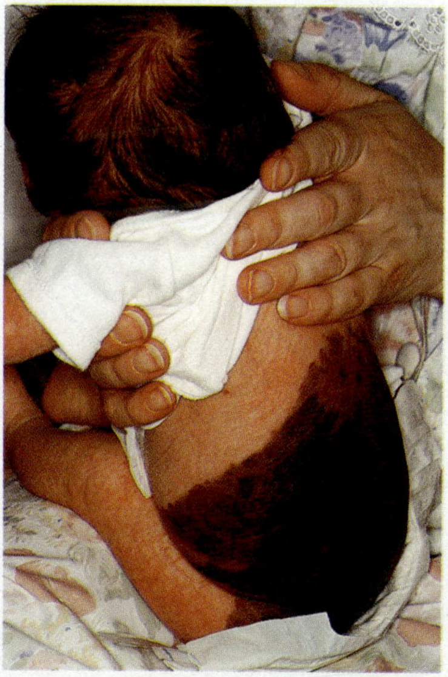

104．新生儿的背部。

a. 是什么疾病？

b. 该疾病的意义是什么？

c. 如何治疗该病？

Back of a newborn infant.

a. What is the lesion?

b. What is the significance of the lesion?

c. How can it be treated?

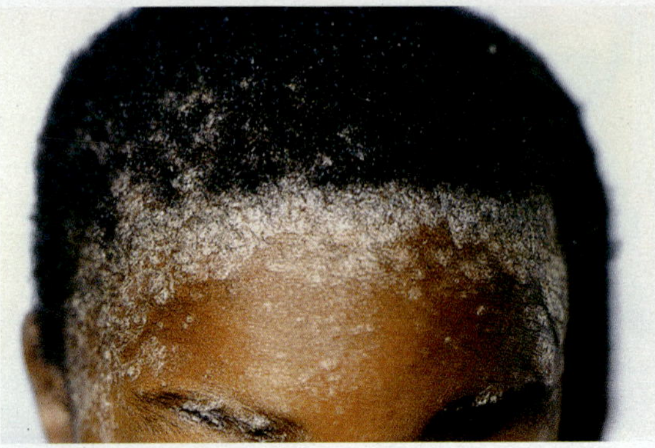

105．12岁男孩的前额。
a. 诊断是什么?
b. 这种疾病的并发症和合并症是什么?
c. 如何治疗?

Forehead of a 12-year-old boy.
a. What is the diagnosis?
b. What are the complications and associations of this condition?
c. What is the treatment?

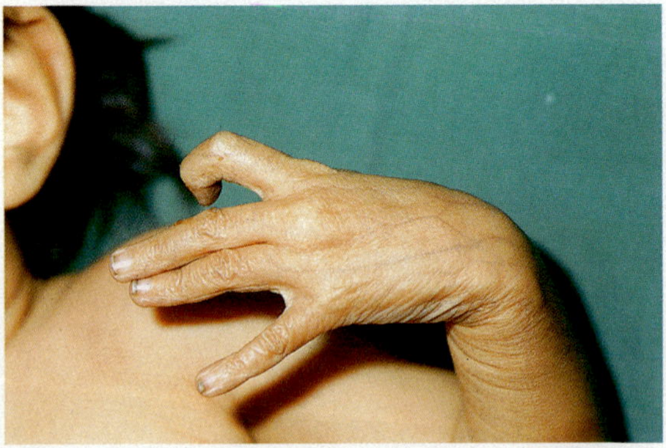

106．一个有高腭弓的婴儿的手。
a. 鉴别诊断是什么?
b. 这种疾病的相关特征是什么?

Hand of an infant with a high arched palate.
a. What is the differential diagnosis?
b. What are associated features?

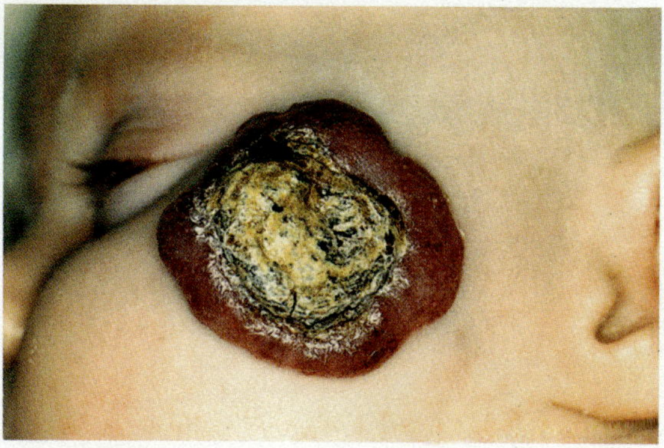

107．健康生长的 8 个月大婴儿面颊部的损伤。

a. 诊断是什么？

b. 如何处理？

c. 预后如何？

Lesion on the cheek of a healthy thriving 8-month-old infant.

a. What is the diagnosis?

b. What is the management?

c. What is the prognosis?

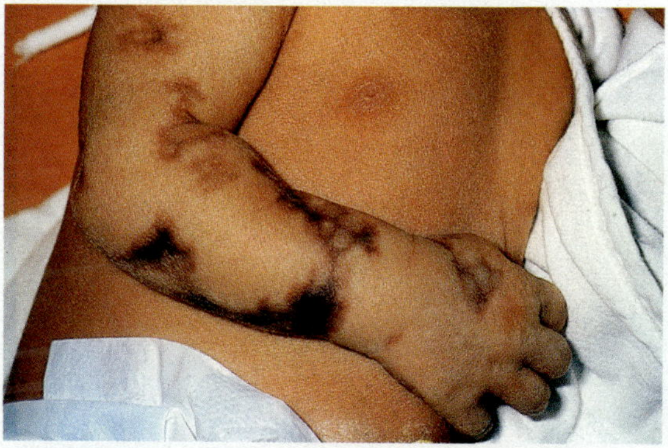

108．健康新生儿的手臂。

a. 诊断是什么？

b. 应该进行什么检查？

c. 长期并发症是什么？

Arm of a healthy newborn infant.

a. What is the diagnosis?

b Which investigations should be performed?

c. What are the long term complications?

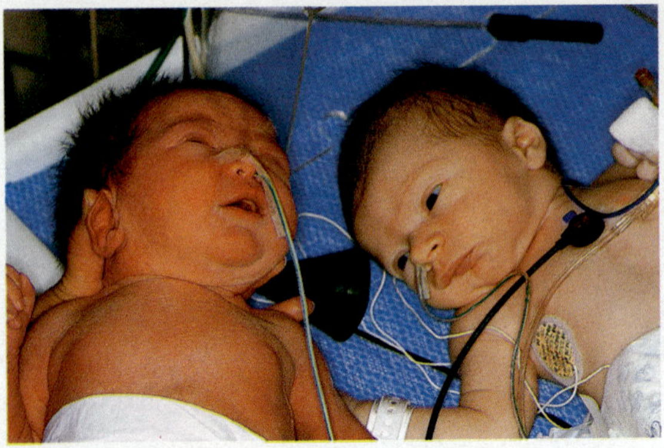

109．双胞胎新生儿。

a. 诊断是什么？

b. 这种疾病的并发症是什么？

These newborn infants are twins.

a. What is the diagnosis?

b. What are the complications of this condition?

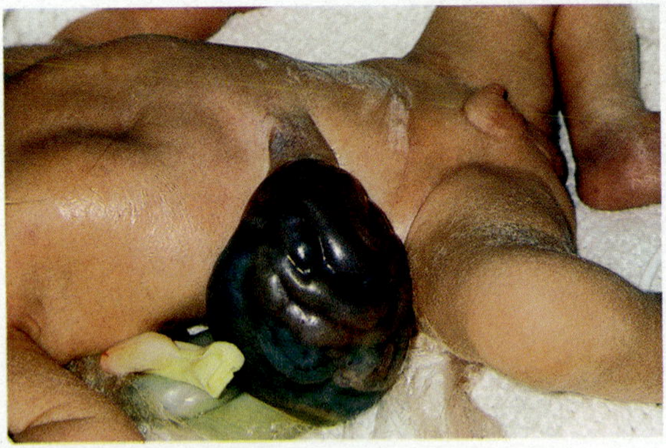

110．新生儿的腹部。

a. 诊断是什么？

b. 如何治疗该病？

c. 这种疾病的染色体异常是哪一种？

Abdomen of a newborn infant.

a. What is the diagnosis?

b. What is the management of this condition?

c. Which chromosome abnormality is associated with this condition?

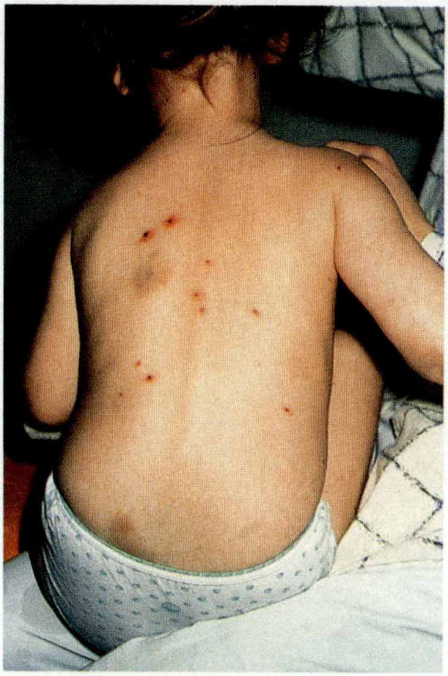

111. 没有外伤史的健康的9岁女孩。

a. 什么检查有助于诊断?

b. 最可能的诊断是什么?

c. 如何治疗该病?

This healthy 9-year-old girl has no history of trauma.

a. Which investigations will be helpful?

b. What is the most likely diagnosis?

c. What is the management of this condition?

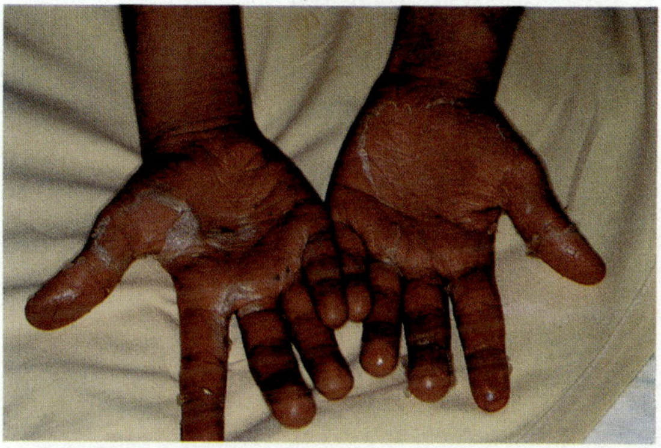

112. 发烧后数周9岁男孩的手。

a. 最可能的诊断是什么?

b. 有什么其他有助于确定诊断的症状和体征?

c. 该病预后如何?

Hands of a 9-year-old boy several weeks after a febrile illness.

a. What is the most likely diagnosis?

b. What other signs and symptoms will help to confirm the diagnosis?

c. What is the prognosis of this condition?

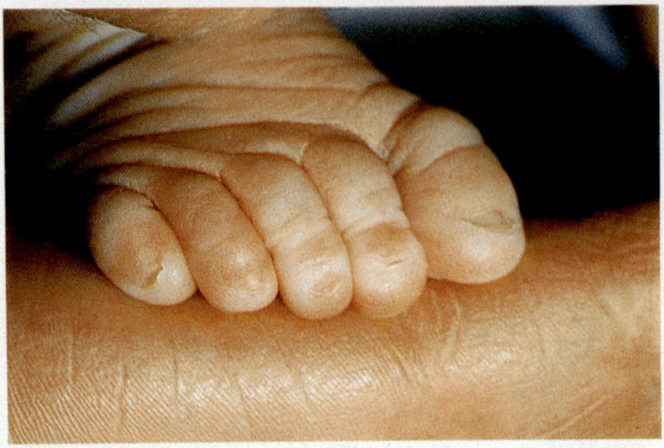

113．膝关节脱位的婴儿。

a. 诊断是什么？

b. 这种疾病的并发症是什么？

c. 该病的遗传模式是什么？

This infant has a dislocated knee.

a. What is the diagnosis?

b. What are the complications of this condition?

c. What is the inheritance of this condition?

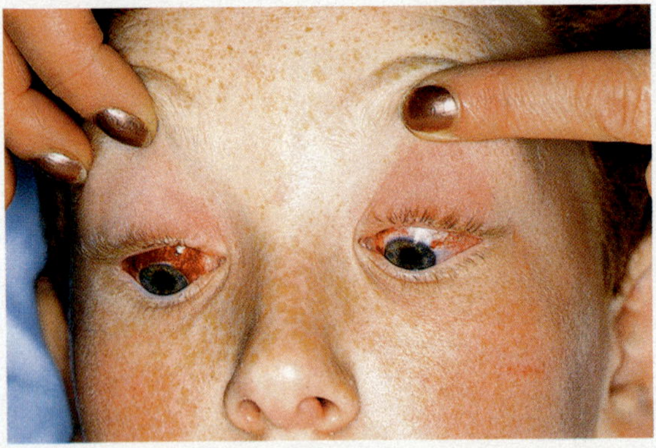

114．一名尿道感染的男孩在使用抗生素后出现了皮疹。

a. 诊断是什么？

b. 这种疾病的临床表现是什么？

c. 如何治疗该病？

This boy developed a rash after being prescribed antibiotics for a urinary tract infection.

a. What is the diagnosis?

b. What are the clinical manifestations of this condition?

c. What is the management of this condition?

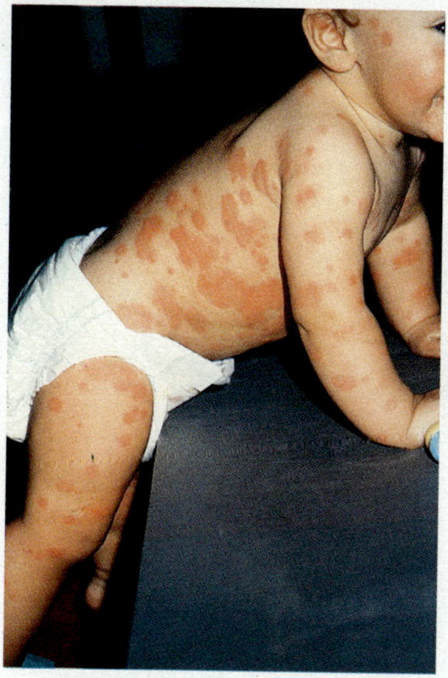

115．有瘙痒性皮疹的刚学走步的小孩。

a. 诊断是什么？

b. 如何治疗该病？

c. 该病最常见的原因是什么？

This toddler has an itchy rash.

a. What is the diagnosis?

b. What is the management of this condition?

c. What are common causes of this condition?

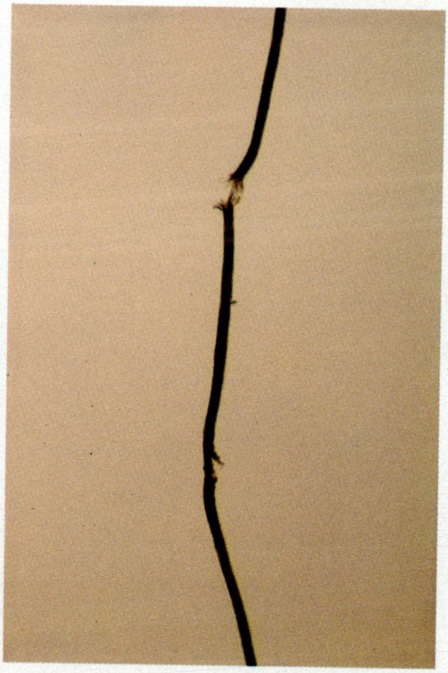

116．有严重发育延迟的孩子的头发。

a. 诊断是什么？

b. 有什么生化学指标异常？

c. 该病的病程和预后如何？

d. 该病在以后出生的孩子中再发率是多少？

Hair of a child with severe developmental delay.

a. What is the diagnosis?

b. What is the biochemical abnormality?

c. What is the course and prognosis of this condition?

d. What is the recurrence risk in future pregnancies?

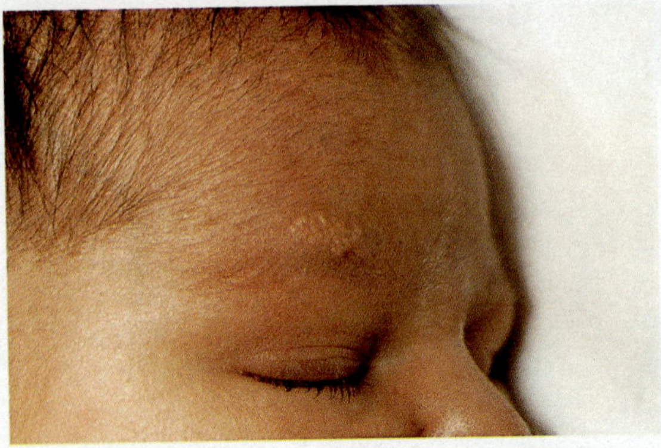

117．自出生后就有的眉毛上方的皮肤损害。

a. 诊断是什么?

b. 病程和预后如何?

c. 如何治疗该皮损?

This skin lesion above the eyebrow has been present since birth.

a. What is the diagnosis?

b. What is the course and prognosis?

c. What is the management of this lesion?

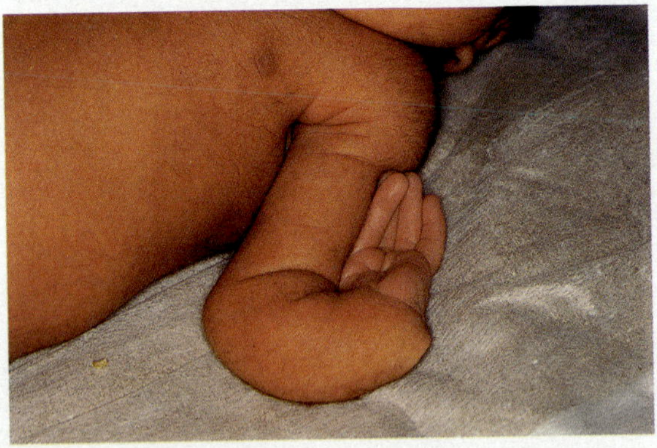

118．有自发性瘀青的3个月大婴儿。

a. 最可能的诊断是什么?

b. 什么检查有助于诊断?

c. 有什么相关的异常?

This 3-month-old infant has spontaneous bruising.

a. What is the most likely diagnosis?

b. Which investigations will be helpful?

c. What are associated abnormalities?

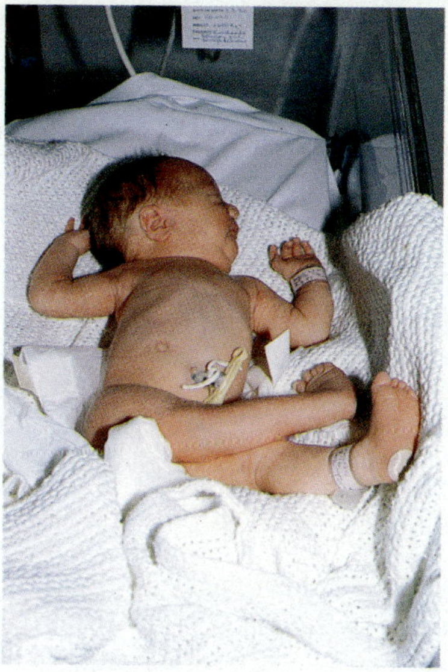

119．一名出生 24 小时的婴儿。
a. 这个婴儿在分娩过程中的先露部位是什么？
b. 有什么相关的并发症？
c. 应进行什么检查？

A 24-hour-old infant.
a. What was the presentation of this baby at birth?
b. What are the associated complications?
c. Which investigations should be undertaken?

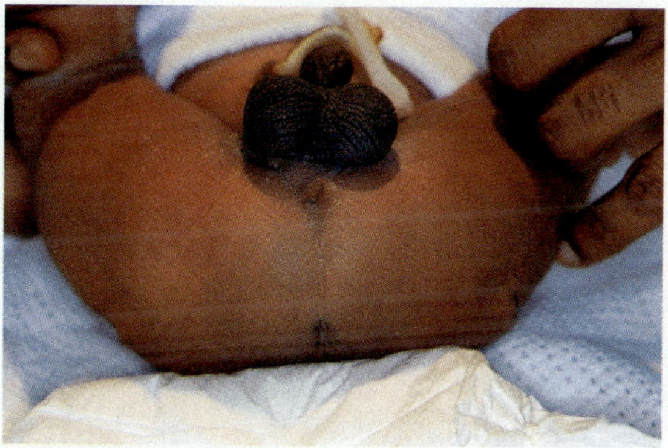

120．新生男婴的会阴。
a. 诊断是什么？
b. 有什么其他相关异常？
c. 如何治疗该病？

Perineum of a newborn male infant.
a. What is the diagnosis?
b. What are other associated abnormalities?
c. What is the management of this condition?

1．a. 分娩时胎儿头部变形、头颅血肿和先锋头。

b. 通过触诊颅骨和软组织肿胀：

- 胎儿头部变形——在正常分娩过程中发生的颅缝重叠。
- 头颅血肿——出血会被骨膜限制，而不会超越骨缝。在肿胀周围可触及一个清楚的骨性边缘。
- 先锋头——胎先露部位软组织的硬化、水肿和青肿。

c. 都会自行消退，没有任何令人焦虑的意义。头颅血肿的消退较为缓慢，并且偶尔会伴有钙化。

a. Moulding, cephalhacmatoma, and caput succedanaeum.

b. By palpation of the skull and soft tissue swelling:

- Moulding — overlapping of cranial sutures which occurs during normal vaginal delivery.
- Cephalhaematoma — Bleeding limited by periosteum and which does not cross suture lines. A distinct bony edge can be palpated around the circumference of the swelling.
- Caput succedanaeum — soft tissue induration, oedema and bruising of presenting part.

c. All disappear spontaneously and are of no worrying significance. Cephalhaematomas resolve slowly and are occasionally accompanied by calcification.

2．a. 脐带与其潮湿的基底部之间正常的分离。没有任何周围红肿（蜂窝织炎）或脓性分泌物等提示感染的征象。

b. 仅需要用清水或酒精拭子轻柔地擦洗，直到它自行分离为止。局部用抗生素粉剂会延迟分离。

a. Normal separation of the umbilical cord with a moist base. There is no sign of any surrounding erythema (cellulitis) or pussy disharge which would be suggestive of infection.

b. Gentle cleaning with water or a spirit swab is all that is required until spontaneous separation occurs. Topical antibiotic powder may delay separation.

3．a. 正常的生理性男性乳房发育。

b. 在生后前几天，男婴和女婴都会分泌少量牛奶样液体。女婴在生后 5～7 天会有黏液样或带血的阴道分泌物。
c. 父母应该对这些现象的生理性质放心，这是由于母亲体内的激素通过胎盘途径进入胎儿体内。

a. Normal physiological gynaecomastia.
b. Discharge of a small amount of milk may occur in both male and female infants in the first few days after birth. Mucousy or blood-stained vaginal secretions are also common in female infants around 5-7 days of age.
c. Parents should be reassured of the physiological nature of these events which are due to placental passage of maternal hormones.

4. a. 脓肿或皮下脂肪坏死。
b. 脓肿通常有触痛，并且会有波动感。皮下脂肪坏死呈现出红斑、硬结样非触痛性皮下肿胀，一般是在骨性突起处。
c. 治疗：
- 脓肿——全身应用抗生素预防局部感染蔓延到其他皮肤或播散到其他部位（如骨髓炎、脑膜炎），以及预防败血症。
- 皮下脂肪坏死——会自行恢复，但是如果累及较广泛，可能需要数月恢复。偶尔会伴有钙化和 / 或高钙血症。

a. Abscess or subcutaneous fat necrosis.
b. An abscess is usually tender and becomes fluctuant over the course of a few days. Subcutaneous fat necrosis presents as an erythematous, indurated non-tender subcutaneous swelling, usually over a bony prominence.
c. Management:
- Abscess — systemic antibiotics prevent local spread to other areas of skin, or dissemination to other sites (e.g. osteomyelitis, meningitis), and septicaemia.
- Subcutaneous fat necrosis — resolves spontaneously but if extensive may take several months. Occasionally associated with calcification and/or hypercalcaemia.

5. a. 外渗的静脉输注液体可能含有刺激性物质（如：钙）。
b. 长期损害可通过以下方式来控制：
- 小心选择外周静脉输液位点，因为关节附近的输液外渗后会因瘢痕形成而发生挛缩。
- 如果担心含有刺激性物质的静脉内液体渗出，就应该从中心静脉导管输入。

- 用大量含有透明质酸酶的稀释液和多孔引流法快速冲洗刚发生的渗出，可以减少组织的损伤。

a. Extravasation of intravenous fluid probably containing an irritant (e.g. calcium).

b. Long term damage may be limited by:
   - Care in siting peripheral intravenous infusions as contractures may occur with scarring after extravasation of fluid near joints.
   - Intravenous fluids containing irritants should be delivered via central venous catheters whenever the risk of extravasation is worrying (e.g. total parenteral nutrition).
   - Prompt irrigation of recent extravasation using large volumes of a diluent containing hyaluronidase and multi-puncture drainage may result in limitation of tissue damage.

6. a. 由于产科操作而引起的创伤性损伤或小的部分厚度头皮缺损。部分厚度头皮缺损可作为一种独立的先天性异常而出现，或是伴随于13三体型帕塔综合征而出现。

   b. 人工破膜，胎儿头皮血采样，胎儿头皮电极。

   c. 产科操作：
   - 人工破膜——促进胎先露部位下降。
   - 胎儿头皮血采样——测量血液pH值和酸中毒程度，并可以帮助监测胎儿的健康状况。
   - 胎儿头皮电极——可以持续监测胎儿的心率。

   a. Traumatic lesion from obstetric procedure or small partial thickness scalp defect. Partial thickness scalp defect may occur as an isolated congenital anomaly or in association with trisomy 13 – Patau syndrome.

   b. Artificial rupture of membranes, fetal scalp sampling, fetal scalp electrode.

   c. Obstetric procedures:
   - Artificial rupture of membranes — facilitates descent of presenting part.
   - Fetal scalp sampling — measurement of blood pH and base deficit, may assist in monitoring fetal well-being.
   - Fetal scalp electrode — allows continuous monitoring of fetal heart rate.

7. a. 不对称颈强直反射。

b. 拥抱反射或惊跳反射，吸吮反射，觅食反射，抓握反射（掌跖反射），眉间轻叩征，放置反射，踏步反射，牵引反射和侧弯反射。

c. 这些反射没有任何特殊的解剖意义，但它们的缺失或延迟出现可能是神经系统问题的早期征象。新生儿反射的存在或缺失必须结合胎龄、病史和神经系统检查的其他方面来考虑。

a. Asymmetric tonic neck reflex.

b. Moro or startle, sucking, rooting, grasp (palmar and plantar), glabellar tap, placing, walking, traction and Galant reflexes.

c. None have any particular anatomical significance but absence or delayed appearance may be an early sign of a neurological problem. The presence or absence of neonatal reflexes must be considered in association with gestational age, history and other aspects of the neurological examination.

8. a. 该婴儿的年龄约为4～6个月大。

b. 这个年龄段婴儿的其他标志性的运动包括：

- 在俯卧位时，孩子可以用前臂作为支撑，抬起头部和胸部。
- 当有人扶着其手臂或抱着其胸部时，开始能够站立起来和负重。
- 开始翻身，从一开始的侧翻身到后来的前后翻。

a. The age of the infant is 4-6 months.

b. Other motor milestones of infants of this age range include:

- In prone position can push up onto forearms and lift head and chest.
- Beginning to rise to standing position and weightbearing when supported under arms or around thorax.
- Starting to roll over, initially from front to side and then on to back.

9. a. 在精确地测量这名儿童的身高。重要的是孩子的脚要平放于地面上，脚后跟要与测量装置底部相接触，并且下颌角要与其头部所顶的测量板相平行。

b. 测距仪。

c. 相似的装置用于在水平位测量婴儿的身长，婴儿的腿必须拉直，即膝部不能弯曲。

a. Obtaining an accurate measurement of the height of the child. It is important that the child's feet are flat on the ground with the heels

touching the base of the measuring device and that the angle of the jaw is parallel to the weighted board touching the head.
b. Stadiometer.
c. A similar device is used with the infant in the horizontal position and the legs of the infant held straight (i.e. knees not flexed).

10. a. 苍白，不均匀的色素沉着或色素脱失，稀疏易折的毛发，有舌苔和水肿。
b. 由于食物蛋白质摄入不足而引起的恶性营养不良症（蛋白质能量营养不良）。
c. 治疗包括：
- 逐步给予营养，充分的饮食。
- 补充维生素。
- 治疗并发的感染。
- 如果孩子有严重的贫血，非常缓慢地输注少量红细胞可能有好处。

a. Pallor, patchy pigmentation or depigmentation, sparse friable hair, coated tongue, and oedema.
b. Kwashiorkor (protein energy malnutrition) due to inadequate dietary protein intake.
c. Treatment includes:
- Gradual reintroduction of a nutritionally adequate local diet.
- Vitamin supplementation.
- Treatment of associated infections.
- If the child is severely anaemic, very slow infusion of small volume red cell infusion may be beneficial.

11. a. 所显示的临床体征包括：
- 粗糙的面部特征。
- 大理石样皮肤外观（大理石样皮肤）。
- 脐疝。
b. 先天性甲状腺功能减退。
c. 其他临床特征包括：大的向外吐出的舌头，嘶哑的哭声，便秘，肌张力减退，黄疸消退延迟，体重增加缓慢，喂养差，自发活动缺少。
d. 如果拖延诊断和治疗，可能会引起发育延迟和长期的智力损害。早期的甲状腺激素替代治疗会改善情况，但是必须终身服用。

a. Clinical signs shown are:
- Coarse facial features.
- Marbled appearance of the skin (cutis marmoris).
- Umbilical hernia.

b. Congenital hypothyroidism.
c. Other clinical features include a large protruding tongue, hoarse cry, constipation, hypotonia, prolonged jaundice, poor weight gain, poor feeding, and paucity of spontaneous activity.
d. Delay in diagnosis and treatment may result in developmental delay and long term intellectual impairment. Early thyroid hormone replacement improves the outlook but must be continued for life.

12. a.上皮珠
b. 这种皮损是表皮囊肿。它们是无症状的，由于它们可以在出生后几天或几周自行消退，所以不需要治疗。
c. 上皮珠最常以成串的形式出现于新生儿硬腭和软腭交汇处的中线部位（Epstein小结）。它们也可以出现于牙槽缘，但较少见。

a. Epithelial pearl.
b. The lesions are epidermal cysts. They are asymptomatic and no treatment is required as they resolve spontaneously within a few days or weeks after birth.
c. Epithelial pearls most commonly occur as a cluster in the midline at the junction of the soft and hard palate (Epstein's pearls) in newborn infants. They also occur less commonly on the alveolar margin.

13. a. 逐渐消退的草莓样痣，其中心灰白，提示将要复原。
b. 草莓样痣在生后第1年中快速生长，然后在以后的几年中逐渐消退，仅留下扁平、灰白的色素脱失区域。
c. 出血、溃疡、感染和消耗性的血小板减少都是较罕见的并发症。偶尔如果草莓样痣对重要脏器造成了压迫（如眼睛或气道），口服类固醇有助于促进草莓样痣的消退。

a. Resolving strawberry naevus which shows central pallor indicating involution.
b. Strawberry naevi grow rapidly over the first year of life and then regress over the next few years, leaving only a flat pale depigmented area.
c. Bleeding, ulceration, infection and consumption thrombocytopenia are rare complications. Occasionally if the naevus causes pressure on a vital organ (e.g. eyes or airway) oral steroids will help to hasten involution.

14. a. 单纯性肥胖或库欣综合征。

b. 临床特征：

- 躯干性肥胖、生长阻滞、多毛、智力缺陷、紫纹、骨质疏松和肌肉萎缩都提示有库欣综合征。
- 肥胖的儿童肢体皮褶厚度和躯干脂肪过多，他们通常要比同龄孩子高很多。单纯性肥胖具有遗传因素。

c. 生化检查。在库欣综合征中由于肾上腺腺瘤或肾上腺癌，ATCH水平受到抑制，在地塞米松负荷剂量治疗后升高的尿类固醇代谢产物不能下降（抑制试验）。

a. Simple obesity or Cushing's syndrome.

b. Clinical features:

- Truncal obesity, growth retardation, hirsutism, apnoea, striae, osteoporosis and muscle wasting are suggestive of Cushing's syndrome.
- Obese children have excess limb skin fold thickness as well as truncal fat and they are often quite tall for their age. Simple obesity has a genetic component.

c. Biochemical investigations. In Cushing's syndrome due to an adrenal adenoma or carcinoma, ACTH levels are suppressed and elevated urinary steroid metabolites fail to decrease after a dexamethasone load (suppression test).

15. a. 佝偻病中长骨干骺端肿大。

b. 胫骨弓形弯曲，肋软骨交界处肿胀（串珠肋），颅骨软化和囟门闭合延迟，骨触痛，肌无力，易激惹和烦躁。

c. 生化学改变包括低钙血症、低磷酸盐血症、碱性磷酸酶升高、维生素D水平降低。佝偻病的放射学改变包括长骨干骺端外张、骨骺骨化延迟和病理性骨折。

a. Swelling of the long bone metaphyses in rickets.

b. Bowing of the tibia, swelling of the costochondral junctions (rachitic rosary), craniotabes and delayed closure of fontanelle, bone tenderness, muscle weakness, irritability and fretfulness.

c. Biochemical changes include hypocalcaemia, hypophosphataemia, elevated alkaline phosphatase, low vitamin D levels.
Radiological signs of rickets include splaying of the metaphyses of long bones, delayed epiphyseal ossification, and pathological fractures.

16. a. 带状疱疹病毒引起的水痘。

b. 潜伏期是12～21天。感染期开始于皮疹出现前2天，在所有皮损结痂后结束。

c. 对于这个暴露于病毒而没有免疫力的母亲应给予超免疫性水痘带状疱疹球蛋白(VZIG),以减少新生儿出现严重水痘的危险性。如果母亲在产前7天到产后28天内出现皮疹，就应该给予婴儿VZIG。由于新生儿肺炎有很高的致死率，所以婴儿若在生后48小时内出现水痘，建议口服阿昔洛韦。

a. Chicken pox (varicella) caused by herpes zoster virus.

b. Incubation period is 12-21 days. The period of infectivity begins 2 days before the the rash appears and ends when all the lesions have crusted.

c. Exposed, non-immune mothers should be given hyperimmune zoster globulin (VZIG) to reduce the risk of severe varicella in the newborn baby. The baby should be given VZIG if the mother develops the rash between 7 days prior to delivery and 28 days post-delivery. Oral acyclovir is also recommended for infants who develop varicella within 48 h of birth as neonatal pneumonitis has a high mortality.

17. a. 大量右侧气胸。

b. 空气进入减少，有过清音和肝大。在早产儿用冷光源进行透照法可以发现。

c. 复苏，新生儿透明膜病，新生儿暂时性呼吸急促，肺发育不良，机械通气（包括持续的正压通气)。足月儿自发性气胸的发生率接近1%。

d. 张力性气胸需要在适当的麻醉后，进行肋间插管引流。小的自发性气胸一般不需引流就会自己愈合。高浓度的氧气吸入会促进愈合，但在早产儿不应使用此法，因为有发生早产儿视网膜病的危险。

a. Large right pneumothorax.

b. Reduced air entry, hyper-resonance and hepatomegaly. May be detected in preterm infants by transillumination with cold light.

c. Resuscitation, hyaline membrane disease, transient tachypnoea of the newborn, pulmonary hypoplasia, and mechanical ventilation including continuous positive-airways pressure. Spontaneous pneumothoraces occur in up to 1% of term babies.

d. Tension pneumothorax requires insertion of an intercostal drain after appropriate analgesia. Small spontaneous pneumothoraces usually resolve without drainage. A high oxygen environment will hasten resolution, but should not be used in preterm infants at risk of retinopathy of prematurity.

18. a. 无脑畸形——前脑和颅骨穹窿缺失，并继发脸部的扭曲。
   b. 中线缺陷（如腭裂和颈椎异常）。
   c. 虽然可以存活数小时或数天，但最终会死亡。无脑畸形很容易通过产前超声检查诊断出来，这可以使父母决定是否继续妊娠。生后将这孩子进行适当的包裹，送给家长看。偶尔，当无脑畸形儿是活产儿且出生体重大于2.2kg时，其心脏可以进行器官捐赠。

   a. Anencephaly — absence of forebrain and skull vault with secondary distortion of face.
   b. Mid-line defects, (e.g. cleft palate and abnormal cervical vertebrae).
   c. Incompatible with life, although may survive for several hours or days. Anencephaly is easily recognizable on antenatal ultrasound scan, and this enables parental choice over continuation of the pregnancy. After birth, the infant can be suitably wrapped for the parents to view the baby. Occasionally, when an anencephalic infant is liveborn and birthweight >2.2 kg, the heart may be suitable for organ donation.

19. a. 小的脑脊膜膨出。
   b. 脊柱的X线片会显示椎弓缺陷。超声检查将显示囊性损伤，并且一般与脊椎管有潜在的连接。在手术前进行MRI和CT检查有助于了解完整的解剖情况。
   c. 若一个孩子有神经管畸形，那么在以后出生的孩子中就会有1/20的再发危险。
   d. 母亲怀孕前后口服叶酸可以降低再发危险。

   a. Small meningocele.
   b. Plain X-ray of the spine will show a defect in the vertebral arch. Ultrasound scan will demonstrate a cystic lesion and usually an underlying connection with the spinal canal. Magnetic resonance imaging or computed tomography scan will help to demonstrate the full anatomy before surgery.
   c. 1 in 20 risk of recurrence for subsequent pregnancies after one child with any neural tube defect.
   d. Periconceptual maternal folic acid reduces the recurrence risk.

20. a. 尿道口在阴茎体上的尿道下裂。

b. 由于腹侧包皮不能融合而形成冗长的背侧包皮，阴茎向腹侧弯曲（痛性阴茎勃起），以及泌尿系统异常。

c. 大多数需要外科手术。包皮环切术应该在外科矫正手术完成后再进行，因为包皮有可能被用于尿道成形术中。阴茎竖立时，应该对痛性阴茎勃起进行评估；如果存在痛性阴茎勃起，则需要释放牵扯的皮肤。肾脏超声检查可以排除其他肾脏畸形。

a. Hypospadias with the urethral orifice on the shaft of the penis.

b. Redundant dorsal hooded prepuce due to failure of fusion of the ventral foreskin, ventral curvature of the penis (chordee), and renal tract anomalies.

c. Most will require surgery. Circumcision should be delayed until corrective surgery has been performed, as the prepuce may be required for the urethroplasty. Chordee should be assessed when the penis is erect and, if present, release of the tethering skin may be required. Renal ultrasonography will exclude other renal anomalies.

21. a. 脐疝，双侧腹股沟疝，双侧睾丸鞘膜积液。

b. 腹股沟疝发生于30%～40%的早产男婴中。脐疝在黑人婴儿中更为常见。

c. 大多数脐疝会在生后前几年内恢复。很少情况下，需要在3岁左右进行外科整形手术。先天性睾丸鞘膜积液通常会自行恢复。腹股沟疝因为在婴儿期有较高的嵌顿绞窄的危险，所以需要在确诊后即进行外科修补手术。

a. Umbilical hernia, bilateral inguinal herniae and bilateral hydroceles.

b. Inguinal herniae occur in 30-40% preterm male infants. Umbilical herniae are more common in black infants.

c. The majority of umbilical herniae resolve within the first few years. Occasionally, cosmetic surgery at around 3 years of age may be required. Congenital hydroceles always resolve spontaneously. Inguinal herniae require surgical repair soon after diagnosis as there is a high risk of strangulation in infancy.

22. a. 瘢痕疙瘩——通常只要很小的损伤就会形成过多的瘢痕组织。

b. 瘢痕疙瘩在黑皮肤的人群中较为常见。

c. 对于已形成的瘢痕疙瘩尚没有满意的治疗方法，也没有限制瘢痕疙瘩进一步发展的方法。由于瘢痕疙瘩的形成有不断增加的趋势，所以要进行外科切除很困难。

a. Keloid — excessive scar formation often following minimal trauma.
b. Keloid scar formation is more common in people with black skin.
c. There is no satisfactory treatment for established keloid scars and no way to limit the development of further keloid. Surgical excision is difficult because of the tendency to increasing keloid formation.

23. a. 颈部肿胀的鉴别诊断：
- 水囊状淋巴管瘤。
- 淋巴结病。
- 淋巴结炎（脓肿形成）。

b. 水囊状淋巴管瘤可以用透照法来检查。
脓肿/淋巴结炎有触痛，并且有波动感。

c. 水囊状淋巴管瘤——外科切除，但是较困难。
脓肿——全身应用抗生素，当有波动感时进行外科引流。
淋巴结肿大——检查可能存在的潜在病因（如结核病、淋巴瘤）。

a. Differential diagnosis of neck swelling:
- Cystic hygroma.
- Lymphadenopathy.
- Lymphadenitis (abscess formation).

b. Cystic hygroma will transilluminate.
An abscess/lymphadenitis will be tender and may become fluctuant.

c. Cystic hygroma — surgical excision but may be difficult.
Abscess — systemic antibiotics and surgical drainage when it becomes fluctuant.
Lymphadenopathy — investigation will depend on the most likely underlying cause (e.g. tuberculosis, lymphoma).

24. a. 颈蹼，乳头间距宽，无乳房发育。
b. 特纳综合征（XO型）。
c. 相关的问题：
- 主动脉缩窄。
- 卵巢发育不全导致无第二性征发育和不育症。

d. 治疗：
- 重组生长激素可被用来改善身材矮小。
- 周期性的雌激素替代治疗将会促进青春期第二性征的发育，但是不育症的情况不能改变。

a. Webbing of the neck, wide-spaced nipples, and absence of breast development.
b. Turner syndrome (XO).
c. Associated problems:
- Coarctation of the aorta.
- Ovarian dysgenesis leading to failure of secondary sexual development and infertility.

d. Management:
- Recombinant growth hormone can be used to improve short stature.
- Cyclical oestrogen replacement will promote secondary sexual characteristics in adolescence, but infertility is invariable.

25. a. 斯特奇-韦伯综合征，有过多的面部血管瘤或葡萄酒色痣，特征性地按照三叉神经走向分布。
b. 癫痫；大头畸形；在面部血管瘤的同侧会有脑膜血管瘤，并且偶尔可能会引起对侧偏瘫；脑萎缩和脑钙化。
c. 脑电图检查常常显示有异常病灶。神经影像学检查（如CT增强扫描或MRI脑血管造影）可以进一步确定是否有脑膜血管瘤。

a. Sturge-Weber syndrome with extensive facial haemangioma or port-wine stain, characteristically in the distribution of the trigeminal nerve.
b. Epilepsy, macrocephaly, meningeal haemangioma on the same side as the facial haemangioma which may occasionally cause a contralateral hemiplegia, cerebral atrophy, and cerebral calcification.
c. Electroencephalogram will often show an irritable focus. Neuro-imaging (e.g. computed tomography with contrast or magnetic resonance imaging angiogram brain scan) will confirm the presence of a meningeal haemangioma.

26. a. 福尔克曼缺血性挛缩，表现为前臂废用性萎缩、腕部屈曲畸形和手部爪样畸形。
b. 这种畸形常继发于肱骨下段髁上骨折后的动脉缺血。髁上骨折复位应该在适当的麻醉下，由经验丰富的小儿整形外科医生来进行。仔细监测肢体末端到肘部的循环情况，能提醒临床医生骨折复位术后缺血的早期症状。

a. Volkmann's ischaemic contracture with wasting of forearm, flexion deformity of wrist and claw deformity of the hand.
b. The deformity is secondary to arterial ischaemia secondary to supracondylar fracture of lower end of humerus. Reduction of a supracondylar fracture should always be undertaken with appropriate anaesthesia and by an experienced paediatric orthopaedic surgeon. Careful monitoring of the circulation of the limb distal to the elbow will alert clinicians to early signs of ischaemia post-reduction of the fracture.

27. a. 拇指缺失，前臂短。
b. 前臂的X线片将会进一步提示有无桡骨的缺失。
全血细胞计数和血涂片——拇指和桡骨缺失有时会伴随有血小板减少症和/或贫血。血小板减少症伴拇指缺失是TAR综合征(即血小板减少及桡骨缺失综合征)。也有其他综合征伴随有贫血和拇指和桡骨缺失（如范康尼贫血，即先天性骨髓发育不全)。拇指缺失也可作为一种独立的畸形而存在。

a. Absent thumb and short forearm.
b. X-ray of the forearm will confirm presence or absence of the radius. A full blood count and blood film — absent thumb and radius is sometimes associated with thrombocytopenia and/or anaemia. Thrombocytopenia associated with absence of the radius is TAR syndrome. There are also other syndromes associated with anaemia and absent thumb and radius (e.g. Fanconi anaemia). Absence of the thumb may also occur as an isolated anomaly.

28. a. 肛门闭锁和高位直肠闭锁，并有肛门外括约肌和皮赘的不透X线标志。
b.通常会在新生儿出生后即行的常规体检中发现。如果有高位直肠闭锁和肛门外括约肌存在，偶尔会在以后因发生肠梗阻和胎粪排出延迟而发现。
c. 直肠-生殖器-尿瘘较常见，尤其是有高位直肠损害。在进一步进行放射学检查以明确其解剖状况之前，预防性进行泌尿系统抗菌有助于防止尿道感染。

a. Imperforate anus and high rectal atresia with a radiopaque marker demonstrating the external anal sphincter or skin tag.
b. Usually diagnosed on routine neonatal examination soon after birth. If there is a high rectal atresia, and the external anal sphincter is

present, may occasionally present later as intestinal obstruction or delayed passage of meconium.

c. Recto-genito-urinary fistulae are common, particularly with high rectal lesions. Prophylactic urinary antisepsis will help to prevent urinary tract infections until the anatomy is clarified by further radiological investigations.

29. a. 膈疝，表现为肠疝入左半侧胸腔。心脏和纵隔都向右侧移位。

b. 通常需要复苏，包括机械通气。用大的鼻胃管（赖尔管，Ryle's tube）进行持续肠道减压。在进行外科修补手术前必须先稳定病情，包括用血管扩张剂（如NO）治疗肺高压。

c. 外科根治手术一般在技术上没有困难。是否存活取决于肺发育不良和肺高压的严重程度。尽管手术前病情稳定情况进一步改善，该病的生存率仍仅有约60%。

a. Diaphragmatic hernia with herniation of bowel into left hemi-thorax. Heart and mediastinum are displaced to the right.

b. Resuscitation, including mechanical ventilation, is usually required. Continuous decompression of the gut with a large bore nasogastric tube (Ryle's tube). Stabilization prior to surgical repair is essential, including management of pulmonary hypertension with vasodilators, including nitric oxide.

c. Definitive surgery is not usually technically difficult. Survival depends on severity of pulmonary hypoplasia and pulmonary hypertension. Despite advances in pre-surgical stabilization, survival rate is still only around 60%.

30. a. 脐疝和直肠分离。

b. 不需要处理。

c. 这两种情况在生后前3年会逐渐改善。脐疝不会发生嵌顿或导致肠箝闭，但是在哭吵时体积会增大。腹部或脐部绷带法不能促进其恢复。偶尔当脐疝到3岁时还不能恢复，就需要进行外科整形手术。

a. Umbilical hernia and divarication of the recti.

b. Nil required.

c. Both conditions improve over the first 3 years of life. Umbilical herniae do not become trapped or result in incarceration of the bowel, but they often increase in size on crying. Strapping of the abdomen or umbilicus does not hasten resolution. Cosmetic surgery is only occasionally required if an umbilical hernia has not resolved by 3 years of age.

31. a. 干梅状腹综合征。
b. 临床特征包括腹壁肌肉组织松弛或缺失、低位耳、生殖器异常和继发于因胎儿尿液排出减少而导致羊水过少的关节弯曲（关节和肢体的屈曲挛缩）。
c. 由于肺发育不良而导致的呼吸功能不全。
d. 阻塞性尿路疾患可以由产前超声发现肾盂扩大和羊水过少而诊断。

a. Prune-belly syndrome.
b. Clinical features include laxity or absence of the abdominal wall musculature, low set ears, genital anomalies and arthrogryposis (flexion contractures of the joints and limbs) secondary to oligohydramnios due to reduced fetal urine output.
c. Respiratory insufficiency due to pulmonary hypoplasia.
d. Obstructive uropathy can be diagnosed by antenatal ultrasound when there are dilated renal pelves and oligohydramnios.

32. a. 支气管肺发育异常(BPD)或慢性肺病。
b. 在左侧胸腔有一个不透射线的夹子，提示对开放未闭的动脉导管（PDA）进行了外科结扎术。
c. PDA的结扎可能会促进早期脱离机械通气。大多数有BPD的婴儿都能脱离机械通气而存活，但是很多在生后前几年都有反复发生的下呼吸道感染和喘鸣。长期的呼吸系统预后不明确，但是存活的低出生体重儿到青春期后，其呼吸功能似乎是正常的。

a. Bronchopulmonary dysplasia (BPD) or chronic lung disease.
b. There is a radio-opaque clip in the left hemithorax indicating surgical ligation of a patent ductus arteriosus (PDA).
c. Ligation of PDA may hasten weaning from mechanical ventilation. Most infants with BPD who can be weaned survive, but many have recurrent lower respiratory tract infections and wheezing in the first few years of life. Long-term respiratory prognosis is uncertain as survival of low birth weight infants is relatively recent, but respiratory function appears to be normal in adolescence.

33. a. 双侧眼球突出。
b. 眼球突出的鉴别诊断包括Graves病（甲状腺毒症或甲状腺功能

亢进）、累及眼眶的肿瘤（如转移的神经母细胞瘤和视网膜母细胞瘤，一般出现在生后前几年）。脑肿瘤也可能会压迫视路或海绵窦导致眼球突出、视野受损和其他视觉障碍。

a. Bilateral proptosis (protrusion of the eyes).
b. Differential diagnosis of proptosis includes Graves' disease (thyrotoxicosis or hyperthyroidism), tumours involving the orbit (e.g. metastatic neuroblastoma, and retinoblastoma, which usually presents in the first few years of life). Cerebral tumours may also cause pressure on the optic pathway or cavernous sinus resulting in proptosis, visual field defects and other visual disturbance.

34. a. 外侧角皮样囊肿——右眼上外侧肿胀。
b. 沿着颅骨骨缝处的囊性发育异常，典型的围绕于眼眶或从枕部到鼻基底部中线处。
c. 其大小通常缓慢增加，并且有时会有感染。一般由于美容原因或反复发生的感染而进行外科手术切除皮样囊肿。

a. External angular dermoid — there is a swelling superior and lateral to the right eye.
b. Cystic developmental anomaly found along the suture line of the skull, typically around the orbit or midline from the occiput to the base of the nose.
c. Usually increase slowly in size and sometimes become infected. Surgery to remove the dermoid cyst is usually done for cosmetic reasons or because of recurrent infection.

35. a. 草莓样痣（毛细血管瘤）。
b. 出生时并没有，但是会在生后前几个月中出现鲜红色的皮损。在生后第一年会迅速长成突起的、有凹痕的皮损，然后慢慢自行消退，到3～4岁时仅留下一个平滑、苍白的脱色素斑块。
c. 偶尔有溃疡、出血、消耗性血小板减少或继发感染。全身性应用类固醇有助于减小侵占重要器官（如气道和眼睑）的皮损的体积。
d. 早熟——发生于将近30%的早产儿中。

a. Strawberry naevus (capillary haemangioma).
b. Not present at birth, but appear as a bright red lesion within first few months. Grow rapidly into protuberant, pitted, lesions over the first year, then spontaneously regress slowly leaving only a smooth, pale,

depigmented area by 3-4 years of age.

c. Occasionally may ulcerate, bleed or develop consumption thrombocytopenia or secondary infection. Systemic steroids may help to reduce size of lesions encroaching on vital organs (e.g. airway or eyelids).

d. Prematurity — occurs in approximately 30% preterm infants.

36. a. 后侧外阴或处女膜皮赘——在女婴外阴部位的肉质隆起，有时在生后前几天会伴有黏液样或水样的血性分泌物。

b. 由于母体激素的胎盘转移引起新生儿处女膜肥大。它是正常的生理现象，不必引起过度担心。没有必要治疗，一般会在生后几天或几周自行消退。

a. Posterior vulval or hymenal tag — a fleshy protuberance in the genital area of female infants which is sometimes associated with a mucousy or watery, blood stained discharge in the first few days after birth.

b. Hypertrophy of the newborn hymen resulting from placental transfer of maternal hormones. It is a normal physiological phenomenon which is of no worrying significance. No treatment is necessary and spontaneous involution always occurs within a few days or weeks after birth.

37. a. 表皮和皮下血管瘤和肢体不对称肥大。

b. 克-特-韦综合征。

c.合并动静脉瘘较为常见，有时会有淋巴管瘤异常。外科切除血管瘤和动静脉瘘通常比较困难，但是人为造成连接血管的栓塞有时较易成功。治疗目的通常是限制患侧肢体的血管瘤异常快速生长。

d. 散发发病。

a. Cutaneous and subcutaneous hemangiomata and asymmetric limb hypertrophy.

b. Klippel-Trenaunay-Weber syndrome.

c. Associated arteriovenous fistulae are common and lymphangiomatous anomalies sometimes occur. Surgical excision of the haemangiomata and fistulae is often difficult, but embolization of connecting vessels is sometimes successful. The aim of treatment is usually to limit abnormally rapid growth of the affected limb.

d. Sporadic occurrence.

38. a. 鱼鳞癣——是一种皮肤异常角质化的遗传性疾病，有特征性的鳞屑形成。

b. 轻度形式可只用润肤剂或温和的角质软化剂（如水杨酸亲水软膏）即可。较为严重的形式在新生儿期可呈现出火棉胶样皮肤，需要精心的护理和监护以预防继发感染，并补充丢失的水分、电解质和蛋白质。
c. 鱼鳞癣一般会持续终生，但是并非所有在新生儿期有火棉胶样皮肤的婴儿在以后的儿童期都会发展成为鱼鳞癣。

a. Ichthyosis — an inherited skin condition with abnormal keratinization characterized by visible scaling.
b. Mild forms may be treated with simple emollients or mild keratolytics (e.g. salicylic acid in aqueous cream). More severe forms may present as collodion skin in the neonatal period, and careful nursing and medical care will be required to prevent secondary infection and to compensate for losses of water, electrolytes and protein.
c. Ichthyosis usually persists throughout life, but not all infants with collodion skin in the newborn period develop ichthyosis in later childhood.

39. a. 腹部疾病或对谷蛋白敏感。
b. 对饮食中的小麦、黑麦，有时是大麦和燕麦，有持久性的不耐受。
c. 大多数孩子在2岁前表现为慢性腹泻、呕吐、腹胀、双臀消瘦、易激惹和肌张力减退。粪便苍白，有泡沫和恶臭味（脂肪痢），难以在马桶中冲走。可能也会有口腔溃疡、光舌、杵状指、外周水肿和佝偻病的体征。

a. Coeliac disease or gluten sensitivity.
b. Permanent intolerance of dietary wheat, rye and sometimes barley and oats.
c. Most children present before 2 years of age with chronic diarrhoea, vomiting, abdominal distension, wasted buttocks, irritability and hypotonia. The stools are pale, frothy, foul-smelling (steatorrhoea) and difficult to flush away in the toilet. There may also be mouth ulcers, smooth tongue, finger clubbing, peripheral oedema and signs of rickets.

40. a. 母乳喂养的营养是适当的，除非早产儿，需要额外补充营养，尤其需要蛋白质、钙、钠和磷。母乳喂养可以预防感染，尤其是大肠杆菌感染和胃肠炎，减少婴儿猝死的危险，促进母婴关系健康发展，并且母乳喂养既方便又经济。

b. 母乳喂养的禁忌证很少，包括母亲偶尔服药（如四环素或肿瘤化疗药）。

a. Breast-feeding is nutritionally appropriate unless the infant is extremely premature, when supplementation, especially of protein, calcium, sodium and phosphate may be required. Breast-feeding provides protection against infection, especially *Escherichia coli* and gastroenteritis, reduces the risk of cot death, facilitates development of healthy maternal/infant relationship, and is convenient and economical.

b. There are very few contra-indications to breast-feeding which include occasional maternal drugs (e.g. tetracycline, or cancer chemotherapy).

41. a. 摇篮样脚，有脚后跟突起和脚背面隆起。

b. 染色体异常，尤其是三体性［如 18 三体（Edward）综合征；13 三体（帕塔）综合征］

c. 低出生体重和宫内发育迟缓，小头畸形，面部中线缺陷，肢体屈曲畸形，手指重叠的手部畸形，肺发育不良和先天性心脏病。在一些新生儿期存活下来的婴儿中，癫痫和严重的神经发育延迟是不可避免的。

a. Rocker-bottom feet with protuberant heel and convex dorsum of the feet.

b. Chromosomal abnormalities, particularly trisomies (e.g. trisomy 18, Edward's syndrome; trisomy 13, Patau syndrome).

c. Low birth weight and intrauterine growth restriction, microcephaly, midline facial defects, flexion deformities of the limbs, abnormal posture of the hands with overlapping fingers, pulmonary hypoplasia and congenital heart disease. Epilepsy and severe neurodevelopmental delay are inevitable in the few infants who survive beyond the neonatal period.

42. a. 脐周蜂窝织炎——脐周皮肤红斑和脱皮，有时有化脓性、黄色分泌物。

b. 细菌感染，最常由金黄色葡萄球菌引起。

c. 在正确的采样和培养之后即静脉内使用广谱抗生素（如头孢呋辛或氟氯西林和庆大霉素）。不充分或延迟的治疗会导致播散性脓毒血症，包括败血症、骨髓炎或中毒性上皮坏死（葡萄球菌性烫伤样皮肤综合征）。

a. Periumbilical cellulitis — erythema and desquamation of the skin surrounding the umbilicus. There is sometimes a purulent, yellowish discharge.

b. Bacterial infection most commonly due to *Staphylococcus aureus.*

c. Prompt intravenous broad spectrum antibiotics (e.g. cefuroxime, or flucloxacillin and gentamicin) after appropriate swabs and cultures. Inadequate or delayed treatment can lead to disseminated sepsis including septicaemia, osteomyelitis or toxic epidermal necrosis (staphylococcal scalded skin syndrome).

43. a. 宫内带状疱疹（水痘）的瘢痕。

b. 对未经免疫的母亲应给予水痘带状疱疹免疫球蛋白(VZIG)，以限制感染对发育过程中的胎儿的影响。如果母亲在分娩的一周内出现皮疹，那么新生儿在出生后也应该给予VZIG。当母亲在分娩一周内出现水痘，为了降低新生儿发生致命并发症（如肺炎）的危险，应该给予新生儿阿昔洛韦。

a. Scars of intrauterine herpes zoster (chickenpox).

b. The non-immune mother should be given hyperimmune zoster globulin (VZIG) to limit the effects of the infection on the developing fetus. If the maternal rash occurs within a week of delivery, the newborn infant will also require VZIG. Acyclovir should be given to newborn infants when maternal chickenpox develops within a week of birth in order to reduce the risk of life-threatening neonatal complications (e.g. pneumonitis).

44. a. 严重的口腔念珠菌感染（鹅口疮，念珠菌病）。

b. 鹅口疮在婴儿期是极其常见的，并且一般是良性疾病。它更常见于使用抗生素之后。如果鹅口疮反复发作或难以根治，就要怀疑是否有免疫缺陷性疾病。在婴儿期以后，口腔念珠菌感染通常与免疫缺陷性疾病相关（如HIV感染、严重的联合性免疫缺陷性疾病或为治疗恶性肿瘤而使用免疫抑制剂）。在大一些的患有哮喘的儿童中，喷雾吸入皮质类固醇也可引起麻烦的鹅口疮。

a. Severe oral candidiasis (thrush, moniliasis).

b. Thrush in infancy is an extremely common and usually benign condition. It is more common after the administration of antibiotics. If thrush is recurrent or is difficult to eradicate, an underlying immunodeficiency disorder should be suspected. Beyond infancy, oral candidiasis is usually associated with an immunodeficiency disorder (e.g. HIV or severe combined immunodeficiency disorder or immunosuppressive treatment for malignancy). Inhaled corticosteroids may also cause troublesome oral thrush in older asthmatic children.

45. a. 脂溢性皮炎——出现于头皮的称为乳痂。
b. 在眉毛、耳朵、发际和会阴周围的油脂性斑块或有鳞屑的皮疹。偶尔盘状皮损会从尿布周围向上蔓延到躯干部位（尿布牛皮癣）。
c. 乳痂一般可以简单使用角质溶解洗剂。脂溢性皮炎一般到1岁左右会自愈。温和的皮质类固醇软膏（如1%的氢化可的松乳膏）在较为严重的脂溢性皮炎中可能较有效，但是应该少量使用，尤其是在脸上。

a. Seborrhoeic dermatitis — on the scalp it is called cradle cap.
b. Greasy plaques or scaly rash around eyebrows, ears, hairline and in the perineum. Occasionally discoid lesions spreading up the trunk from the napkin area (napkin psoriasis).
c. Cradle cap usually responds to a simple keratolytic shampoo. Seborrhoeic dermatitis always improves spontaneously towards the end of the first year of life. A mild corticosteroid cream (e.g. 1% hydrocortisone cream) may be helpful in more troublesome seborrhoeic dermatitis, but should be used sparingly, particularly on the face.

46. a. 是佝偻病肋软骨连接处肿胀（串珠肋）。
b. 口服维生素D对于纠正生化和放射学异常是必要的，并且可以预防长期骨畸形，尤其是承重的肢体。家庭的饮食宣教和长期饮食摄入维生素D的改善，对于预防佝偻病复发和保护其他家庭成员是很重要的，尤其是未来的婴儿。
c. 吸收不良，肝疾病，肾小管功能不良，长期服用抗惊厥药和遗传性X连锁低磷酸盐血症性佝偻病。

a. Swelling of the costo-chondral junctions in rickets (rachitic rosary).
b. Oral vitamin D supplementation will be necessary to correct the biochemical and radiological abnormalities and to prevent long-term bony deformity, particularly of weight-bearing limbs. Dietary education of the family and improved long-term dietary intake of vitamin D will be important to prevent recurrence of rickets and to protect other family members, especially future infants.
c. Malabsorption, liver disease, renal tubular dysfunction, long-term anticonvulsants and hereditary X-linked hypophosphataemic rickets.

47. a. 由于宫内受压而导致的体位性畸形足。
  b. 对于轻度体位性畸形足，足和踝关节可以进行充分的被动运动，并会自行恢复正常。偶尔对于较严重的体位性畸形足，可用足部夹板固定法，虽然尚没有证据表明这种治疗的效果如何。
  c. 相关的异常：
  - 先天性髋关节脱位。
  - 脊髓脊膜膨出。

  a. Postural talipes is due to intrauterine compression.
  b. In mild postural talipes, there is a full range of passive movement of the foot and ankle and spontaneous resolution will occur. Occasionally, splinting of the feet is used for more severe postural talipes, although there is no evidence for efficacy of this treatment.
  c. Associated anomalies:
  - Congenital dislocation of the hip.
  - Meningomyelocele.

48. a. 唇裂和腭裂的并发症包括喂养困难、体重增加缓慢和口腔正畸的问题。牛奶反流入鼻咽部会导致反复发作的中耳感染和听力缺陷。如果腭裂是在9～12个月大小以后才关闭，就会出现语言问题，尤其是鼻音。
  b. 大约有1/600的活产儿发生唇裂和腭裂。如果有一个同胞患此病，那么在以后出生的孩子中再发的危险性就较高。

  a. Complications of cleft lip and palate include feeding difficulties, poor weight gain and orthodontic problems. Regurgitation of milk into the nasopharynx may lead to recurrent middle ear infections and hearing deficit. Speech problems, especially nasal voice, occur if palate closure is after 9-12 months of age.
  b. Cleft lip and palate occur in approximately 1 in 600 livebirths. After one affected sibling, there is a higher risk of recurrence in future children.

49. a. 枕部脑膨出。
  b. 并发症包括脑（脊）膜炎和癫痫。神经系统缺陷的严重性取决于为使颅骨关闭而切除的脑组织的数量和部分。
  c. 母亲如果在怀孕前后未补充叶酸，那么在以后的每一次妊娠中有1/20的神经管畸形再发危险。

a. Occipital encephalocele.
b. Complications include meningitis and epilepsy. The severity of the neurological deficit will be dependent upon the amount and part of brain which has to be excised to allow skull closure.
c. In the absence of peri-conceptual maternal folic acid supplementation, there is a 1 in 20 risk of recurrence of a neural tube defect in each subsequent pregnancy.

50. a. 白癜风——色素沉着和脱色素皮肤区。
b. 白癜风一般合并有瓦尔登伯格综合征——白色额发和感觉神经性耳聋存在。瓦尔登伯格综合征通常是一种常染色体显性遗传性疾病。患有瓦尔登伯格综合征的成人可能难以被识别，因为他们常将其白色额发染色。与成人相比，患有白癜风的儿童具有自身免疫性疾病的可能较为少见。
c. 化妆用乳膏可以用来掩盖脱色素皮肤，但是结果往往不令人满意。

a. Vitiligo — areas of pigmented and depigmented skin.
b. Vitiligo is sometimes associated with Waardenburg syndrome — white forelock and sensorineural hearing loss. Waardenburg syndrome is often inherited as an autosomal dominant condition. Adults with Waardenburg syndrome may be difficult to recognize as they often dye the white forelock. Underlying autoimmune disorders are much less common in children with vitiligo than adults.
c. Cosmetic creams may be used to disguise the depigmented skin, but the result is often unsatisfactory.

51. a. 腹部细纹或白纹。
b. 细纹在儿童中并不常见。在儿童期可能的原因包括库欣综合征(Cushing's syndrome)和单纯性肥胖。对于一些有满月脸、躯干性肥胖、多毛症、痤疮、肌肉萎缩和生长缓慢的孩子，应怀疑其是否有库欣综合征。库欣综合征可能是由于垂体腺瘤导致肾上腺增生而产生过多的氢化可的松引起(库欣病)，或继发于外源性使用过多的皮质类固醇药物而引起。

a. Striae or stretch marks on the abdomen.
b. Striae are uncommon in children. Underlying causes in childhood include Cushing's syndrome and simple obesity. Cushing's syndrome should be suspected in those with moon facies, truncal obesity, hirsutism, acne, muscle wasting, and slow growth. Cushing's syndrome

may be due to excessive cortisol produced by adrenal hyperplasia caused by pituitary adenomata (Cushing's disease) or secondary to excessive exogenous corticosteroid administration.

52. a. 亨－舍紫癜(HSP)，即过敏性紫癜。

b. 检查：

- 检查尿液有无血尿和蛋白尿。
- 肾功能检查，包括血清肌酸酐。
- 监测血压。
- 即使HSP皮疹的分布通常是有特征性的，也要进行血小板计数和凝血测试，以排除血小板减少症和出血性疾病。

c. HSP一般过了几周后有自限性倾向。HSP复发和再发的危险性大约为30%。少数病例会发生肾小球肾炎（＜1%），但发生长期慢性肾功能衰竭的危险较低。

a. Henoch-Schönlein purpura (HSP).

b. Investigations:

- Test urine for haematuria and proteinuria.
- Renal function tests including serum creatinine.
- Monitor blood pressure.
- Platelet count and clotting studies to exclude thrombocytopenia and bleeding disorders, although distribution of rash in HSP is usually characteristic.

c. HSP usually runs a self-limiting course over weeks. Relapse or recurrence occurs in approximately 30% cases of HSP. Glomerulonephritis occurs in a minority of cases (<1%), but there is a low risk of long term chronic renal failure.

53. a. 鉴别诊断是坏死性皮肤炎症损伤，包括结节性多动脉炎和严重的过敏性紫癜(HSP)。

b. 结节性多动脉炎在儿童是一种很罕见的疾病，但是当HSP很严重、反复发病或者出现非典型性皮损或症状时，就应该怀疑结节性多动脉炎。结节性多动脉炎和HSP最令人担忧的长期并发症是肾功能衰竭和肠道梗塞。

a. The differential diagnosis of necrotic inflammatory skin lesions include polyarteritis nodosa and severe Henoch-Schönlein purpura (HSP).

b. Polyateritis nodosa is rare in childhood, but should always be suspected when HSP is severe, recurrent or presents with atypical lesions or symptoms. The most worrying long-term complications of both polyarteritis nodosa and HSP are renal failure and bowel infarction.

54. a. 湿疹。

b. 屈曲部位，尤其是腘窝、肘窝、腕关节和躯干是最常被累及的部位。

c. 湿疹有很强烈的瘙痒感，并且由于搔抓而使表皮脱落后常常发生继发性感染。疱疹性湿疹（单纯疱疹病毒）是一种不常见的并发症，有时在临床上较难与细菌性感染区分，但是一旦诊断，应及时口服阿昔洛韦。慢性未经治疗的湿疹可能会导致皮肤苔癣样变和色素沉着，且难以根治。

a. Eczema.

b. Flexures particularly the popliteal and antecubital fossae, wrists and trunk are most commonly affected.

c. Eczema is intensely itchy and secondary infection often occurs after there has been excoriation of the skin from scratching. Eczema herpeticum (herpes simplex virus) is an uncommon complication which is sometimes difficult to distinguish clinically from bacterial infection, but once diagnosed responds rapidly to oral acyclovir. Chronic untreated eczema may result in lichenification and hyperpigmentation of the skin which can be difficult to eradicate.

55. 一名喂养困难的4周大的婴儿大腿。

a. 骨髓炎或骨肿瘤。骨髓炎发病在新生儿中比较隐袭，在临床体征变得明显之前，可能已经累及很广泛了。

b. 全血细胞计数、血培养、红细胞沉降率或C反应蛋白一般可确诊有无感染或炎症。MRI骨扫描可以帮助整形外科医师进行细针穿刺或骨活组织检查从而获得组织学诊断。锝的骨扫描可以显示早期急性骨髓炎位点处有“热”点显现，但是在小婴儿可能就难以解释了。

c. 全身应用广谱抗生素，包括抗葡萄球菌治疗，至少3周。

a. Osteomyelitis or bone tumour. Osteomyelitis presents insidiously in neonates and may be quite extensive before clinical signs become apparent.

b. Full blood count, blood cultures, erythrocyte sedimentation or C-reactive protein usually confirm infection/inflammation.

MRI bone scan will assist the orthopaedic surgeon in obtaining a tissue diagnosis by needle aspirate or bone biopsy. Technetium bone scan will show a hot spot at an early stage in acute osteomyelitis but may be difficult to interpret in very young infants.

c. Broad-spectrum systemic antibiotics including anti-staphylococcal cover for at least 3 weeks.

56. a. 白化病——皮肤和毛发的色素缺乏。

b. 虹膜色素沉着不足和视网膜异常导致对亮光（包括阳光）极度敏感。

c. 一些有白化病的儿童仅仅只是皮肤色素缺乏。如果视网膜受累及，就要防止亮光照射以减少损害，但是视力损伤较常见，并且是进行性的，经常会在生命后期变得较严重。

a. Albinism — absence of pigmentation in the skin and hair.

b. Hypopigmentation of the iris and retinal abnormality leading to extreme sensitivity to bright light including sunlight.

c. Some children with albinism have lack of pigmentation only in the skin. If the retina is affected, protection from bright sunlight will help to limit damage, but visual impairment is common, progressive and often severe in later life.

57. a. 长骨干骺端分离（“芹菜杆样外观”）。

b. 先天性风疹综合征（风疹性胚胎畸形）。

c. 在孕早期（< 12 周）感染风疹病毒的婴儿将会受到严重影响。可能会发生小头畸形、先天性心脏病、颅内钙化、肝脾大、淋巴结肿大、发育停滞、神经发育延迟、癫痫、耳聋和白内障。在孕晚期发生感染仍可能引起感觉神经性耳聋，并且进行性加重即使在出生后。

a. Metaphyseal streaking of the long bones (‘celery stalk appearance’).

b. Congenital rubella syndrome (rubella embryopathy).

c. Infants infected with the rubella virus in early gestation (<12 weeks) will be most severely affected. Microcephaly, congenital heart disease, intra-cranial calcification, hepatosplenomegaly, lymphadenopathy, failure to thrive, neurodevelopmental delay, epilepsy, deafness and cataracts may occur. Infection later in pregnancy may still cause sensorineural hearing loss which is progressive, even after birth.

58. a. 并趾畸形——左脚的第 2 和第 3 脚趾蹼化。

b. 脚趾的并趾畸形是常见的小的先天性外观异常，没有功能上的影响。一般为常染色体显性遗传。

a. Syndactyly — webbing of the second and third toes of the left foot.
b. Syndactyly of the toes is a common minor cosmetic congenital anomaly and is of no functional significance. It is often inherited as an autosomal dominant.

59. a. 口内和口周的溃疡和大水疱可能会有剧烈的疼痛，引起进食和饮水困难，多涎和流涎，轻度发热和易激惹。在治疗方面进行止痛和充分补水是较重要的。
b. 单纯疱疹性口炎。
c. 单纯疱疹性口炎一般是自限性疾病，但是如果孩子很小或是免疫减弱，就可能会发生致命的脑炎或播散性单纯疱疹感染。

a. Ulcers and blisters in and around the mouth are likely to be extremely painful and will cause difficulty in eating and drinking, excessive salivation and dribbling, mild fever, and irritability. Analgesia and adequate hydration will be important in the management.
b. Herpes simplex stomatitis.
c. Herpes simplex stomatitis is usually a self-limiting condition, but if the child is very young or immunocompromised, encephalitis or disseminated herpes infection can be life-threatening.

60. a. 努南综合征——特纳综合征的表型特征，但是核型正常。患有努南综合征的孩子一般是男孩，但是偶尔也有女孩患病。
b. 努南综合征的临床体征有生长缓慢、身材矮小、颈蹼、低位耳和器官距离过远（两眼间距宽）。
c. 在努南综合征中肺动脉瓣狭窄是最常见的心脏异常。在特纳综合征中主动脉缩窄是最常见的心脏异常。
d. 一般是散发发病，但是偶尔作为常染色体显性遗传病进行遗传。

a. Noonan syndrome — phenotypic features of Turner syndrome, but normal karyotype. Children with Noonan syndrome are usually male, but occasionally females also affected.
b. Clinical signs of Noonan syndrome are slow growth, short stature, webbed neck, low-set ears and hypertelorism (widely-spaced eyes).
c. Pulmonary stenosis is the most common cardiac abnormality in Noonan syndrome. Coarctation of aorta is the most common cardiac lesion in Turner syndrome.
d. Usually sporadic, but occasionally may be inherited as an autosomal dominant.

61. a. 左侧髋关节脱位。左侧髋关节的髋臼较浅，左股骨头向上外侧移位。

b. 髋关节先天性脱位在臀位产的婴儿中较常见，在有畸形足、脊柱裂、关节弯曲和有髋关节发育不良家族史的婴儿中也较常见。

c. 用固定带或石膏绷带进行外展夹板固定疗法至少6周。如果在新生儿期未能做出诊断，那么就很可能需要进行外科手术治疗。

a. Dislocation of the left hip. The acetabulum of the left hip is shallow and the head of the left femur is displaced upwards and laterally.

b. Congenital dislocation of the hip is more common after breech presentation, and in infants with talipes, spina bifida, arthrogryposis and in those with a family history of developmental dysplasia of the hip.

c. Abduction splinting in a harness or plaster cast for at least 6 weeks. If the diagnosis is not made in the newborn period, surgery is more likely to be required.

62. a. 广泛的肺实质性病变。

第6、7、8肋骨的双后侧骨折。

b. 慢性肺病(CLD)或支气管肺发育不良，出现于将近40%的极低出生体重儿中。早产儿骨质减少，一般是由于磷酸盐或维生素D缺乏。

c. CLD的原因是多因素的，并且目前也没有明确的预防方法。充分的摄入磷酸盐和维生素D，尤其是对于需要长期胃肠外营养的婴儿，将会减少早产儿骨质减少的危险性。

a. Widespread parenchymal lung disease.

Bilateral posterior fractures of 6,7 and 8th ribs.

b. Chronic lung disease (CLD) or bronchopulmonary dysplasia which occurs in up to 40% extremely low birth weight infants. Osteopenia of prematurity which is usually due to phosphate or vitamin D deficiency.

c. The cause of CLD is multi-factorial and there is no clear method of prevention as yet. Adequate intake of phosphate and vitamin D, particularly in babies requiring prolonged parenteral nutrition, will reduce the risk of osteopenia of prematurity.

63. a. 纵隔积气——在胸廓中央气体聚集。

b. 机械通气（包括持续的正压通气）、新生儿透明膜病和胎粪吸入综合征都是诱发因素。偶尔有已在出生时建立了自主呼吸的新生儿发生气体渗漏（如纵隔积气或气胸）。

c. 在足月儿，给予吸入高浓度的氧将会促进气体渗漏的愈合，包括纵隔积气。外科引流则很少需要。

a. Pneumomediastinum — central collection of air in the thorax.
b. Mechanical ventilation including continuous positive airways pressure, hyaline membrane disease, and meconium aspiration syndrome are predisposing factors. Occasionally a newborn infant who has established spontaneous onset of respiration at birth may develop an air leak (e.g. pneumomediastinum or pneumothorax).
c. In a term infant, a high inspired oxygen concentration will hasten resolution of air leaks, including pneumomediastinum. Surgical drainage is rarely required.

64. a. 脑积水——头部大，有突出的额头和眼睛的落日征。
b. 头颅超声或脑部的CT检查将会显示侧脑室扩大。第3和第4脑室的增大取决于梗阻的水平。
c. 治疗要根据潜在的原因。当存在有头围迅速增大或颅内压增高的症状，就需要进行脑室腹膜分流术。早产儿脑室内出血导致的脑室扩大只是暂时的，会自行消退。

a. Hydrocephalus — large head with a prominent forehead and setting sun eye sign.
b. Cranial ultrasound scan or computed tomograph brain scan will show dilatation of the lateral ventricles. Enlargement of the third and fourth ventricles will depend on the level of the obstruction.
c. Management depends on the underlying cause. When there is a rapid increase in head circumference or symptoms of raised intracranial pressure, a ventriculoperitoneal shunt may be required. After intraventricular haemorrhage in a preterm infant, ventriculomegaly may be transient and resolve sponateously.

65. a. 双侧踝关节肿胀——反应性关节炎，青少年慢性关节炎（JCA），过敏性紫癜，风湿热，系统性红斑狼疮（SLE）和炎性肠病。
b. 检查——全血细胞计数，咽喉拭子，血培养， 炎症标志物如CRP，ESR，抗链球菌溶血素滴度（AST）和自身抗体测试。
c. 非甾体抗炎药物，如阿司匹林和布洛芬，可以帮助减轻症状。无论何时都要尽可能地坚持运动。理疗、水疗和夹板固定法可以减轻症状，减少慢性关节炎所致的残疾。有时在严重的病例中需要应用免疫抑制剂或皮质类固醇。

a. Bilateral swollen ankles — reactive arthritis, juvenile chronic arthritis (JCA), Henoch-Schönlein purpura, rheumatic fever, systemic lupus erythematous (SLE) and inflammatory bowel disease.
b. Investigations — full blood count, throat swab, blood cultures, inflammatory markers e.g. CRP, ESR, antistreptolysin titre (AST), and autoantibody tests.
c. Non-steroidal inflammatory drugs e.g. aspirin and ibuprofen help to relieve symptoms. Activity should be maintained whenever possible. Physiotherapy, hydrotherapy, and splinting provide symptomatic relief and reduce disability in chronic arthritis. Sometime immunosuppressive drugs or corticosteroids are required in severe cases.

66. a. 并指畸形——左手第2和第3手指蹼化。
b. 不像脚趾的并趾畸形那样，只是常见的小的先天性外观异常而功能上不受什么影响，手指的并指畸形需要进行外科整形手术以改善手的功能和外观。手指的并指畸形比脚趾的并趾畸形较为少见。

a. Syndactyly — webbing of the second and third fingers of the left hand.
b. Unlike syndactyly of the toes which is a common minor cosmetic congenital anomaly of no functional significance, syndactyly of the fingers will require plastic surgery to improve hand function as well as cosmetic appearance. Syndactyly of the fingers is much less common than syndactyly of the toes.

67. a. 通贯手——单根横穿手掌的褶纹。
b. 通常伴随于21三体综合征（唐氏综合征）。通贯手也可见于18%的正常儿童中。
c. 肌张力减退，扁平的满月形脸，宽鼻梁，内眦赘皮，上斜的眼睛，布拉什菲尔德点，第三囟门，短颈，低发际，枕部扁平（短头畸形），小耳伴耳轮发育不良，宽的铲形手，小指中指骨短小弯曲（先天性指侧弯），以及第1与第2脚趾间间隔明显(sandalgap)。

a. Simian crease — a single transverse palmar crease.
b. Often associated with trisomy 21 (Down syndrome). Simian creases are also found in 18% normal children.
c. Hypotonia, flat moon shaped facies, broad nasal bridge, epicanthic folds, upward slanting eyes, Brushfield spots, third fontanelle, short neck, low hairline, flattened occiput (brachycephaly), small ears with

an immature helix, broad spade-shaped hands, short incurved middle phalanx of the little finger (clinodactyly), and a wide gap between first and second toes (sandal gap).

68. a. 凉鞋趾缝——在脚的跖面第1与第2脚趾之间有深而宽的褶纹。

b. 先天性心脏病、甲状腺功能减退、希施斯普龙病(Hirschsprung's disease，即先天性巨结肠)、十二指肠闭锁、白内障、暂时的异常骨髓细胞生成和髓性白血病在唐氏综合征的儿童中都是较常见的。唐氏综合征的患儿即使没有心脏病的临床体征，也应该在新生儿期进行超声心动检查，因为大约30%的患儿有房室间隔缺损。

a. Sandal gap — deep, wide crease on the plantar surface of the foot, between the first and second toes.

b. Congenital heart disease, hypothyroidism, Hirschsprung's disease, duodenal atresia, cataracts, transient abnormal myelopoiesis and myeloid leukaemia are more common in children with Down syndrome. Infants with Down syndrome should have an echocardiogram in the neonatal period even if there are no clinical signs of cardiac disease as approximately 30% will have an atrio-ventriculo-septal defect.

69. a. 人乳头状瘤病毒感染引起的肛门生殖器疣（尖锐湿疣）。

b. 疣可能在感染后将近2年形成，小年龄儿童可能在分娩时通过母亲的产道感染此病毒。在大于2岁的儿童中还应考虑性虐待的可能。

c. 应该进行其他性传播疾病的检查，如果是阳性，性虐待的诊断就成立。需要通过多学科的方法进行机构间合作以评估孩子和家庭。

a. Anogenital warts (condyloma acumanta) caused by human papilloma virus.

b. Warts may develop up to 2 years after exposure and young children may acquire the virus from the genital tract of the mother during delivery. In children >2 years of age, sexual abuse should always be suspected.

c. Tests for other sexually transmitted diseases should be performed and, if positive, the diagnosis of sexual abuse is confirmed. A multi-disciplinary approach with inter-agency collaboration will be necessary to assess the child and family.

70. a. 腱膜下或骨膜下血肿，可能伴有潜在的颅骨骨折。

b. 头颅X线片可以确定有无骨折。婴儿至少应在医院留诊观察24小时以确保没有颅内出血的体征或症状，颅内出血可导致硬膜下或硬膜外积血。小婴儿的颅骨骨折是由于遭受到明显的外伤。评估损伤是否是意外事故时，了解病史和受损的情况很重要。

a. Subaponeurotic or subperiosteal haematoma which may be associated with an underlying fracture of the skull.

b. Skull X-ray will confirm the diagnosis of fracture. The infant should remain under observation in hospital for at least 24 h to ensure that there are no signs or symptoms of intracranial haemorrhage resulting in a subdural or extradural collection. Skull fracture in a young infant results from significant trauma. The history and circumstances of the injury will be important in assessing whether the injury was accidental.

71. a. 18三体综合征(Edward 综合征)——伴有手指重叠的钳握样手。

b. 小于胎龄儿，小头畸形，肺发育不良，髋关节和肢体的屈曲畸形，摇篮脚，隐睾，多毛，小颌，短睑裂，低位耳，小口，面瘫和先天性心脏病。

c. 大多数会在生后前几个月内死亡。少于10%的病例会存活超过1年，而且他们通常有严重的智力和发育延迟。

a. Trisomy 18 (Edward syndrome)— denched hand with overlapping of the fingers.

b. Small for gestational age, microcephaly, pulmonary hypoplasia, flexion deformities of the hips and limbs, rocker-bottom feet, cryptorchidism, hirsutism, micrognathia, short palpebral fissures, low-set ears, microstomia, facial plasy and congenital heart disease.

c. Most die within the first few months after birth. Fewer than 10% survive beyond the first year of life and they are always severely mentally and developmentally delayed.

72. a. 耳前皮赘。

b. 单独的皮赘通常只作为单独的先天性畸形而存在，仅仅是外观上的异常。多发皮赘可能合并有其他的头部和颈部先天性异常。应该用耳镜确定外耳道是否通畅和中耳是否存在。因为在一小部分儿童中多发皮赘会伴随有听力缺陷，所以应该进行听力测试。

c. 散发发病。

a. Pre-auricular skin tags.
b. Single skin tags are usually an isolated congenital anomaly and of cosmetic significance only. Multiple skin tags may be associated with other congenital anomalies of the head and neck. Patency of the external meatus and presence of the middle ear should be confirmed using an auriscope. Hearing tests should be undertaken as multiple skin tags are associated with hearing deficit in a small proportion of children.
c. Sporadic occurrence.

73. a. 杵状趾。
b. 发绀性先天性心脏病，囊性纤维化病，支气管扩张症，炎性肠病，肝病，胃肠道吸收不良和感染性心内膜炎。
c. 囊性纤维化病——胸部X线片和发汗试验。
支气管扩张——CT检查。
心脏缺陷和心内膜炎——超声心动图。
心内膜炎、溃疡性结肠炎和克隆病——发热和炎性标志物升高（如C反应蛋白）。
结肠镜检查、钡餐、随访或肠道活检对于确诊炎性肠病或吸收不良是有必要的。

a. Clubbing of the toes.
b. Cyanotic congenital heart disease, cystic fibrosis, bronchiectasis, inflammatory bowel disease, liver disease, gastrointestinal malabsorption and infective endocarditis.
c. Cystic fibrosis – chest X-ray and sweat test. CT scan – bronchiectasis. Echocardiogram – heart defects and endocarditis. Fever, raised inflammatory markers (e.g. C-reactive protein) – endocarditis, ulcerative colitis and Crohn's disease. Colonoscopy, barium meal and follow-through or bowel biopsy will be necessary to make a definitive diagnosis of inflammatory bowel disease or malabsorption.

74. a. 脓疱病——离散存在的周围发红的大水疱，以后会结痂。它具有高度传染性，可通过手或密切接触而传播。
b. 由金黄色葡萄球菌引起的细菌感染。
c. 在做了表皮拭子和血培养之后，至少要全身应用抗生素7天。在药敏结果出来以前，至少要联合应用2种抗葡萄球菌的抗生素（如氟氯西林和庆大霉素或万古霉素）。

a. Impetigo — discrete blisters with a surrounding flare and which later become crusted. It is highly infectious and transferred by hands or close contact.
b. Bacterial infection caused by *Staphylococcal aureus.*
c. Systemic antibiotics for at least 7 days, after taking superficial swabs and blood cultures. A combination of at least two anti-staphylococcal antibiotics (e.g. flucloxacillin and gentamycin or vancomycin) should be used until sensitivities of the organism are known.

75. a. 由于周围皮下组织的血管收缩效应而引起的静脉周围明显苍白。静脉输液中含有血管收缩性药物（如多巴胺或多巴酚丁胺）。
b. 含有血管收缩性药物的外周静脉输液应该立即停止，以防止组织坏死。血管收缩性药物的静脉输液应该由中心静脉导管输入。

a. Intense pallor around the vein due to the effects of vasoconstriction in the surrounding subcutaneous tissue. The intravenous infusion contains an inotropic drug (e.g. dopamine or dobutamine).
b. The peripheral infusion containing the inotrope should be ceased immediately to prevent tissue necrosis. Infusions of inotropes should always be given through a central venous catheter.

76. a. 严重贫血可能是由于胎儿-母体输血、从脐带急性失血（如帆状附着或脐带未钳闭）、严重的溶血性疾病、血红蛋白病（如α重型地中海贫血）、宫内病毒感染、先天性白血病或红细胞发育不良。
b. 在分娩48小时内在母体血中通过Kleihauer试验检测胎儿细胞。母体和婴儿血型和间接抗球蛋白试验（Coomb试验）。对病毒感染进行IgM或PCR检测。骨髓穿刺对于诊断白血病或输血依赖性贫血的潜在原因是很有必要的。

a. Severe anaemia may be due to a feto-maternal transfusion, acute blood loss from the umbilical cord (e.g. velamentous insertion or unclamped cord), severe haemolytic disease, haemoglobinopathy (e.g. alpha thalassaemia major), intra-uterine viral infection, congenital leukaemia or erythroid dysplasia.
b. A Kleihauer test for fetal cells in maternal blood within 48 h of delivery. Maternal and infant blood group and an indirect antiglobulin (Coomb's) test. IgM or PCR tests for viral infections. Bone marrow aspirate will be necessary to diagnose leukaemia or the underlying cause of transfusion-dependent anaemia.

77. a. 上背部大的不规则的色素痣或鲨革斑，在左下背部有3个直径大于1cm的咖啡牛奶斑，许多其他较小的色素痣以及在腰骶部的胎斑。

b. 多发性神经纤维瘤（Von Recklinghausen病）。

c. 常染色体显性遗传疾病，但是许多病例是作为一个新的突变而出现。

a. Large irregular pigmented naevus or shagreen patch on the upper back, 3 café au lait patches >1 cm diameter on the left lower back, numerous other smaller pigmented naevi and a Mongolian blue spot in the lumbosacral region.

b. Neurofibromatosis (von Recklinghausen's disease).

c. Autosomal dominant inheritance, but many cases occur as a new mutation.

78. a. 撕裂的上唇系带。

b. 因强行将乳头或其他物体塞入婴儿嘴里而引起。有时照看者会提供婴儿喂养困难的病史。

c. 应该怀疑非意外伤害。应该通过多学科儿童保护团体调查社会和家庭环境。

a. Torn frenulum of the upper lip.

b. Caused by aggressively forcing a teat or other object into the infant's mouth. A history of poor feeding by the infant is sometimes given by the carers.

c. Non-accidental injury should be suspected. The family and social circumstances should be investigated by a multi-disciplinary child protection team.

79. a. 腓肠肌肥大。

b. Duchenne肌营养不良。

c. 孩子从地板上爬起时会有Gower征；近端肌肉无力，包括肩胛带；渐进性肌无力和萎缩；心肌病；语言和教育不同程度的延迟。

d. 血清肌酸磷酸激酶将会明显升高。肌电图、肌肉超声将会有异常。肌肉活检会显示抗肌萎缩蛋白缺乏或异常。已确定抗肌萎缩蛋白基因在Xp21。

a. Hypertrophy of the calf muscles.

b. Duchenne muscular dystrophy.

c. Gower sign on rising from the floor, proximal muscle weakness including shoulder girdle, increasing muscle weakness and atrophy, cardiomyopathy, and variable speech and educational delay.
d. Serum creatinine phosphokinase will be markedly elevated. Electromyography, muscle ultrasound will be abnormal. Muscle biopsy will show absent or abnormal dystrophin. The dystrophin gene has been identified at Xp21.

80. a. 牙龈瘤——在新生儿期牙槽缘的一种罕见的肉芽肿样病变。
b. 病变是无症状的，并且不会影响喂养。
c. 不需要治疗，因为其会在几周内自行恢复。

a. Epulis — a rare, granulomatous lesion on the alveolar margin in the newborn period.
b. The lesion is asymptomatic and does not interfere with feeding.
c. No treatment is required as spontaneous resolution always occurs within a few weeks.

81. a.有多余皮褶的短颈，发际低。
b. 短颈和发迹低通常会合并有染色体异常疾病（如唐氏综合征、特纳或努南综合征、克利佩尔－费尔综合征）。
c. 染色体分析。颈部和背部的X光片可以揭示骨骼异常（如半脊椎畸形或脊柱侧凸）。

a. Short neck with redundant skin folds and a low hairline.
b. Short neck and low hairline is often found in association with chromosomal abnormalities (e.g. Down syndrome, Turner or Noonan's syndrome, and Klippel-Feil syndrome).
c. Chromosome analysis. X-ray of the neck and back may reveal skeletal anomalies (e.g. hemivertebrae or scoliosis).

82. a. 眶周蜂窝织炎。
b. 在进行了浅表拭子检测和血培养之后，至少要全身应用广谱抗生素7天。还需要进行止痛。
c. 全身扩散可能会导致菌血症或败血症。局部扩散会引起眼眶脓肿形成，导致眼肌麻痹、失明、眼球突出、海绵窦血栓形成和颅神经麻痹。如果蜂窝织炎治疗后没有迅速起效，或如果出现任何新的眼部体征，那么应立即咨询小儿眼科医师的建议。

a. Peri-orbital cellulitis.
b. Broad spectrum systemic antibiotics for at least 7 days, after taking

superficial swabs and blood cultures. Analgesia will be required.

c. Systemic spread may result in bacteraemia or septicaemia. Local spread can lead to abcess formation in the orbit, resulting in ophthalmoplegia, loss of vision, proptosis, cavernous sinus thrombosis and cranial nerve palsy. The advice of a paediatric ophthalmologist should be sought immediately if the cellulitis does not respond rapidly, or if any new eye signs develop.

83. a. 剪刀腿。

b. 大脑性瘫痪。

c. 一般无法明确确切的原因。大约有10%的病例在胎儿期或新生儿早期有缺氧性脑损伤。痉挛性双瘫在早产儿中较为常见。在生后前几周可以通过颅脑超声检查或MRI脑扫描识别出大多数大脑性瘫痪高危早产儿。通过脑部CT和MRI检查，那些偏瘫或轻偏瘫的儿童可能有脑梗死表现，在一些病例可能存在有凝血障碍。

a. Scissoring of the legs.

b. Cerebral palsy.

c. The precise cause is usually not identifiable. In approximately 10%, it is due to hypoxic brain damage in fetal or early neonatal life. Spastic diplegia is more common in preterm infants. Cranial ultrasound or a magnetic resonance imaging (MRI) brain scan in the first few weeks after birth will identify most preterm infants at high risk of cerebral palsy. Children with a hemiplegia or hemiparesis may have a cerebral infarct on computed tomography or MRI brain scan and, in some, an underlying coagulopathy will be identified.

84. a. 脂肪瘤、神经瘤或海绵状血管瘤。

b. 出于外观原因以及为了做出确切诊断，一般有必要进行外科切除。

c. 复发的危险性较低，但这取决于外科切除是否彻底以及病变的性质。海绵状血管瘤通常很难完全切除。

a. Lipoma, neuroma or cavernous haemangioma.

b. Surgical excision will usually become necessary for cosmetic reasons and to make a precise diagnosis.

c. Recurrence risk is low, but will depend on the completeness of surgical excision and the nature of the lesion. Cavernous haemangiomas are often difficult to excise completely.

85. a. 明显的新生儿头部抬起迟缓。
    b. 颈部肌张力减退可能是由于先天性肌营养不良或肌病、脑瘫或代谢性疾病。
    c. 颅脑超声或MRI脑扫描，甲状腺功能试验，肌肉活检和超声扫描，肌电图，常规生化检查（包括肝、肾功能），血氨和乳酸，血清肌酸酐磷酸激酶，尿氨和有机酸。

a. Marked head lag.
b. Hypotonia of neck muscles may be due to a congenital muscular dystrophy or myopathy, cerebral palsy, or metabolic disorders.
c. Cranial ultrasound or a magnetic resonance imaging brain scan, thyroid function tests, muscle biopsy and ultrasound scan, electromyography, routine biochemical tests including liver and renal function, plasma ammonia and lactate, serum creatinine phosphokinase, and urinary amino and organic acids.

86. a. 由于细菌感染引起的新生儿乳腺炎。
    b. 在获得表皮拭子检测和血培养之后，至少全身应用广谱抗生素7天。偶尔如果有波动性脓肿形成，应进行外科切开引流脓液。在外科操作过程中要小心以免损伤乳腺组织。
    c. 及时应用抗生素治疗会彻底恢复。

a. Neonatal mastitis due to bacterial infection.
b. Broad spectrum systemic antibiotics for at least 7 days, after taking superficial swabs and blood cultures. Occasionally, surgical incision may be required to drain the pus if a fluctuant abscess develops. Care should be taken to avoid damage to the breast tissue during surgical incision.
c. Complete resolution occurs with prompt antibiotic treatment.

87. a. 颈部中线损伤通常是甲状舌管囊肿或甲状舌管瘘。
    b. 一般应该进行甲状腺功能试验。颈部的超声检查可以帮助鉴别囊肿或瘘。放射性同位素检查会对功能性甲状腺组织进行精确的定位。为了获得明确的组织学诊断和出于外观原因，通常有必要进行外科探查和切除，但是外科手术应该等到甲状腺检查结果出来之后再进行。

a. Midline neck lesions are usually thyroglossal cysts or fistulae.
b. Thyroid function tests should always be performed. An ultrasound scan of the neck may help to identify a fistula or cyst. A radio-isotope

scan will show the precise location of functioning thyroid tissue. Surgical exploration and excision will usually be necessary for a definitive histological diagnosis and for cosmetic reasons, but surgery should always be delayed until the results of thyroid investigations are known.

88. a. 胎斑。
b. 胎斑最常出现于背部的腰骶部区域。
c. 青灰色或瘀青样皮肤色素沉着区域在婴儿长大后逐渐变得不那么明显，而其余部分皮肤颜色会随着年龄增长变深。胎斑在亚洲婴儿尤其多见，并且在非高加索人群新生儿中非常普遍，但是在 1 岁以后就很少看到。

a. Mongolian blue spot.
b. Mongolian blue spots most commonly occur over the lumbosacral region of the back.
c. The slate-grey or bluish pigmented area of skin gradually becomes less obvious as the infant grows older and the rest of the skin becomes darker with age. Mongolian blue spots are particularly common in Asian infants and almost universal in non-Caucasian neonates, but are rarely seen beyond the first year of life.

89. a. 副乳头，在正常乳头位置的正下方。有时会误诊为色素痣。
b. 无须治疗，但如果当孩子长大后，副乳使其感到难堪，那么出于外观原因可以进行外科切除手术。副乳头可能会有潜在的乳腺芽，由于孕期经胎盘转移的母体雌激素或青春期正常的生理性雌激素产生会使其增大，但这种情况较为罕见。

a. Accessory nipple, below and in line with the normally placed nipple and breast bud. Sometimes mistakenly diagnosed as a pigmented naevus.
b. No treatment is necessary, but surgical excision can be performed for cosmetic reasons if the lesion causes the child embarassment when he is older. Occasionally, accessory nipples may also have an underlying breast bud which will enlarge in response to placental transfer of maternal oestrogen during gestation or normal physiological oestrogen production at puberty.

90. a. 伴随于严重先天性贫血的巨型肝大，最可能的原因是髓外造血和心力衰竭。
b. α 重型地中海贫血或严重的溶血（如恒河猴溶血病）。

c. 母亲血涂片显示有小红细胞和血红蛋白过少，有可能是缺铁性贫血或α地中海贫血。父亲也应进行筛查，如果他是携带者，便应对胎儿进行产前检测。母亲的血型和抗体检查将会提醒有恒河猴溶血病或其他溶血性疾病的可能。

a. Massive hepatomegaly, which in association with profound congenital anaemia, is most likely to be due to extra-medullary haemopoiesis and heart failure.
b. Alpha thalassaemia major, or severe haemolysis (e.g. rhesus haemolytic disease).
c. A microcytic, hypochromic maternal blood film which is likely to be due to either iron deficiency anaemia or alpha thalassaemia trait. The father should also be screened to allow antenatal testing of the fetus if he is also a carrier. Maternal blood group and antibody testing will alert to the possibility of rhesus and other haemolytic disease.

91. a. 蜂窝织炎，可能是由于潜在的淋巴结炎或淋巴结脓肿。
b. 金黄色葡萄球菌，溶血性链球菌，流感嗜血杆菌，以及任何定殖在鼻咽部或上呼吸道的细菌。
c. 在进行表皮拭子检测和血培养之后，全身应用广谱抗生素至少7天。偶尔当有波动性脓肿形成，就需要外科切开进行脓液引流。

a. Cellulitis, probably due to an underlying lymphadenitis or lymph node abscess.
b. *Staphlyococcal aureus*, *Haemolytic streptococcus, Haemophilus influenzae*, and any bacteria which colonize the nasopharynx or upper respiratory tract.
c. Broad-spectrum systemic antibiotics for at least 7 days, after taking superficial swabs and blood cultures. Occasionally, surgical incision may be required to drain pus if a fluctuant abscess develops.

92. a. 发亮、膨胀的腹部，伴有皮肤紫癜或瘀青，浅表静脉显著，透过腹壁可见肠管呈浅蓝色。
b. 坏死性小肠结肠炎。
c. 较差的预后：
- 穿孔。
- 持续性血小板减少。
- 持续性代谢性酸中毒。

- 异常血凝块。
- 在开始常规治疗的48h内腹部膨胀仍不能得到改善——禁食；开始用广谱抗生素，包括甲硝唑以防止厌氧菌对肠粘膜的侵袭；循环支持。

a. Shiny distended abdomen with purpura/bruising of skin, prominent superficial veins and faint bluish discoloration of bowel visible through the abdominal wall.

b. Necrotizing enterocolitis.

c. Poor prognosis:

- Perforation.
- Persistent thrombocytopenia.
- Persistent metabolic acidosis.
- Abnormal blood clotting.
- Failure of abdominal distension to improve within 48 h of commencing conventional mangement — ceasing enteral feeds, starting broad-spectrum antibiotics including metronidadazole to cover invasion of the bowel mucosa by anaerobic organisms, and circulatory support.

93. a. 膈疝，肠疝入左侧胸腔，心脏向右侧移位。

b. 临床体征包括呼吸窘迫、发绀、舟状腹、右位心和左侧胸腔通气减少。

c. 紧急处理包括气管插管和机械通气。用大号鼻胃管（Ryle管）进行持续的胃肠减压是必要的。

肺动脉高压较常见，并且需要在纠治手术实施前进行治疗。服用肺血管扩张药（如前列环素、硫酸镁和NO吸入）可能有所帮助。

a. Diaphragmatic hernia with bowel in left hemithorax and heart displaced to the right.

b. Clinical signs will include respiratory distress, cyanosis, a scaphoid abdomen, dextrocardia and reduced air entry in left hemithorax.

c. Emergency treatment will be intubation and ventilation. A large bore naso-gastric (Ryle's) tube on continuous drainage is essential to deflate the stomach.

Pulmonary hypertension is common and will need to be treated before definitive surgery is undertaken. Pulmonary vasodilators (e.g. prostacyclin, magnesium sulphate and nitric oxide) may be helpful.

94. a. 腮腺肿胀（腮腺炎）。
b. 急性细菌或病毒感染，最常见的是流行性腮腺炎病毒。HIV 感染的儿童在出现其他免疫缺陷相关的感染之前，经常有慢性或反复发作的腮腺炎。
c. 流行性腮腺炎在那些对生后 12~18 个月的小孩接种 MMR（麻疹、腮腺炎、风疹）疫苗的社区中已较少见。细菌性腮腺炎可以用广谱抗生素治疗。对反复发生腮腺炎的儿童应该考虑进行 HIV 检查。

a. Swelling of the parotid gland (parotitis).
b. Acute bacterial or viral infection, most commonly mumps virus. Chronic or recurrent parotitis is often found in children with HIV infection before they develop other immunodeficiency-related infections.
c. Mumps is now uncommon in communities where the MMR vaccine is given at 12-18 months of age. Bacterial parotitis will respond to broad spectrum antibiotics. An HIV test should be considered in children with recurrent parotitis.

95. a. 意外伤害性的耳后瘀青在婴儿期以后非常少见。
b. 用握住的拳头（拳击）反复击打耳朵所引起的非意外伤害是最可能的原因。
c. 凝血检查和血小板计数将会排除出血异常性疾病引起自发性出血的可能。如果与一名有经验的富有同情心的儿科医师进行交谈，孩子可能会揭发受伤害的过程。还应该通过多学科团体对家庭和社会环境进行调查。

a. Bruising behind the ear of a child beyond infancy is very rarely related to accidental trauma.
b. Non-accidental injury caused by repeated hitting of the ears with a closed fist (boxing) is the most likely cause.
c. Clotting studies and a platelet count will exclude the unlikely possibility of a bleeding disorder giving rise to spontaneous bleeding. The child may reveal the nature of the assault if he is interviewed by an experienced, sympathetic paediatrician. The family and social circumstances should be investigated by a multi-disciplinary team.

96. a. 中毒性红斑（新生儿荨麻疹、中毒性红斑、嗜酸性皮疹）。
b. 婴儿没有什么症状。

c. 在生后第 1 周末和第 2 周这种皮疹极其常见。皮疹一般分布广泛且有变化性，会自行消失。它没有临床意义，有经验的临床医生可以通过临床检查将其与败血病性皮疹相鉴别。

a. Erythema toxicum (urticaria of the newborn, toxic erythema, eosinophil rash).
b. The infant will have no symptoms attributable to this rash.
c. The rash is extremely common towards the end of the first week and in the second week of life. It is usually widespread and fluctuating and disappears spontaneously. It is of no clinical significance and can usually be distinguished from septic spots on clinical examination by an experienced clinician.

97. a. 很有可能是由于在儿童早期服用了四环素而引起的牙齿染色。
b. 骨骼系统。
c. 口服四环素在儿童恒牙列还未全部长出之前（即小于 10 岁）是禁忌的。一般可以选择其他抗生素进行用药，即使在那些有已知药物过敏史的儿童。

a. Staining of the teeth most likely due to the administration of the antibiotic tetracycline in early childhood.
b. The bones of the skeletal system.
c. Oral tetracycline is contra-indicated in children in whom full permanent dentition has not erupted i.e. under the age of 10 years. There is always an alternative antibiotic which can be prescribed, even in those who have known drug allergies.

98. a. 面容粗糙，具有高的突起前额（额部隆起），宽颧骨，下颌骨增大，很可能是由于神经变性疾病或贮积病引起（如黏多糖贮积症或黏脂贮积症）。
b. X 光片可以有特征性表现，包括脊椎椎体呈喙样改变、宽肋骨、骨盆髂嵴的骨质溶解和颅骨增厚。
c. 根据白细胞内特异性酶缺陷，以及黏多糖贮积症中尿液中排泄糖胺聚糖，来做出诊断。

a. Coarse facial features with a high protuberant forehead (frontal bossing), broad cheek bones and an enlarged mandible most likely to be due to a neurodegenerative or storage disorder (e.g. mucopolysaccharidosis or mucolipidosis).
b. X-rays may show characteristic features including beaking of the vertebral bodies of the spine, broad ribs, osteolucent whirls in the iliac

crest of the pelvis and thickening of the skull bones.

c. The diagnosis is made by identifying the specific enzyme defect in leucocytes, and the excretion of glycosaminoglycogans in the urine in mucopolysaccharidoses.

99. a. 颅骨骨干发育异常，是一种严重毁损面容的进行性骨病，主要累及颅骨、锁骨和胸骨。颅骨干骺端发育异常与之相似，但是严重程度较轻，进展较为缓慢。

b. 颅神经麻痹，耳聋，视觉障碍，骨痛，出牙、张嘴、咀嚼和进食困难。在疾病的终末期，由于骨的过度生长而导致枕骨大孔狭窄，可能会出现神经系统症状和脑干功能障碍。

c. 常染色体隐性遗传。有 1/4 的再发危险率。

a. Craniodiaphyseal dysplasia, a severely disfiguring and progressive disorder of bone, mainly affecting the skull, clavicles and sternum. Craniometaphyseal dysplasia is a similar, but much less severe, more slowly progessive disorder.

b. Cranial nerve palsies, deafness, visual disturbance, bone pain, difficulties with dentition and jaw opening, mastication and eating. Neurological symptoms and brain stem dysfunction may develop in the terminal stages when the foramen magnum is narrowed by bony overgrowth.

c. Autosomal recessive inheritance. There will be a 1 in 4 risk of recurrence.

100. a. 头皮发育不全或小的脑膨出。

b. 有经验的医师一般比较容易做出诊断。如果存在脑膨出，在颅骨 X 线片中可见有骨缺损。颅脑超声、CT 或 MRI 脑扫描可明确脑膨出的程度。

c. 头皮发育不全可以通过自身的肉芽形成而治愈，即使当缺损较大时。很少需要进行外科修补手术。脑膨出需要在充分的神经影像检查后进行切除和皮肤关闭。

a. Cutis aplasia of the scalp or a small encephalocele.

b. The diagnosis can usually be readily distinguished by an experienced clinician. If an encephalocele is present, there will be a bony defect visible on skull X-ray. Cranial ultrasound, computed tomography or magnetic resonance imaging brain scan will define the extent of the brain protrusion.

c. Cutis aplasia heals by spontaneous granulation even when the lesion is large. Surgical repair is rarely required. Encephaloceles require excision and skin closure after appropriate neuro-imaging.

101. a. 紫癜和蓝莓松饼斑——宫内病毒感染（如风疹病毒、CMV或弓形体）。

b. 生长阻滞，小头畸形，肝脾大，淋巴结肿大，小眼畸形，白内障，脉络膜视网膜炎，听力受损，溶骨性骨损伤，颅内钙化和癫痫。

c. 血液特异性IgM和PCR检测。小婴儿抗体检测阳性（IgG）不能诊断为感染，因为可能是母亲的抗体。眼科检查和听力测验将有所帮助。长骨的X光片可能会显示有芹菜茎样特征，这可诊断为先天性风疹。颅脑超声会显示出颅内钙化。

a. Purpura and blueberry muffin spots — intrauterine viral infection (e.g. rubella, CMV or toxoplasmosis).

b. Growth restriction, microcephaly, hepatosplenomegaly, lymphadenopathy, microphthalmia, cataracts, chorioretinitis, hearing deficit, osteolytic bone lesions, intracranial calcification, and epilepsy.

c. Blood for specific IgM or PCR testing. Positive antibody tests (IgG) in young infants are not diagnostic of infection and may be maternal antibodies. Ophthalmological examination and hearing tests will be helpful. X-ray of long bones may show a celery-stalk appearance which is diagnostic of congenital rubella. Cranial ultrasound scan will demonstrate intracranial calcification.

102. a. 小颌和低位耳。

b. 当婴儿有小颌症时，检查腭部很重要。第一鳃弓综合征便是腭裂伴有小颌畸形。

c. 泌尿系统的超声检查会在大约10%有低位耳的婴儿中发现肾脏泌尿道异常。一旦有耳部异常或多发性副耳（皮赘），就应该进行听力检查。

a. Micrognathia and low-set ears.

b. Examination of the palate is important when an infant has micrognathia. The Pierre-Robin syndrome is cleft palate in association with microcephaly.

c. Ultrasound scan of the renal tract will reveal renal tract anomalies in approximately 10% of infants with low-set ears. Hearing tests should be done whenever there is an abnormality of the ears or multiple accessory auricles (skin tags).

103. a. Graves 病——由于甲状腺毒症（甲状腺功能亢进）而导致的双侧眼球突出。

b. 甲状腺功能亢进的症状包括持续性心动过速、反复发作的室上性心动过速、震颤、易激惹、多汗、体重减轻和甲状腺肿。

c. 服用抗甲状腺药物（如卡比马唑），直到症状自行减轻为止，一般要在症状出现后的几年内服用。偶尔有必要进行甲状腺切除，然后需要终生进行甲状腺激素替代治疗。

a. Graves disease — bilateral proptosis due to thyrotoxicosis (hyperthyroidism).

b. Symptoms of hyperthyroidism include persistent tachycardia, recurrent supraventricular tachycardia, tremor, irritability, sweating, weight loss and goitre.

c. Antithyroid drugs (e.g. carbimazole) until spontaneous remission occurs, usually within a few years of onset of symptoms. Occasionally, thyroidectomy may be necessary, and then life-long thyroid hormone replacement therapy will be required.

104. a. 在背部分布的巨大色素痣。

b. 若不进行治疗会有外观上的影响，并且在青春期前会有较高的恶性变可能。

c. 皮肤摩擦术或激光治疗将会去除表面痣细胞，改善外观。外科手术切除对于降低恶性变可能是有必要的，但是手术难度较大，可能需要多次手术、皮肤移植和输血。

a. Giant pigmented naevus in the bathing trunk distribution.

b. The untreated naevus will be of cosmetic significance. There is also a high risk of malignant transformation before puberty.

c. Dermabrasion or laser therapy will remove superficial naevus cells and improve the appearance. Surgical excision is necessary to reduce the risk of malignant transformation, but is often difficult and may require multiple procedures, skin grafting and blood transfusions.

105. a. 银屑病（牛皮癣）——似珍珠样的红斑，最常见于发际、躯干部、肘部和膝部。

b. 指甲凹痕，甲剥离，关节炎，但通常不累及远端的指（趾）节间关节。

c. 局部应用水杨酸、蒽三酚、口服焦油或维生素 D 类似物（如钙泊三醇）对于控制银屑病都有帮助。偶尔进行紫外线光照疗法可以减轻和缓解严重的病情。

a. Psoriasis — erythematous pearly plaques most commonly around the hairline, and on the trunk, elbow and knees.
b. Pitting of the nails, oncholysis, and arthritis but not usually affecting the distal interphalangeal joints.
c. Topical salicylic acid, dithranol, coal tar, or vitamin D analogues (e.g. calcipotriol) are helpful in keeping psoriasis under control. Occasionally, a course of ultraviolet light may induce remission in severe cases.

106. a. 埃–当综合征(Ehlers-Danlos syndrome)或马方综合征(Marfan's syndrome)中的长而细的手指（趾），即蜘蛛足样指（趾）。
b. 胶原性疾病导致关节运动过度——拇指和小指能够过度伸展到前臂。马方综合征还会有身材较高、高腭弓、严重近视、眼部晶状体移位、胸部畸形、脊柱侧凸、主动脉瘤、主动脉瓣和二尖瓣脱垂和返流。

a. Long thin digits (arachnodactyly) of Ehlers Danlos or Marfan's syndrome.
b. Collagen disorders resulting in hypermobility of joints — the thumb and little finger can be hyper-extended onto the forearm. Tall stature, high arched palate, severe myopia, dislocation of the lenses of the eyes, chest deformity, scoliosis, aortic aneurysm, and aortic and mitral valve prolapse and regurgitation also occur in Marfan's syndrome.

107. a. 草莓样痣，它可以自行消退。皮损的中央会坏死。
b. 不需要积极治疗，除非有继发性感染或出血过多。
c. 草莓样痣会在几个月后彻底消退，只留下很浅的皮肤白色斑痕。自然消退会产生最好的美容学效果，所以不需要进行外科手术。如果有令人烦恼的出血，可以口服类固醇以促进消退。

a. Strawberry naevus which is showing signs of spontaneous involution. The centre of the lesion has become necrotic.
b. No active management is required unless there is secondary infection or excessive bleeding.
c. The naevus will resolve completely over a period of months and will leave only a faint white mark on the skin. Natural involution provides the best cosmetic result and surgery is never indicated. Oral steroids will hasten resolution if there is troublesome bleeding.

108．a. 由动脉栓塞或严重的长期痉挛而引起的前臂脂肪和皮肤的缺血性坏死。

b. 因为许多有缺血性坏死的婴儿有蛋白 C 或蛋白 S、抗凝血酶Ⅲ。或 V 因子 Leiden 的缺失，所以应进行血栓形成倾向的筛查。

c. 受影响的组织和肢体会有瘢痕形成，但是通常正常的功能，如肌肉很少受累及。如果确定有血栓形成的倾向，在成年后或手术时就有静脉血栓形成的危险。

a. Ischaemic necrosis of the fat and skin of the forearm caused by arterial thrombosis or severe prolonged spasm.

b. A thrombophilia screen should be performed as many infants with ischaemic necrosis have protein C or S, anti-thrombin 3 or factor V Leiden deficiency.

c. There may be scarring of the affected tissue and limb, but usually normal function, as muscle is rarely involved. If a thrombotic tendency is identified, there will be a risk of venous thrombosis in adult life and in association with surgery.

109．a. 单卵双生双胞胎的双胎输血；一个是多血症，而另一个是苍白的。

b. 大约 15% 的单卵双生双胞胎共享胎盘血管。急性输血在供体可能会引起贫血和低血容量症，在受体会引起红细胞增多症。症状有赖于输血量和输血速率。缓慢的慢性胎儿-胎儿输血可能会导致供体宫内生长限制，受体也会有心力衰竭和水肿的危险。羊水过多较常见，并且两个双胞胎都有发病和致死的危险。

a. Twin-to-twin transfusion in monozygotic twins; one is plethoric and one is pale.

b. Approximately 15% monozygotic twins have shared placental blood vessels. An acute transfusion may cause anaemia and hypovolaemia in the donor, and polycythaemia in the recipient. Symptoms depend on the volume and rate of transfusion. Slow chronic feto-fetal transfusion may result in intra-uterine growth restriction in the donor. The recipient will be at risk of heart failure and hydrops. Polyhydramnios is common and both twins are at risk of morbidity and mortality.

110．a. 脐疝（脐膨出）——脐部腹壁缺损，而由一层腹膜囊覆盖，并有腹部内容物疝入脐带。

b. 在仔细检查以排除肠闭锁和肠狭窄后进行外科关闭手术。如果缺损较大，可将肠管放在一个人工膜袋中，经过几周后，将内容物慢慢地回纳入腹腔中。

c. 13 三体（帕塔综合征）。

a. Exomphalos (omphalocele)— an abdominal wall defect at the umbilicus covered by a sac of peritoneum, or herniation of abdominal contents into the umbilical cord.

b. Surgical closure after careful inspection to exclude bowel atresias and stenoses. With large defects, the bowel is suspended in an artificial membrane and the contents are slowly returned into the abdominal cavity over a period of weeks.

c. Trisomy 13 (Patau syndrome).

111. a. 全血细胞计数，包括血小板计数和凝血检查。

b. 特发性血小板减少性紫癜是健康儿童出现自发性瘀青和紫癜最常见的原因。

c. 大多数能够自愈。口服类固醇和静脉输注免疫球蛋白将会使血小板计数轻微的上升，但是对预后没有帮助。如果有黏膜出血、神经系统症状或最近有头部损伤史，就应该考虑治疗了。对那些有长期的、持续性血小板减少症的患者，进行脾切除一般是治愈的方法。

a. Full blood count, including platelet count and coagulation studies.

b. Idiopathic thrombocytopenic purpura is the most common cause of spontaneous bruising and purpura in healthy children.

c. Most will resolve spontaneously. Oral steroids and intravenous immunoglobulin administration will cause a slightly faster rise in platelet count, but does not affect the prognosis. Treatment should be considered if there is mucosal bleeding, neurological signs or a history of recent head injury. Splenectomy is usually curative and performed in those with prolonged, persistent thrombocytopenia.

112. a. 川崎病（黏膜皮肤淋巴结综合征）。

b. 发热持续 5 天，并且至少有下列 5 项中的 4 项：

- 明显的颈部淋巴结肿大。
- 手掌和足跖红斑和水肿，以及脱皮。
- 多形性皮疹。

- 双侧结膜充血。
- 嘴唇潮红而皲裂。

通常在病程的第二周会有血小板增多症。

c. 如果在病程早期服用阿司匹林和静脉输注免疫球蛋白，可以减少冠状动脉瘤的危险。

a. Kawasaki disease (mucocutaneous lymph node syndrome).

b. Fever persisting for 5 days and at least 4 of 5 of the following:
- Marked cervical lymphadenopathy.
- Erythema and oedema of palms and soles, and desquamation of the skin.
- Polymorphous rash.
- Bilateral conjunctival congestion.
- Reddening and cracking of the lips.

Thrombocytosis is common in the second week.

c. Aspirin and intravenous immunoglobulin reduce the risk of coronary aneurysms if given in the early stages of the disease.

113. a. 指甲膝盖综合征—— 一种很罕见的疾病，通常在进行新生儿常规体检的过程中检出。婴儿指（趾）甲缺乏或发育不良，缺乏膝部隆凸，或有时甚至有膝关节先天性脱位。膝关节的X光片将会证实有髌骨的缺失。

b. 髌骨缺失易造成膝关节反复脱位。在成人经常发生膝部骨关节炎。

c. 散发发病。

a. Nail-patella syndrome — a rare condition which can usually be diagnosed at the time of the routine neonatal examination. The infant will have absent or hypoplastic finger and toe nails and there will be an absence of the prominence of the knee or sometimes even congenital dislocation. X-ray of the knee will confirm the absence of the patella.

b. Absent patella predisposes to recurrent dislocation of the knees. Osteoarthritis of the knees is common in adult life.

c. Sporadic occurrence.

114. a. 双侧结膜充血——斯-约综合征。

b. 多形性红斑，皮肤以及口腔、直肠、阴道、或结膜的黏膜有广泛分布的水疱-大疱性皮损。会发生广泛的皮肤脱落和体液丢失，并且有很高的继发性感染发生的危险。

c. 停止使用刺激性抗生素。隔离护理以预防感染、充分的液体摄入和电解质补充都是治疗的重要方面。严重的病例由于出现败血症的可能较大，所以死亡率较高。

a. Bilateral conjunctival hyperaemia — Stevens-Johnson syndrome.
b. Erythema multiforme, widespread vesiculo-bullous lesions of the skin and mucous membranes of the mouth, rectum, vagina, or conjunctiva. Extensive skin and fluid loss occurs and there is a high risk of secondary infection.
c. Discontinue the offending antibiotic. Barrier nursing to prevent infection and adequate fluid and electrolyte replacement therapy is the mainstay of treatment. Severe cases have a high mortality from septicaemia.

115. a. 多形性红斑——广泛的荨麻疹。
b. 如果早期全身应用抗组胺药可以减轻瘙痒和缩短病程。在少数发生严重呼吸道梗阻并伴有口、舌水肿的病例，皮下应用肾上腺素可能是挽救生命的措施。
c. 令人烦恼的过敏源一般不明确，但是药物（如青霉素）是常见的原因。反复发作的荨麻疹可能是由于对食物添加剂或色素敏感。很少情况下，可能会有家族性乙酰胆碱酯酶缺乏。

a. Erythema multiforme — widespread urticaria.
b. Systemic antihistamines reduce itching and limit the course if commenced early. Subcutaneous adrenaline may be life-saving in the few who develop severe respiratory obstruction with associated oedema of the mouth and tongue.
c. The offending allergen is often not identifiable, but drugs (e.g. penicillin) are a common cause. Recurrent urticaria may be due to food additives or coloring sensitivity. Rarely, there may be a familial acetylcholinesterase deficiency.

116. a. 门克斯卷发综合征——特征性的稀疏、卷曲纠结的毛发，在显微镜检查下呈现部分断裂和扭曲形态。所有的身体毛发都有异常。
b. 可能有铜结合金属蛋白的缺陷。
c. 还会有严重的神经系统退行性变和发育停滞。在儿童早期便会死亡。
d. 门克斯综合征是X连锁隐性遗传疾病。母亲若为携带者，其所生的男婴中有50%的发病几率。

a. Menkes kinky hair syndrome — characteristic sparse, twisted kinky hair with partial breakages and twists on microscopic examination. All body hair is abnormal.
b. Probably a defect of copper-binding metalloprotein.
c. There is also profound neurological deterioration and failure to thrive. Death occurs in early childhood.
d. Menkes syndrome is an X-linked recessive condition. Male infants of a carrier mother have 50% chance of inheriting the syndrome.

117. a. 皮脂腺痣——一种不常见的先天性皮损，其表面呈浅黄色、腊样、有凹痕且无毛发。通常见于头皮和发际周围。
b. 一些病例到了成人期会有恶性转变，但是该并发症的危险还难以确定。
c. 如果该皮肤损害持续到青春期，那么建议进行切除术。

a. Sebaceous naevus — an uncommon congenital lesion with a yellowish, waxy, pitted, hairless surface. Usually found on the scalp or around the hairline.
b. Malignant transformation occurs in some of these lesions in adult life, but the risk of this complication is difficult to determine.
c. Excision is advisable if the lesion persists into adolescence.

118. a. TAR综合征，即血小板减少及桡骨缺失综合征。
b. 手臂的X光片会证实是否有桡骨的缺失，以及全血细胞计数，包括血小板计数。
c. 相关异常包括有心脏异常（Holt-Oram综合征）、Fanconi全血细胞减少综合征和VACTERL合并症（脊椎异常、肛门闭锁、先天性心脏病、气管缺陷、肾异常、桡骨缺失和肺发育不全）。

a. TAR (thrombocytopenia and absent radius) syndrome.
b. X-ray of the arm will confirm the presence or absence of the radius, and a full blood count, including platelet count.
c. Associated abnormalities include cardiac anomalies (Holt-Oram syndrome), the Fanconi pancytopenia syndrome, and the VACTERL association (Vertebral abnormalities, Anal atresia, Congenital heart disease, Tracheal defects, Renal anomalies, absent Radius, and Lung hypoplasia).

119. a. 臀先露，伴有伸展的双腿。

b. 相关并发症包括分娩性损伤、会阴和臀部的水肿和瘀青、发育不良危险性的增加和先天性髋关节脱位。

c. 在生后24小时的新生儿常规检查中应该仔细检查髋关节。臀先露分娩的新生儿即使髋关节在临床检查中是正常的，也应该接受超声检查以排除先天性脱位。

a. Breech presentation with extended legs.

b. Associated complications include traumatic delivery, oedema and bruising of the genitals and buttocks, and an increased risk of developmental dysplasia and congenital dislocation of the hips.

c. The hips should be carefully examined during the routine neonatal examination at around 24 h of age. After breech presentation, ultrasound examination should be always be performed to exclude congenital dislocation even if the hips appear normal on clinical examination.

120. a. 肛门闭锁。

b. 肾脏泌尿道异常（如会阴、直肠阴道瘘和闭锁）、脊椎异常、其他闭锁（如气管食管闭锁）和尿道感染。

c. 高位异常应该先行一期的结肠造口术，以后再进行外科修补（肛门直肠成形术或拖出术）。低位异常可能仅仅是单纯的皮瓣覆盖于肛门口而形成，所以只要在此处切开皮肤即可治愈。排便节制性在高位异常中很罕见，因为内括约肌发育不良或受损。

a. Imperforate anus (anal atresia).

b. Renal tract anomalies (e.g. perineal, rectovaginal fistula and atresias), vertebral abnormalities, other atresias (e.g. tracheo-oesophageal atresia), and urinary tract infections.

c. High lesions require a preliminary colostomy and later surgical repair (anorectoplasty or pull-through procedure). Low lesions may have a simple skin flap over the anus and incision will be curative. Continence is rarely achieved in high lesions because of hypoplasia or damage to the internal sphincter.

A

abscess	脓肿
abuse	虐待
achondroplasia	软骨发育不全
acute lymphoblastic leukemia(ALL)	急性淋巴母细胞性白血病
adenoma sebaceum	皮脂腺瘤
abrasion	擦破，磨损
adrenal hyperplasia	肾上腺增生
AIDS(acquired immune deficiency syndrome)	艾滋病（获得性免疫缺陷综合征）
albinism	先天性色素缺乏，白化病
allergic reaction	变应性反应，过敏反应
alopecia areata	局限性脱发，斑秃
amblyopia	弱视
ammoniacal dermatitis	氨皮炎(尿布皮炎的一种)
amniotic bands	羊膜索
amputation	截肢术
anaemia	贫血
aplastic	再生障碍性
sickle cell disease	镰刀形红细胞(贫)血病
anencephaly	无脑畸形
angular cheilitis	口角炎
ankles	踝关节
Ankylostoma(hookworm)	钩虫
anus	肛门
imperforate	闭锁的
patulous	张开的
tags and sinuses	皮赘和窦道
aplastic anemia	再生障碍性贫血
arthritis	关节炎
arthrogryposis multiplex congenital	先天性多关节弯曲，先天性多关节挛缩
ascaris lumbricoides (roundworm)	蛔虫

asphyxiating thoracic dysplasia	窒息性胸廓发育异常
asthma	哮喘
asymmetry	不对称
auditory meatus	耳道
auricle	耳廓

B

Bacille Calmet e-Guerin(BCG) vaccination	卡介苗
bat ear	横位耳甲(招风耳)
bathing trunk nevus	躯干下部痣
Beckwith's syndrome	Beckwith 综合征
bilirubinaemia	胆红素血症
unconjugated	未结合的
birth injury	产伤
blast cell	原始细胞，母细胞，胚细胞
leukaemia	白血病
bleeding disorders	出血障碍
blood disorders	血液病
bone marrow transplantation	骨髓移植
bow leg	弓形腿，膝内翻
branchial arch (facio-auriculo-vertebral) syndrome	鳃弓综合征（面－耳－脊椎综合征）
breast	乳房
accessory nipple	副乳头
breast development	乳房发育
breast feeding	母乳喂养
breech delivery	臀位分娩
brittle bone disease(osteogenesis imperfecta)	脆骨病(成骨不全)
bronchiolitis	细支气管炎
bronchopulmonary dysplasia(BPD)	支气管肺发育不良
bronze baby syndrome	青铜综合征婴儿
bruising	擦伤，瘀伤
idiopathic thrombocytopenic purpura	特发性血小板减少性紫癜
non-accidental injury	非意外伤害
sexual abuse	性虐待
spontaneous	自发的，特发的

Brushfield spots	布鲁什菲尔德点
bullae	大(水)疱

C

café-au-lait spot	咖啡牛奶斑
candida(monilial) infection	白色念珠菌感染
caput succedaneum	先锋头，胎头水肿
cataracta	白内障
cellulitis	蜂窝织炎
haemophilus	嗜血杆菌(属)
periorbital	眼眶周围的
periumbilical	脐周围的
staphylococcal	葡萄球菌属的
cephalhematoma	头颅血肿
cerebral palsy	脑性麻痹
cerebral tumor	脑肿瘤
chickenpox(varicella)	水痘
intrauterine	子宫内的
child abuse	儿童虐待
chlamydia trachomatis	沙眼衣原体
choanal atresia	鼻后孔闭锁
chondrodysplasia	软骨发育不全
chromosomal abnormalities	染色体异常
chronic lung disease	慢性肺病
circumcision	包皮环切术
claw deformity	爪样畸形
cleft lip and palate	唇裂和腭裂
club foot(talipes equinovarus)	畸形足(马蹄内翻足)
clubbing	杵状变
finger	指
toes	趾
coarctation of aorta	主动脉缩窄
cockayne syndrome	科凯恩综合征(视网膜退变、听力受损、皮肤薄且对光敏感)
coeliac disease	腹部疾病
collodion skin	火棉胶皮肤
coloboma	缺损

condylomata acuminate(anogenital wart)	尖锐湿疣(肛门生殖器疣)
congenital heart disease	先天性心脏病
conjunctivitis	结膜炎
cradle cap	乳痂
cranial nerve palsies	颅神经麻痹
craniodiaphyseal/craniometaphyseal dysplasia	颅骨骨干发育异常或发育不全(颅骨干骺端发育不良)
craniosynostosis	颅缝早闭
Crohn's disease	克隆病
croup(acute laryngotracheobronchitis)	哮吼(急性喉气管支气管炎)
cryptorchidism	隐睾
Cushing's syndrome	库欣综合征
cutis marmorata	大理石样皮肤
cyanosis	发绀
cystic fibrosis	囊性纤维化病
cystic hygroma	水囊状淋巴管瘤
cytomegalovirus	巨细胞病毒

D

de Lange's syndrome	德朗热综合征（智力迟钝伴多种先天畸形）
dehydration	脱水
delivery	分娩
dermatitis	皮炎
diaper rash	尿布疹
diaphragmatic hernia	膈疝
diet	饮食的
dimples	浅凹
Down syndrome(21 trisomy)	唐氏综合征(21 三体综合征)
duchenne muscular dystrophy	进行性假肥大性肌营养不良
dwarfism	侏儒症

E

ectodermal dysplasia	外胚层发育不良
ectopia vesica	膀胱外翻
eczema	湿疹
Edward syndrome（trisomy 18）	Edward 综合征（18 三体综合征）

Ehlers Danlos syndrome	埃-当综合征（全身弹性纤维发育不良综合征）
encephalitis	脑炎
encephalocele	脑膨出
enterocolitis	小肠结肠炎
erythema toxicum	中毒性红斑
epidermal necrolysis	表皮坏死松解
epidermolysis bullosa	大疱性表皮松解症
epiglottis	会厌
Epithelial's pearl	上皮珠
Epstein's pearls	爱泼斯坦小结
epulis	牙龈瘤
Erb palsy	Erb 麻痹
erysipelas	丹毒
erythema multiforme	多形性红斑
erythema nodosum	结节性红斑
erythema toxicum	中毒性红斑
Escherichia coli	大肠埃希杆菌
exfoliatin	脱叶霉素
exomphalos	脐疝
extremely low birth weight	极低出生体重

F

facial palsy	面瘫
factor VIII deficiency(haemophilia A)	Ⅷ因子缺乏(A 型血友病)
failure to thrive	发育停滞
femur	股骨
feto-fetal transfusion	胎儿-胎儿输血
floppy baby	婴儿松软症
fracture	骨折
fungal infection	霉菌感染

G

Galant reflex	侧弯反射
gangrene	坏疽
gastrointestinal	胃肠的
genital warts	生殖器疣

genitalia	外生殖器
genu valgum(knock-knee)	膝外翻
german measles	风疹
Giardia lamblia	肠兰伯鞭毛虫
Gingivostomatitis	龈口炎
glabellar tap sign	眉间叩击征
glandular fever	腺热
glaucoma	青光眼
glomerulonephritis	肾小球性肾炎
glossoptosis	舌下垂
gluten-sensitivity	谷蛋白敏感
goiter	甲状腺肿
gonococcal ophthalmia	淋球菌性眼炎
Gower's sign	Gower 征(光刺激时,虹膜有间隙性迅速颤动)
Granuloma	肉芽肿
grasp reflex	抓握反射
graves disease	Graves 病（突眼性甲状腺肿，毒性弥漫性甲状腺肿）
growth hormone deficiency	生长激素缺乏
gynaecomastia	男性乳房发育

H

haemangioma	血管瘤
haematological disoders	血液病
haemolytic disease	溶血病
Haemophilus influenzae	流感(嗜血)杆菌
hammer toe	槌状趾
harlequin fetus	斑色胎，先天性鱼鳞癣胎儿，花斑胎
head circumference	头围
henoch-schonlein purpura	亨－舍紫癜，过敏性紫癜
hepatomegaly	肝大
hernia	疝
herpes simplex	单纯性疱疹
herpes zoster	带状疱疹
Hirschsprung's disease	希施斯普龙病（先天性巨结肠）
histiocytosis	组织细胞增多病

hookworm	钩虫
human immunodeficiency virus(HIV)	人类免疫缺陷病毒
human papilloma virus	人乳头状瘤病毒
humerus	肱骨
Hunter syndrome	Hunter 综合征(Ⅱ型黏多糖病)
Hurler syndrome	Hurler 综合征(Ⅰ型黏多糖病)
hyaline membrane disease	新生儿透明膜病
hydrocele	阴囊水囊肿
hydrocephalus	脑积水
hydrops fetalis	胎儿水肿
hygroma cystic	囊状水囊瘤
hymen	处女膜
hyperbilirubinaemia	高胆红素血症
hyperthyroidism	甲状腺功能亢进
hypoglycaemia	低血糖
hypospadias	尿道下裂
hypothyroidism	甲状腺功能减退
Hypotonia	张力减退

I

ichthyosis	鱼鳞病
idiopathic thrombocytopenic purpura(ITP)	特发性血小板减少性紫癜
impetigo	脓疱病
In-toeing	趾朝内
incontinentia pigmenti	色素失调症
infestation	侵袭，感染
inflammatory bowel disease	炎性肠病，肠炎
inguinal hernia	腹股沟疝
intestinal parasites	肠寄生虫
intrauterine growth retardation	宫内发育迟缓
intravenous fluids	静脉内输液
intussusception	套叠

J

jaundice	黄疸
juvenile chronic arthritis	青少年慢性关节炎

K

Kawasaki disease	川崎病
keloid	瘢痕疙瘩
kernicterus	核黄疸
Kippel-Feil syndrome	克利佩尔–费尔综合征（先天性短颈畸形）
knock knee	膝外翻
Koplik's spots	Koplik 斑（麻疹黏膜斑）
kwashiorkor(protein-energy malnutrition)	恶性营养不良症(蛋白质–能量营养不良)

L

lactation	哺乳期
Langerhans cell histiocytosis	朗格汉细胞组织细胞增生症
lanugo hair	胎毛
laryngo-tracheo-bronchitis	喉气管支气管炎
Lesch-Nyhan syndrome	莱–尼综合征（自毁容貌症）
Leukaemia	白血病
lichen sclerosus et atrophicus	硬化萎缩苔癣
limbs	肢
lipoma	脂(肪)瘤
Listeriosis	李斯特菌病
low birth weight infant	低出生体重婴儿
Lowe syndrome	洛氏综合征（眼脑肾综合征）
lymphadenitis	淋巴结炎
lymphadenopathy	淋巴结病
lymphoedema	淋巴管性水肿

M

malabsorption	吸收不良
malignancy	恶性，恶性肿瘤
malnutrition	营养不良
Mantoux reaction	芒图反应，结核菌素反应试验
marasmus	消瘦，消耗
marfan's syndrome	马方综合征（指趾过长综合征）
mastitis	乳腺炎

measles	麻疹
measles,mumps and rubella(MMR) vaccine	麻疹、流行性腮腺炎和风疹三联疫苗
meconium	胎粪
medulloblastoma	成神经管细胞瘤
meningitis	脑（脊）膜炎
meningocele	脑（脊）膜膨出
meningococcus	脑膜炎双球菌
meningomyelocele	脊髓脊膜膨出
Menkes syndrome	门克斯综合征（遗传性铜吸收异常）
metaphyses	干骺端
metatarsus varus	内翻跖
microcephaly	小头
micrognathia	小颌
microphthalmos	眼过小
milia	粟粒疹
milk spot	乳样斑
molluscum contagiosum	传染性软疣
Moro reflex	莫罗反射(婴儿拥抱反射)
Morquio syndrome	Morquio 综合征（Ⅳ型多糖病）
motor skill	运动技能
moulding	(分娩时)胎头变形
muco-cutaneous lymph node syndrome	皮肤黏膜淋巴结综合征
mucolipidosis	黏脂贮积症
mucopolysaccharidosis	黏多糖贮积症
mucus	黏液
muscular dysgenesis	肌肉发育不全
myasthenia gravis	重症肌无力
mycobacterium tuberculosis	结核分支杆菌
mycoplasma pneumoniae	肺炎支原体

N

naevus	痣
nail-patella syndrome	指甲－髌骨综合征
napkin psoriasis	尿布皮炎
neck reflex	颈反射
necrotising enterocolitis(NEC)	坏死性小肠结肠炎

Neisseria gonorrhoea	淋病奈瑟球菌
Neisseria meningitidis	脑膜炎奈瑟球菌
nephroblastoma	肾母细胞瘤
nephrotic syndrome	肾病综合征
neural tube defect	神经管缺损
neuroblastoma	神经母细胞瘤
neurofibromatosis	多发性神经纤维瘤
neuroma	神经瘤
neuromuscular disorders	神经肌肉障碍
nipples	乳头
non-accidental injury(NAI)	非意外伤害
Noonan syndrome	努南综合征
nutrition	营养

O

obesity	肥胖症
obstructive uropathy	阻塞性尿路疾患
oculo-cerebro-renal syndrome	眼-脑-肾综合征
oedema	水肿
omphalocele	脐膨出
ophthalmia	眼炎
opisthotonus	角弓反张
osteogenesis imperfecta	成骨不全
osteomyelitis	骨髓炎

P

palate	腭
parasite	寄生虫
paronychiae	甲沟炎
parotitis	腮腺炎
Patau syndrome（trisomy 13）	帕塔综合征（13 三体综合征）
patella	髌骨，膝盖骨
patent ductus arteriosus(PDA)	动脉导管未闭
penis	阴茎
Perthes' disease	佩尔特斯病（骨骺的骨软骨病）
phocomelia	短肢畸形
phototherapy	光疗

Pierre-Robin syndrome	第一腮弓综合征
pinna	耳廓
pituitary hormone	垂体激素
placing reflex	放置反射
plagiocephaly	斜形头
pneumatosis intestinalis	肠壁囊样积气症
pneumococcus	肺炎球菌
pneumomediastinum	纵隔积气
pneumonia	肺炎
pneumothorax	气胸
poliomyelitis	脊髓灰质炎
polyarteritis nodosa	结节性多动脉炎
polydactyly	多指，多趾
portwine stain	葡萄酒色痣
postural deformity	姿态性畸形
Potter syndrome	波特综合征
progeria	早老综合征
proptosis	突出，凸出（尤指眼球凸出）
prune-belly syndrome	干梅状腹综合征
psoriasis	牛皮癣，银屑病
ptosis	下垂，上睑下垂
puberty	青春期
pyloric stenosis	幽门狭窄

R

rachitic rosary	佝偻病性串珠，串珠肋
radius	桡骨
ranula	舌下囊肿
rectal atresia	直肠闭锁
renal agenesis	肾发育不全，肾缺如
respiratory distress syndrome	呼吸窘迫综合征
retinoblastoma	视网膜母细胞瘤
rheumatic fever	风湿热
rib fracture	肋骨骨折
rickets	佝偻病
ringworm	癣菌病，癣

Ritter disease	里特尔病,婴儿剥脱性皮炎（葡萄球菌性烫伤样皮肤综合征）
rooting reflex	觅食反射
Rubella	风疹
roundworm	蛔虫，线虫
Russell-Silver syndrome	拉－西综合征

S

Sanfilippo's syndrome	Sanfilippo 综合征（Ⅶ型黏多糖病）
scabies	疥疮
scalded skin syndrome	皮肤烫伤综合征
scald	烫伤
scalp	头皮
scarring	瘢痕形成，瘢痕化
scoliosis	脊柱侧凸
self-mutilation	自残
sexual abuse of child	儿童性虐待
shagreen patch	鲨革斑
shingles	带状疱疹
short-limbed dwarfism	短肢性侏儒症
short stature	身材矮小症
sickle-cell disease	镰形细胞(贫血)病
skin disorder	皮肤病
skin tag	皮赘
skull	颅骨
small for gestational age(SGA)	小于胎龄儿
social behaviour	社会行为
spasticity	痉挛状态，僵直状态
speech	言语,语言
spina bifida occulta	隐性脊柱裂
spinal muscular atrophy	脊髓性肌萎缩
squint	斜视, 斜眼
staphylococcal infection	葡萄球菌感染
staphylococcus aureus	金黄色葡萄球菌
startle reaction	惊跳反应
stem cell transplantation	干细胞移植

Stevens-Johnson syndrome	斯－约综合征(多形糜烂性红斑的一型)
still disease	斯蒂尔病，系统性幼年型类风湿关节炎(儿童多发性关节炎伴发热、脾及淋巴结肿大)
stomatitis	口炎
stool	粪,粪便
stork bite naevus	毛细血管扩张痣
strabismus	斜视,斜眼
strawberry naevus	草莓样痣
streptococcus pneumoniae	链球菌性肺炎
striae	纹
Sturge-Weber syndorme	斯特奇－韦伯综合征（脑三叉神经血管瘤病）
subcutaneous fat necrosis	皮下脂肪坏死
sucking pad	吸吮垫
sucking reflex	吸吮反射
supracondylar fracture	髁上骨折
surfactant deficiency	表面活性物质缺乏
syndactyly	并指，并趾
synovitis	滑膜炎

T

talipes	畸形足
talipes equinovalgus	马蹄外翻足
TAR syndrome	TAR 综合征（血小板减少及桡骨缺失综合征）
tetracycline	四环素
thalassanemia	地中海贫血
thelarche	乳房初发育
thrombocytopaenia	血小板减少
thrombocytopenia and absent radius(TAR) syndrome	血小板减少及桡骨缺失综合征
thrombocytopenia purpura	血小板减少性紫癜
thrush	真菌性口炎
thyroglossal cyst	甲状舌管囊肿
thyroid disorder	甲状腺疾病

thyrotoxicosis	甲状腺毒症
tinea	癣
torticollis	斜颈
toxoplasmosis	弓形体病
traction	(肌肉)牵引
trauma	创伤，外伤
trisomy 13	13 三体
tuberculosis	结核病
tumour	肿瘤
Turner syndrome	特纳综合征（性腺发育障碍症）
twin-to-twin transfusion syndrome	双生胎儿血液交换综合征

U

ulceration	溃疡形成，溃疡
ulcerative colitis	溃疡性结肠炎
umbilical cord	脐带
umbilical hernia	脐疝
urethral valve	尿道瓣膜
urinary tract infection(UTI)	泌尿道感染
uropathy	尿路病
urticaria	荨麻疹

V

vaccination	接种疫苗
vagina	阴道
varicella	水痘
ventriculoatrial	有关（或连接）脑室与心房的
ventriculo-peritoneal shunt	脑室－腹腔分流术
vernix membrane	胎脂膜
vesicoureteric reflux	膀胱输尿管回流现象，膀胱输尿管反流
virilization	男性化
vitamin D deficiency	维生素 D 缺乏
vitiligo	白斑，白斑病，白癜风
Von Recklinghausen's disease	冯 · 雷克林豪森病(多发性神经纤维瘤)

W

Waardenburg syndrome	瓦尔登伯格综合征
walking reflex	踏步反射
warts	疣
Werdnig-Hoffmann disease	韦-霍病（脊髓性肌萎缩症）
Wilms tumor	肾母细胞瘤
‘wind-swept’ deformity	“风蚀样”畸形
witch's milk	Witch 乳，新生儿乳
wry neck	斜颈